FOOD AND BEVERAGE CONSUMPTION AND HEALTH

BERRIES: PROPERTIES, CONSUMPTION AND NUTRITION

FOOD AND BEVERAGE CONSUMPTION AND HEALTH

Additional books in this series can be found on Nova's website
under the Series tab.

Additional E-books in this series can be found on Nova's website
under the E-book tab.

FOOD AND BEVERAGE CONSUMPTION AND HEALTH

BERRIES: PROPERTIES, CONSUMPTION AND NUTRITION

CARLO TUBEROSO
EDITOR

Nova Biomedical Books
New York

For permission to use material from this book please contact us:
Telephone 631-231-7269; Fax 631-231-8175
Web Site: http://www.novapublishers.com

NOTICE TO THE READER

Additional color graphics may be available in the e-book version of this book.

LIBRARY OF CONGRESS CATALOGING-IN-PUBLICATION DATA

Berries : properties, consumption, and nutrition / editor, Carlo Tuberoso.
p. ; cm.
Includes bibliographical references and index.
ISBN 978-1-61470-257-3 (hardcover : alk. paper) 1. Fruit in human nutrition. 2. Berries. I. Tuberoso, Carlo.
[DNLM: 1. Fruit. 2. Nutritive Value. WB 430]
QP144.F78B465 2011
613.2--dc23

2011022166

Published by Nova Science Publishers, Inc. + New York

Contents

Preface

The purpose of this book is to fulfill the need for accurate state-of-the art information and perspectives regarding the most recent studies on berries. Edible berries have been part of the human diet for thousands of years and today numerous studies suggest that their regular dietary consumption may be beneficial in decreasing the risk for chronic diseases and for age-related pathologies. Over the past ten years, the scientific literature on berries' characteristics and properties has rapidly matured from sporadic articles to a solid body of information. However, sometimes access to such data is not easy.

The eleven chapters of the book cover different topics, from chemical composition and biological properties to marketing of the small edible fruits commonly defined as "berries". Special emphasis has been placed on bioactive constituents extracted from berries and their important biological activities.

Chapter I – Epidemiological studies in different countries have identified fruits and vegetables as key components in a healthy diet; they are good sources of dietary fiber, essential nutrients and phytochemicals. Consumption of fruits and vegetables delays the ageing process and reduces the risk of various lifestyle diseases, mainly cardiovascular and anti-degenerative diseases, cancer, rheumatoid arthritis, cataract, Parkinson, Alzheimer, among other biological effects on human beings. Fruits, but in particular berries, have been the focus among researchers and health professionals and now it is known that the intake of berries has a positive impact on human health, principally in disease prevention. Berries must be one of the main components of healthy diets, particularly because they are a rich source of phytochemicals, especially a wide variety of phenolic compounds (phenolic acids, anthocyanins, flavonols, flavones, flavanols, flavanones, isoflavonoids, stilbenes and tannins), and also contain vitamins, mainly vitamin C, and minerals. The effects of phenolic compounds on health have been mostly attributed to their antioxidant properties; berries are a particularly rich source of antioxidants, but the biological activities exhibited by berries phytochemicals *in vivo* extend beyond antioxidation. Besides a positive influence on oxidative status, they also have a mechanism associated with the low-grade systemic inflammation that helps to control many diseases. On the other hand, the phenolic profiles of berries species are quite diverse and, therefore, expected to have different biological activities. The diversity of bioactive compounds is reflected in the broad spectrum of their biological and medicinal properties, and such differences are observed in the content and the qualitative composition of the compounds. In recent years, several berries such as strawberry, blueberry, cranberry, and black raspberry have been extensively studied and the observations on the health benefits of their constituents are well documented. In this chapter we analyze the bioactive constituents, biological properties and human health benefits of berries, and their importance in the prevention of various diseases.

Chapter II - Resveratrol is a polyphenolic compound found in several plant tissues and organs which is mainly detected in berries. In plants resveratrol acts as a phytoalexin, that is, plant metabolites produced against pathogen attacks or certain environmental stress factors. This compound possesses diverse biochemical and physiological properties including anti-inflammatory and immunomodulatory activities plus a wide range of health benefits ranging from chemoprevention to cardioprotection. Furthermore, recent studies have suggested that resveratrol also possesses antiaging properties. The present review describes and compares the occurrence of resveratrol in berries including data on the origin of the samples analyzed, the incidence observed, and the range of concentrations reported. A brief description of resveratrol biosynthesis and its biotechnological implication is also included.

Chapter III - In recent years, polysaccharides and their conjugates, which are present in plant materials, have emerged as an important class of compounds that possess biological activities. Polysaccharide conjugates isolated from a variety of plant sources have been identified as bioactive components. Polysaccharides-protein conjugates (i.e. glycoproteins) from wolfberry (*Lycium barbarum* L.), commercially called goji berry, have been reported to possess important bioactive functions, including hypoglycemic and hypolipidemic activities, immuno-modulating action, and antioxidant activity. Conjugated polysaccharides isolated from sweet cherries (*Prunus avium* L.) and cranberries (*Vaccinium macrocarpon* Aiton) have been shown to possess antioxidant activity. Polysaccharide-lipid conjugates (i.e. glycolipids) represent another class of conjugated polysaccharides that exhibit bioactive properties. Galactolipids, a specific type of glycolipid, have been shown to possess in vitro and in vivo anti-tumour promoting activity. Galactolipids have been reported to be present in edible plants such as common beans (*Phaseolus vulgaris*), bell peppers (*Capsicum annuum*), kiwi (*Actinidia deliciosa*), grapes (*Vitis vinifera*) and strawberries (*Fragaria x ananassa*). The bioactivity of polysaccharide conjugates depends on their chemical and structural characteristics. This chapter focuses on: the state of knowledge of different types of conjugated polysaccharides, the bioactivity of naturally occurring conjugated polysaccharides, different types of isolation and purification techniques, the relationships between their bioactive functions, chemical composition, and the structure of conjugated polysaccharides along with the distribution of conjugated polysaccharide in berries and cherries in comparison to other plant sources.

Chapter IV - Consumption of blueberries has increased rapidly over the past decade, as have the numbers of studies suggesting health benefits. Now the blueberry is a commonly consumed berry in the United States. They are used in jellies, jams, and pies, baked into muffins, and are an ingredient of many other snacks and delicacies or baby foods. The major phytochemicals in blueberries are polyphenols, including anthocyanins, proanthocyanidins, other flavonoids, phenolic acids and stilbene derivatives. A diet rich in fruits and vegetables has long been recognized to reduce the risk of cardiovascular diseases. In recent years, evidence has emerged suggesting that some phytochemicals in plant foods, polyphenols in particular, may be largely responsible for their protective activities against cardiovascular diseases, mainly through antioxidant and anti-inflammatory activities. Blueberries are rich in polyphenols and exhibit extremely high antioxidant capacity. They have been implicated in preventing cardiovascular diseases for many years. Recent studies, including animal and human studies, have found the beneficial effects of blueberries in cardiovascular diseases from different aspects: preventing development of atherosclerotic lesions, protecting the myocardium from induced ischemic damage, having positive effects on the course of chronic heart failure, lowering blood pressure and improving selected features of metabolic syndrome and related cardiovascular risk factors. The possible underlying mechanisms included but not limited to reducing oxidation of lipoproteins, improving serum antioxidant status and lipid levels, improving endothelial dysfunction and inhibiting inflammation on the vascular system.

Chapter V - Flavour is a combination of odour, taste and chemesthesis. Various volatile and non-volatile chemical compounds are contributing to berry flavour. To understand the role of those compounds in sensory perception of berries, it is necessary to connect chemico-physical analyses to sensory evaluation. Trained sensory panel is sensitive to describe and rate the intensity of different flavours, but not able to identify the compounds causing the properties. Many factors such as berry genus, variety, growing conditions, stage of ripeness and processing affect flavour. Berries are very sensitive material to quality changes. Different headspace techniques are useful tools to extract the volatile berry compounds. Gas chromatography coupled to sniffing system for instance makes it possible to study the odour active compounds. In the case of non-volatile orosensory contributing compounds the modern methods using liquid chromatography coupled with mass spectrometry are very important. Moreover, it is very important to optimise the sample preparation to be similar both in sensory studies and instrumental measurements. Multiregression methods should be applied to investigate the interaction between perceived flavour and chemical composition. This chapter reviews studies concerning berry odour, taste and astringency. It demonstrates the complexity of berry flavour. The berry samples investigated here are strawberry, black currant, bilberry, crowberry and sea buckthorn and they have been growing in North Europe.

Chapter VI - A full evaluation of elderberry botany, production, orchard establishment and technology together with chemical composition of flowers, berries and elder products is presented. The uses of American and European Elderberry are discussed and medical reports on both elder flowers and berries highlighted. The antioxidant, antimicrobial, anti-inflammatory and cancer-chemo preventive properties of elderberry products are reported. Chemical composition of elderberry consists of primary metabolites (organic acids, sugars), secondary metabolites (phenols) and several other constituents (vitamins A and C, cytokines). Elder flowers are distinguished by their intensive, pleasant odor and serve as a basis for industrially produced soft drinks and extracts. They are a rich source of potential bioactive flavonoids and phenolic acids; quercetin-3-rutinoside (rutin), quercetin-3-glucoside (isoquercitrin), kaempferol-3-rutinoside, isorhamnetin-3-rutinoside and isorhamnetin-3-glucoside were identified among flavonoids and among derivates of phenolic acids, caffeic and *p*-coumaric acid were identified. Flavonol glycosides rutin, kaempferol-3-rutinoside and isorhamnetin-3-rutinoside are the major flavonoids in elder flowers, present in much higher concentrations than in elder fruit. Elder flowers exhibit a much stronger neutralizing activity of free radicals compared to elderberry fruit, which is characterized by high organic acids levels, particularly citric acid, and the most abundant sugars in berries, fructose and glucose. These make the ripe berries ideal for processing to juices, candy and concentrates. Among phenolic compounds in elder berries, anthocyanins, quercetins and other polyphenolic flavonoids are of great interest due to their health-beneficial properties. Cyanidin-3-glucoside and cyanidine-3-sambubioside are the prevalent anthocyanins in elder berries, characterizing their purple color and particularly important for natural pigment industry. Other anthocyanins, such as cyanidin-3-sambubioside-5-glucoside, cyanidin-3,5-diglucoside and cyanidin-3-rutinoside are only presented in minor concentrations. In the group of quercetins, quercetin, rutin and quercetin 3-glucoside were detected; with rutin the predominant one. In elderberry extracts and wine, a high content of both primary and secondary metabolites has also been reported. Anthocyanins, as well as other flavonoids, exhibit antioxidant, immune-stimulating, antibacterial, antialergic and antiviral properties; therefore, their consumption may contribute to prevention of several degenerative diseases such as cardiovascular disease, cancer, inflammatory disease and diabetes.

Chapter VII - Myrtle (*Myrtus communis* L.) berries are very popular fruits in the Mediterranean area. They are used for food aromatization and for the preparation of characteristic alcoholic products such as liqueur, eau-de-vie and wine. The berries are spherical in shape, dark red to violet in color, and contain organic acids, carbohydrates, phenolic compounds, volatiles, lipids, anions and cations. Their distinctive flavor and color are due to their volatiles and polyphenols content, respectively. The main compounds in myrtle berries' volatile fraction are α-pinene, limonene and 1,8-cineole. The phenolic compounds fraction is characterized by gallic acid, flavonoids and anthocyans that represent the most abundant phytochemicals in myrtle berries. The anthocyanin profile shows five anthocyanin glucosides and four anthocyanin arabinosides with malvidin-3-*O*-glucoside, delphinidin-3-*O*-glucoside, and petunidin-3-*O*-glucoside as major peaks. Flavonoid profile is characterized by myricetin-3-*O*-galactoside, myricetin-3-*O*-rhamnoside, myricetin and quercetin. Myricetin and gallic acid derivatives are thought to be the most efficient molecules in inhibiting free radical and lipid peroxidation. Myrtle berry extracts prepared using solvents with different polarity (water, ethanol, and ethyl acetate) were analyzed using several in vitro tests to investigate their antioxidant properties. The strongest antiradical and antioxidant activities (measured with DPPH and FRAP tests, respectively) were found in ethanol and ethyl acetate extracts. These same extracts also showed the highest content of phenolic compounds. The ethyl acetate extract had the strongest protective effect in assays of thermal (140°C) cholesterol degradation and Cu^{2+}-mediated LDL oxidation, inhibiting the reduction of polyunsaturated fatty acids and cholesterol, and the increase of their oxidative products. These results suggest that besides the well-established food use, myrtle berries could be used in dietary supplement preparation or as food additives. Therefore, because of their multiple possible uses, a cultivar selection programme has been recently started with the aim of providing berries with the best nutritional properties for industrial use.

Chapter VIII - *Vaccinium meridionale* Swartz is a wild shrub belonging to the family of Mirtaceae and native to the country of Colombia. The fruit which is called mortiňo or agraz is a bilberry, 5 -10 mm in diameter, with many small seeds and a sour and tart character. Berries are eaten fresh or processed into dried fruit, sauces, jellies, yogurt bases, wine and jams. The consumption and potential for export of *V. meridionale* is increasing due to the known nutraceutical properties of bilberries (*Vaccinium myrtillus* L.), including management of visual disorders and protection against cancer, age-related neurodegenerative conditions, and inflammatory responses. These nutraceutical properties are strongly associated with the content and profile of anthocyanins and non-anthocyanin polyphenols, which are also partially responsible for the high antioxidant activity of bilberries. Given the supporting information on the potential nutraceutical properties of bilberry, it is of interest to characterize the wild *Vaccinium* species that grow in Colombia. Accordingly, available information on the chemical composition, total anthocyanin and phenolic contents, anthocyanin profile, non-anthocyanin phenolic profile, and antioxidant activity of Colombian bilberry is summarized, discussed and compared with reports for other well-characterized *Vaccinium* species. The reported anthocyanin content of *V. meridionale* ranges between 201 ± 10 and 329.0 ± 28.0 mg cyanidin 3-glucoside equivalents/100 g FW while the total phenolic content varies between 609.0 ± 39.0 and 758.6 ± 62.3 mg gallic acid equivalent/100 g FW. Unlike other bilberries, Colombian bilberries contain only cyanidin and delphinidin. Cyanidin 3-galactoside is the major anthocyanin representing 43% of the total peak area. Non-anthocyanin phenolics include hydroxycinnamic acids and flavonols and the most abundant compound is chlorogenic acid. Berries of *V. meridionale* show high antioxidant activity. The reported ABTS radical scavenging activity is within 45.5 ± 2.3 - 86.9 ± 4.4 µmol Trolox equivalents/g FW. This radical scavenging activity is close to that one of blueberries, which constitute one of the richest reported antioxidants. Similarly, the ferric reducing antioxidant potential (FRAP) (87.0 ± 17.8 µmol Trolox equivalents/g FW or 116.0 ± 23.7 µmol ferric iron reduced/g FW) is close to that one of *V. myrtillus.* Overall, results from available studies show that the anthocyanin composition of Colombian wild bilberry can be differentiated from other bilberries by their unique pattern. Moreover, *V. meridionale* berries are an excellent source of dietary phytochemicals such as anthocyanins and polyphenolics, being comparable to *V. myrtillus*. Consequently, there is potential for the use of *V. meridionale* as a source of phytochemicals in the nutraceutical and functional food market.

Chapter IX - To date, reports on allergenicity of berries are still scarce. Allergies to berries have been mainly associated with similar disorders provoked by fruits that contain proteins that are homologous to those considered to be major fruit allergens: profilins, homologous to Bet v 1 (major birch pollen allergen) and plant nonspecific lipid transfer proteins (ns-LTPs). However, the main factors involved in allergies to fruits have not been well determined due to high variability in the allergen-protein contents of fruits, which are dependent on cultivar, harvest and production systems. It has been observed that clinical reactivity is highly dependent on a variety of factors such as exposure frequency and individual responses to allergens. It is also necessary to determine the actual clinical relevance of *in vitro* assays and to clarify the possible correlation among the results obtained from *in vitro* assays, skin prick tests and oral challenge. Recent research works performed at the molecular level allow the isolation and characterization of those proteins identified as major allergens for allergies to fruits, which is key information for future immunotherapy.

In this chapter we discuss various clinical reports on allergies to *Morus, Vaccinium* and *Fragaria* berries which help clarify the causes and main symptoms associated with this hypersensitive disorder of the immune system.

Chapter X - Berry fruit is highly perishable and it should be marketed soon after picking. When modern storage techniques are applied, fruit harvested in a particular season can be consumed some weeks later, decay is prevented and quality is ensured. In order to maximize storage life, fruit must have a high initial quality. The main factors, that limit the postharvest life of blueberries are excessive softening, water loss which results in fruit shrivelling, and the incidence of postharvest diseases (mainly caused by *Botrytis cinerea* and *Colletotrichum gloeosporioides*). Temperature management is the most critical postharvest factor, and for this reason, after harvesting, blueberries must be rapidly cooled and kept at temperatures close to 0°C for a maximum postharvest life. Cold storage, controlled atmosphere, modified atmosphere packaging, ozonation and innovative atmospheres have been used to extend the marketing season, reduce losses and increase profitability. However, the benefits of most of these treatments have been limited and often inconsistent. According to our experimental results, controlled atmosphere storage can maintain the quality and extend the storage life of blueberries. When added to refrigeration at close to 0°C, the controlled atmosphere maintained fruit firmness, the total soluble solids content and titratable acidity. Storage in plastic films reduced weight loss and slowed down the deterioration of the visual quality. In particular, berries packaged in micro-perforated (1mm ∅) and non-perforated films maintained their high quality attributes (high TSS content and titratble acidity) throughout the cold storage period. Non-perforated films maintained also berry crispness and a good intensity of flavour. Moreover, this treatment was the only one that reduced pathogen-induced decay during cold storage. The air treatment with ozone during the storage period was effective in reducing fungal decay, but little or no quality advantages were noted with the use of ozone on fruit firmness, soluble solids content or acidity.

Chapter XI - The strength of today's global fresh "berry" industry can be attributed to a combination of factors. New production techniques, improved varieties (that taste great) and the growing scientific evidence of the health and nutritional benefits all contribute to build consumer appetite for berries.

Public and private health sector programs have developed consumer education campaigns stressing the importance of fruits and vegetables in our diet. This increased awareness of the "benefits of berries" along with higher quality, better tasting individual berry types has propelled berries to become the leading produce category in US retail supermarkets.

Berry growers and their sales and marketing teams cannot, however, take for granted this favorite fruit status. Consumer eating habits are fragile and ever shifting. Producers and their trading partners - retailers and restaurant operators, must never fall into the trap that there will always be high consumer demad for fresh berries. They must constantly explore how to be efficient and effective marketers, allowing for reasonable profits for those in the supply chain. All the while, the goal is to consistently satisfy the consumer's taste buds and ensure future purchasing.

This is not a passive exercise, engaged producers and marketers must find ways to build value (real and perceived), generate sales velocity (aligned with production and inventories) and perhaps most importantly, ensure viability (through sustainable farming and business practices).

In: Berries: Properties, Consumption and Nutrition
Editor: Carlo Tuberoso
ISBN 978-1-61470-257-3

Chapter I

Berries: Bioactive Constituents and Their Impact on Human Health

María Elena Valverde and Octavio Paredes-López*
Centro de Investigación y de Estudios Avanzados del Instituto Politécnico Nacional. Unidad Irapuato, Irapuato, Gto., México

Abstract

Epidemiological studies in different countries have identified fruits and vegetables as key components in a healthy diet; they are good sources of dietary fiber, essential nutrients and phytochemicals. Consumption of fruits and vegetables delays the ageing process and reduces the risk of various lifestyle diseases, mainly cardiovascular and anti-degenerative diseases, cancer, rheumatoid arthritis, cataract, Parkinson, Alzheimer, among other biological effects on human beings. Fruits, but in particular berries, have been the focus among researchers and health professionals and now it is known that the intake of berries has a positive impact on human health, principally in disease prevention. Berries must be one of the main components of healthy diets, particularly because they are a rich source of phytochemicals, especially a wide variety of phenolic compounds (phenolic acids, anthocyanins, flavonols, flavones, flavanols, flavanones, isoflavonoids, stilbenes and tannins), and also contain vitamins, mainly vitamin C, and minerals. The effects of phenolic compounds on health have been mostly attributed to their antioxidant properties; berries are a particularly rich source of antioxidants, but the biological activities exhibited by berries phytochemicals *in vivo* extend beyond antioxidation. Besides a positive influence on oxidative status, they also have a mechanism associated with the low-grade systemic inflammation that helps to control many diseases. On the other hand, the phenolic profiles of berries species are quite diverse and, therefore, expected to have different biological activities. The diversity of bioactive compounds is reflected in the broad spectrum of their biological and medicinal properties, and such differences are observed in the content and the qualitative composition of the

* E-mail: oparedes@ira.cinvestav.mx, Centro de Investigación y de Estudios Avanzados del Instituto Politécnico Nacional. Unidad Irapuato, Apdo. Postal 629, 36821, Irapuato, Gto., México.

compounds. In recent years, several berries such as strawberry, blueberry, cranberry, and black raspberry have been extensively studied and the observations on the health benefits of their constituents are well documented. In this chapter we analyze the bioactive constituents, biological properties and human health benefits of berries, and their importance in the prevention of various diseases.

Abbreviations

CoA = Co-enzyme A
UV = Ultraviolet
HHDP = Hexahydroxydiphenoyl
ROS = Reactive oxidant species
AOC = Antioxidant capacity
iNOS = Inducible nitric oxide synthase
COX-2 = Cyclooxygenase 2
NO = Nitric oxide
PGE2 = Prostaglandin E2
DNA = Deoxyribonucleic acid
HepG2 = Hepatocellular liver carcinoma cells
LDL = Low density lipoproteins
VEGF = Vascular endothelial growth factor
fw = Fresh weight

Introduction

Dietary guidelines around the world recommend a diet rich in fruits and vegetables as a good source of fiber, essential nutrients, and beneficial phytochemicals, especially because there is increasing evidence that they delay the ageing process and reduces the risk of various lifestyle diseases (i.e., cardiovascular diseases, cancer, rheumatoid arthritis, lung diseases, cataract, Alzheimer's disease) [1-4]. At the present time, consumers expect the foods to be sensory attractive, but also safe and healthy [5].

Bioactive compounds present in foods elicit physiological responses to modulate processes of metabolism, mainly oxidative stress and inflammation; they play a key role in a big number of chronic diseases, promote health and reduce disease risk [63]. Different studies emphasize that the compounds responsible for these protective effects are vitamins, minerals, fiber, and more recently phytochemicals, particularly phenolic compounds [6-10].

Phenolic compounds are widely distributed throughout the plant kingdom; in particular berries contain a wide variety of these phytochemicals and are exceptionally rich sources of antioxidant phenolics compounds [10-12]. Berries contain vitamins A, C, E, and folic acid; calcium and selenium; α- carotene, β-carotene and lutein; phytoesterols as β-sitosterol and stigmasterol and triterpene esters. The majority groups of phenolic compounds are phenolic acids (hydroxibenzoic and hydroxycinnamic acids), flavonoids (flavonols, flavones, flavanols or catechins, flavanones, isoflavonoids and anthocyanins), stilbenes and tannins [13-16].

In recent years many researchers and health professionals have targeted the study of berry bioactive compounds; their characterization and utilization in functional foods and their beneficial properties. Various groups of scientists have firmly established that the dietary intake of berry fruits has a positive and profound impact on human health, performance, and disease control. Berry phenolics contribute to the protection against degenerative diseases, in particular have a huge impact on cardiovascular health. Also, it has been demonstrated by clinical analysis that the bioavailability of the phenolic compounds significantly exceeds the health benefits proportioned by their corresponding supplements in pharmaceutical form [16-19]. And their effects on health have been mostly attributed to their antioxidant properties [5,20]. Berry fruits, such as bilberry (*Vaccinium myrtillus*), blackberry (*Rubus fruticosus*), blueberry (*Vaccinium corymbosum*), chokeberry (*Aronia melanocarpa*), cranberry (*Vaccinium macrocarpon*), grape (*Vitis vinifera*), raspberry (*Rubus idaeus*), and strawberry (*Fragaria x ananassa*) are a particularly rich source of antioxidants [21-31].

In conclusion, berries provide an ideal resource for investigating phytochemicals that influence human health. There is strong evidence that polyphenols from berries deliver positive effects at various levels in the human body; however, more research is needed to fully understand which molecules are effective and what mechanisms are involved in their action [32-34]. In this chapter we discuss berry fruits constituents, biological properties, human health benefits and their importance in prevention of some diseases.

Phenolic Compounds

Polyphenolic compounds are characterized by the presence of one or more six-carbon aromatic ring, benzene, and one or more hydroxyl groups attached directly to the aromatic ring. The term phenolics cover a very large and diverse group of chemical compounds widely distributed throughout the nature [35-37].

They are classified by their structural characteristics [13,35-38]. Flavonoids and phenolic acids are the most abundant polyphenols in the human diet; however, phenolics compounds are ubiquitous in all food plants. They are the products of secondary metabolism and have many diverse biological functions, including roles in plant growth, development, and defense; provide pigmentation, antimicrobial and antifungal functions, insect-feeding deterrence, UV radiation protection, chelation of toxic heavy metals, antioxidant quenching of free radicals generated during photosynthesis, and much more [10-12,39]. On the other hand, there is huge evidence that phenolic compounds have diverse effects on human health.

Phenolic Components in Berries

Berries contain vitamin C and are a rich source of phytochemicals. The phenolic profiles are quite diverse and have different biological activities. Phenolics compounds are the main group of phytochemicals that strongly influence the sensorial attributes and the nutritional value [40]. Berry fruits are rich in phenolic acids, flavonols (quercetin and kaempferol), flavanols (catechins and luteolin), isoflavones (genistein), proanthocyanidins, anthocyanidins (pelargonidin), stilbenes, tannins and in particular anthocyanins which provide the distinctive and vibrant palette of colors found in berries (Figure 1). In general, the anthocyanin profile is characteristic and it has been used in taxonomy, as well as for the detection of adulteration of juices and wines. They also contain ellagitannins, flavan-3-ols, procyanidins, flavonols and hydroxybenzoate derivatives [10,24,26,34,36,41].

The concentration of phenolic compounds in plants might be determined by biotic and abiotic factors [25,33,42,43]. The genotype, species, environment and cultivation conditions have a profound influence on the content of bioactive compounds in berries, and the phenolic composition changes throughout growth and stages of ripening [44-46]. Kellogg *et al.* [47] worked with wild Alaskan berries and reported that the phytochemical content and characterization is very different in each berry analyzed, depending on species and biogeographic location. The authors concluded that the severity of the environment could be a big contributing factor to the overall composition of these particular fruits; this study supported the hypothesis that climate fluctuations affect quantity and quality berries phytochemical composition.

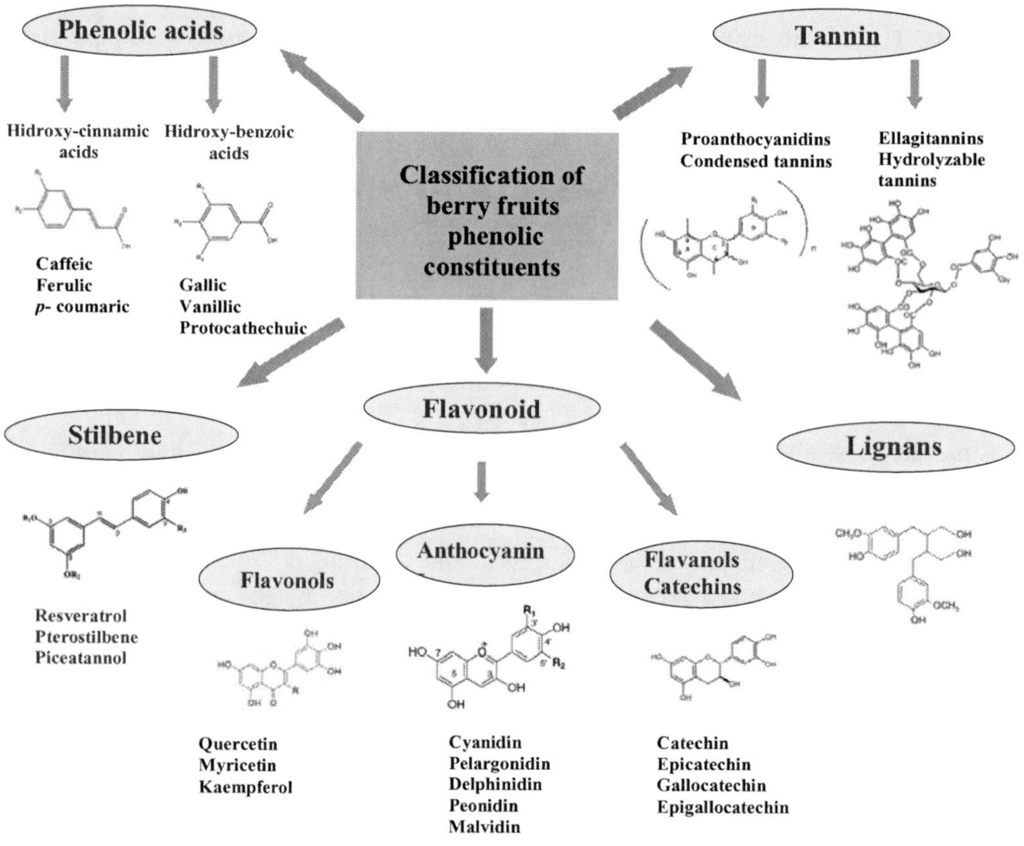

Figure 1. Phenolic constituents in berry fruits.

Thus, the impact of climate change on berries and their bioactive health properties could be significant. On the other hand, wild berries may provide a preferred resource for investigating phytochemicals that can improve human health, because they contain natural inherent levels of compounds that have not been influenced by commercial breeding and selection [32]. Several studies have demonstrated more or distinct antioxidant activity and phenolic composition in wild berries compared to their domesticated relatives [32,44,45,48-51]. However, berry fruits, such as bilberry (*Vaccinium myrtillus*), blackberry (*Rubus fruticosus*), blueberry (*Vaccinium corymbosum*), chokeberry (*Aronia melanocarpa*), cranberry (*Vaccinium macrocarpon*), grape (*Vitis vinifera*), raspberry (*Rubus idaeus*) and strawberry (*Fragaria x ananassa*) are a particularly rich source of antioxidants and polyphenolic compounds (Table 1) [10,29].

Table 1. Total phenolic content in berry fruits

Species	Phenolics (mg/100 g fresh weight)	References
Bilberry (*Vaccinium myrtillus*)	525	[52]
Blackberry (*Rubus fruticosus*)	193–577	[24,29,53]
Blueberry (*Vaccinium corymbosum*)	181–929	[25,52]
Chokeberry (*Aronia melanocarpa*)	662–690	[27,29]
Cranberry (*Vaccinium macrocarpon*)	120–315	[54,55]
Grapes (*Vitis vinifera* L.)	582	[56]
Raspberry (*Rubus idaeus*)	113–517	[57,58]
Strawberry (*Fragaria x ananassa*)	317–443	[30,56,58]

Phenolic Acids

Phenolic acids in berries are represented by cinnamic acid and benzoic acid derivatives [59]. The main benzoic acid derivatives found in berries are *p*-hydroxybenzoic acid, gallic acid, salicylic acid, vanillic acid and ellagic acid; and cinnamic acids derivatives are *p*-coumaric acid, caffeic acid and ferulic acid [10,21,36,60-62]. Caffeic acid and ferulic acids are the most common in berries and generally are esterified with carbohydrates and organic acids. Variation in the phenolic acid contents in berries may be small to moderate, but sometimes big chances are abserved [10,61].

Phenolic acids are plant metabolites widely spread throughout the plant kingdom and has been reported that they have a potential protective role against oxidative damage diseases, like coronary heart disease, stroke, and cancers, such as other polyphenol compounds [5,10,37,63].

Flavonoids

Flavonoids are C15 compounds, all of which have the structure C6-C3-C6. Flavonoids may be grouped into three big classes based on their general structure. In each case, two benzene rings are linked together by a group of three carbons. It is the arrangement of the C3 group that determines how the compounds are classified (Figure 2) [36,37]. Flavonoids have an A-, B- and C-ring, and are typically depicted with the A-ring on the left-hand side. The A-ring originates from the condensation of three malonyl-CoA molecules, and the B-ring originates from *p*-coumaroyl-CoA. These origins explain why the A-ring of most flavonoids is either *meta*-dihydroxylated or *meta*-trihydroxylated [36,37].

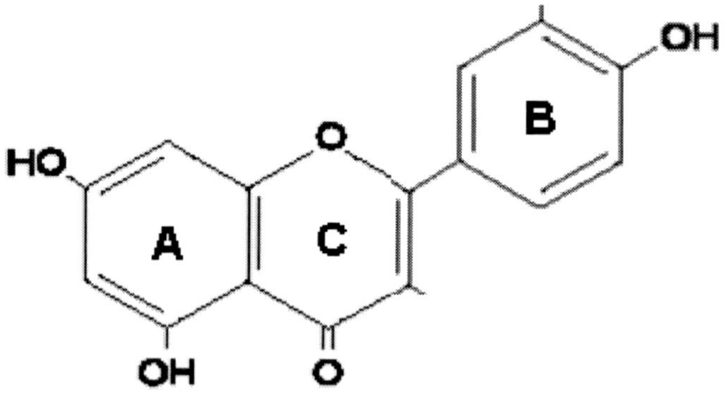

Figure 2. Flavonoid.

Table 2. Flavonols and flavanols content in berry fruits

Species	Total flavonol (mg/100 g fresh weight)	Main flavonol	References
Bilberry (*Vaccinium myrtillus*)	29–44	Quercetin	[21,69]
Blackberry (*Rubus fruticosus*)	366	Catechin	[25]
Blueberry (*Vaccinium corymbosum*)	3–387	Catechin	[25,69]
Chokeberry (*Aronia melanocarpa*)	89	Quercetin	[69]
Cranberry (*Vaccinium macrocarpon*)	83–157	Quercetin	[69,70]
Grapes (*Vitis vinifera* L.)	12	Epicatechin	[56]
Raspberry (*Rubus idaeus*)	6	Quercetin	[69]
Strawberry (*Fragaria x ananassa*)	7–15	Quercetin	[69]

They are commonly divided into: flavonols, flavanols (so called catechins) and anthocyanidins. In berries the flavonols are commonly quercetin, myricetin and kaempferol and the most abundant flavanols are catechin, epicatechin, gallocatechin and epigallocatechin (Table 2) [21,37,64-66].

Berries also can contain the flavan-3-ol monomers (+)-catechin and (-)-epicatechin as well as dimers, trimers and polymeric proanthocyanidins. The concentration of the polymers is usually greater than the monomers, dimers and trimers, and cranberries are a particularly rich source of these compounds [67,68].

Flavonoids may benefit health in cardiovascular diseases by adjusting adhesion of monocytes (large mononuclear leukocytes in the blood) in the inflammatory process of atherosclerosis and it was suggested that metabolites of flavonoids contribute to reduce the risk of cardiovascular diseases [36].

Anthocyanins

Table 3. Anthocyanins content in berry fruits

Species	Total anthocyanins (mg/100g fresh weight)	Main anthocyanins	References
Bilberry (*Vaccinium myrtillus*)	201–611	Delphinidin and cyanidin	[27,34,52,78]
Blackberry (*Rubus fruticosus*)	67–325	Cyanidin and pelargonidin	[25,29,34,79]
Blueberry (*Vaccinium corymbosum*)	63–495	Peonidin, delphinidin, malvidin and petunidin	[29,34,78]
Chokeberry (*Aronia melanocarpa*)	311–461	Peonidin, cyanidin and delphinidin	[29, 34,78]
Cranberry (*Vaccinium macrocarpon*)	19–140	Cyanidin and peonidin	[55,78,79]
Grapes (*Vitis vinifera* L.)	11–27	Malvidin and peonidin	[79]
Raspberry (*Rubus idaeus*)	19–116	Cyanidin and pelargonidin	[34,58,78,80]
Strawberry(*Fragaria x ananassa*)	20–52	Pelargonidin and cyanidin	[34,58,78]

Anthocyanins are water-soluble glycosides of anthocyanidins, and are the most important group of water-soluble pigments throughout the plant kingdom. They are responsible for the red, blue, purple and orange colors in fruits and vegetables [71]. Different plants present anthocyanins also in leaves, flowers and stems. These compounds are found in the vacuole sites called anthocyanoplasts of epidermal cells [36,37,72-74]. Major sources of anthocyanins are bilberries, blueberries, chokeberries, raspberries, cranberries, strawberries, black currants, and purple grapes. And the most abundant anthocyanidins (Table 3) are cyanidin (magenta, red), pelargonidin (orange-red), delphinidin (purple, blue-red), petunidin (purple, blue-red), peonidin (magenta, orange-red) and malvidin (blue-red) (Table 3) [21,34,75-77].

They have differences in their number and positions in the hydroxyl or methoxyl groups, and their basic structures are shown in Figure 3 [41,81]. The principal anthocyanin found in most fruits is cyanidin-3-glucoside and also occupy a special place in the group of polyphenols found in berry fruits. The content of anthocyanins and their qualitative composition in berries are determined by the species; they are particularly diversified in blueberry and bilberry, where more than ten anthocyanins have been found; fewer differences are observed in chokeberry, strawberry and raspberry [10,82].

One important characteristic of anthocyanins and anthocyanidins is the ability to form complexes with metals such as Al, Fe, Cu and Sn, and the stability of blue colors are due to a complexation among anthocyanins and metals [81]. In recent years several studies have shown that anthocyanins display a wide range of biological activities including antioxidant, anti-inflammatory, antimicrobial and anti-carcinogenic activities. In addition, display a variety of effects on blood vessels, platelets and lipoproteins able to reduce the risk of coronary heart diseases and a high consumption of them will reduce the risk of chronic diseases [5,34,63,83].

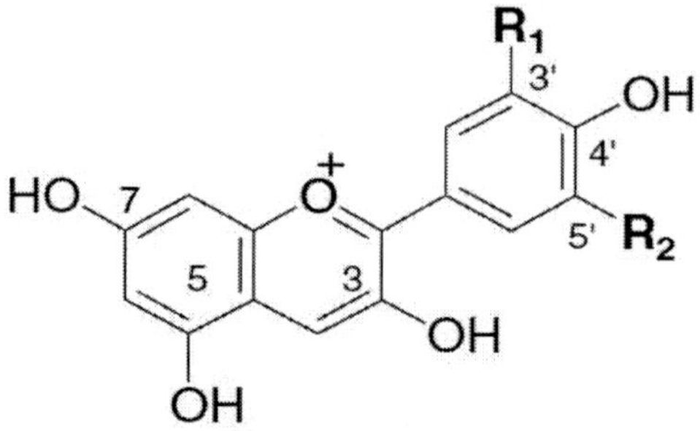

Name	R_1	R_2	Color
Pelargonidin	H	H	Orange-red-salmon
Cyanidin	OH	H	Magenta
Delphinidin	OH	OH	Purple, blue-red
Petunidin	OH	OCH_3	Purple, blue-red
Peonidin	OCH_3	H	Magenta, orange-red
Malvidin	OCH_3	OCH_3	Blue-red

Figure 3. Basic structure of anthocyanins present in berries.

Anthocyanins have been associated with increased neuronal signaling in brain centers, mediating memory function as well as improved glucose disposal, benefits that would be expected to mitigate neurodegeneration [84].

Stilbenes

Stilbenes have a C6-C2-C6 structure and they have a 1, 2-diphenylethylene nucleus (Figure 4). Ring A commonly carries two hydroxyl substituents, while ring B is substituted by methoxy and hydroy groups.

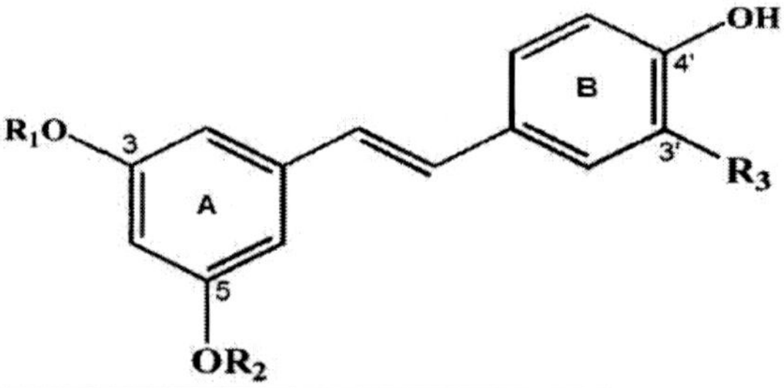

Name	R_1	R_2	R_3
Resveratrol	OH	OH	H
Pterostilbene	CH_3	CH_3	H
Piceatannol	OH	OH	OH

Figure 4. The main structure of berry fruits stilbenes.

They are found in plants as monomeric form and as dimeric, trimeric and polymeric stilbenes, the so-called viniferins, and normally associated with heartwood of trees [36,37,66,85]. The most important is resveratrol and the best known is trans-resveratrol. Piceatannol (also known as astringinin) and pterostilbene are other resveratrol analogues, which have been found in berries [86-89]. The stilbenes possess important biological actions such as antiageing, algicidal activity, antimutagenic activity, anti-inflammatory, cardiovascular protection and chemopreventive/chemotherapeutic effects demonstrated *in vitro* and *in vivo* assays [89-94]. Resveratrol has been shown to have cancer chemopreventive activity in the three major stages of carcinogenesis: promotion, initiation, and progression [95].

Tannins

Tannins comprise a group of compounds with a wide diversity in structure that shares their ability to bind and precipitate proteins. They play an essential role in shaping the sensory properties of fruit and fruit products. They are responsible for the tart taste and changes in the color of fruit and fruit juice [10,36,37].

Tannins can be classified in three groups: condensed tannins, hydrolysable tannins, and complex tannins [96]. However, in berries they can be classified into two groups: condensed tannins (so called proanthocyanidins) and hydrolysable tannins. The hydrolysable tannins consist of gallic acid polymers that include gallotannins, and ellagic acid polymers that include ellagitannins [36,97,98]. The astringency of berries is caused by condensed tannins; they are responsible for the tart taste resulting from interactions among proteins and tannins at the surface of the mouth mucosa [36].

Berries tannins include monomeric units of catechin or epicatechin with a flavan-3,4-diol or flavan-4-ol molecule as its precursor [97]. Figure 5 shows the basic structure of condensed tannins found in berries; however, berries are the richest source of hydrolysable tannins. They are defined as hexahydroxydiphenoyl (HHDP) esters of carbohydrates and cyclitols but also include compounds derived from additional oxidative transformations.

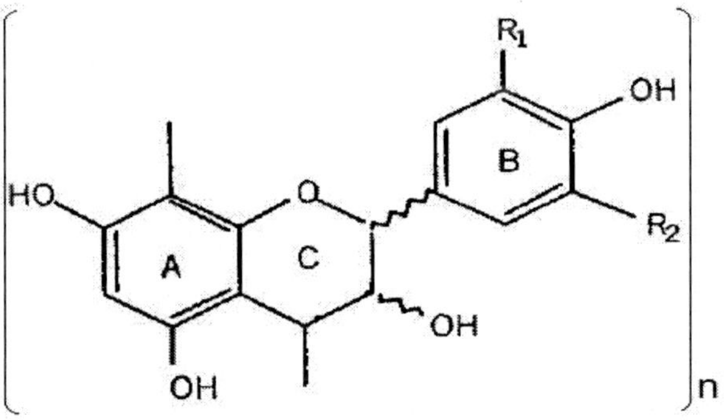

Figure 5. Basic structure of condensed tannins found in berries.

HHDP is a product of the oxidation of galloyl groups [39,99]. They have a wide range of structures and can be present as monomers, oligomers, and complex polymers; also contain organic acids such as ellagic acid, in acylated and glycosylated forms [43,70,100-102].

The hydroxybenzoate ellagic acid has been reported particularly in raspberries, strawberries and blackberries [103]. Indeed, ellagic acid has been described as being responsible for 50% of total phenolics quantified in strawberries and raspberries [75]. In berries, the largest quantity of condensed tannins with a high degree of polymerization is found in chokeberry [104]. Small quantities of tannins were found in honeyberry and blackberry. But blackberry contains only hydrolysable tannins, and condensed tannins were found in chokeberry fruits. Fruit tannins comprise (−)epicatechin and (+)catechin. (−)Epicatechin is the dominant tannin component in chokeberry [10].

Ellagitannins have been often identified as the active principle in medicinal plants [5, 34,96]. Wang *et al.* [105] worked with three berry types and found differences in their content of ellagitannins in this order, black raspberries > strawberries > blueberries. They were looking if ellagitannins contribute to the chemopreventive activity in tumor development in rat esophagus and concluded that the inhibitory effects of the three berry types were not due solely to their content of ellagitannins; they attempted to identify other constituents in the residue fractions of these berries that might be responsible for chemoprevention. On the other hand, tannins have been used to treat a wide array of illnesses, including diarrhea and tumors in the stomach or duodenum. Another application of tannins is in wine and beer production, where they are used to precipitate proteins.

Effects on Human Health of Phenolic Compounds

There is huge evidence that phenolic compounds have effects on human health. Perhaps the oldest medical application of phenolic compounds is the use of phenol as antiseptic; because of its negative side effects, especially at higher concentrations, it is no longer used with this purpose [36]. Another very common use of phenolic compounds is in sunscreens. The presence of the aromatic ring results in the effective absorbance of the UV-B radiation (between 280 and 315 nm) from the sun and thus prevents sunburns. Health benefits of many phenolic phytochemicals have been identified using *in vitro* methods, which may not be relevant *in vivo* due to poor absorption and metabolism. The levels of these compounds appearing in the blood or excreted in urine may be found at very low concentrations and in very different forms from those ingested. On the other hand, there is strong evidence that polyphenols from berry fruits are absorbed to varying degrees and deliver positive effects at various levels in the human body. However, phenolic compounds have been long used as natural remedies in the treatment of various diseases (circulatory, respiratory, digestive and urinary system ailments). They are applied in the production of various pharmaceutical products due to their ability to seal capillary vessels and improve circulation [10]. Figure 6 shows some human health effects of the selected berries constituents. In addition, phenolic compounds may provide benefit to human subjects for several mechanisms; however, the best-described and most well-known mechanism is through their antioxidant properties and modulation of biological oxidative stress to prevent damage to cellular lipids, proteins and DNA [63].

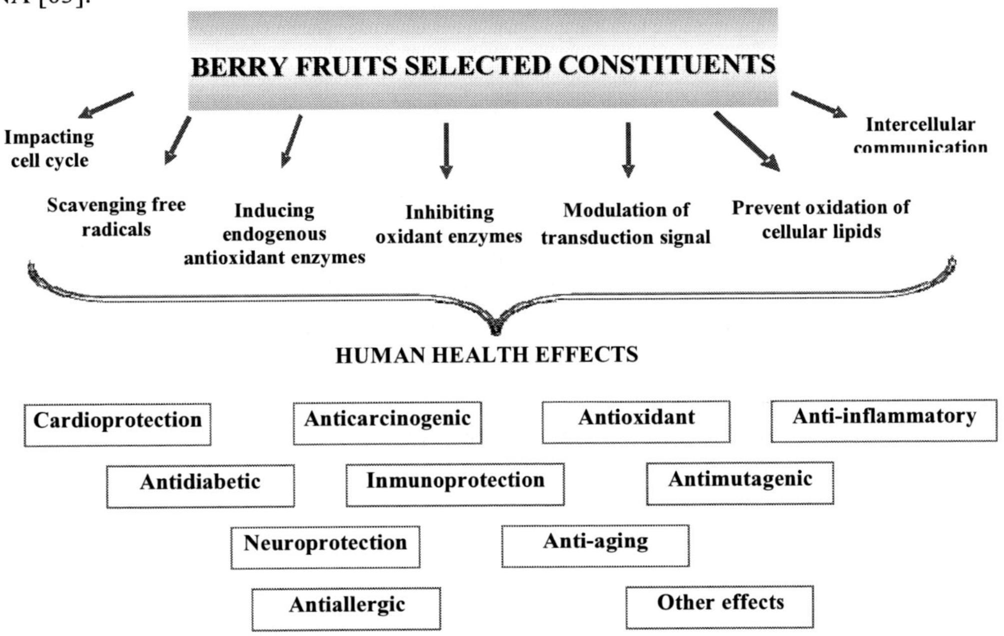

Figure 6. Human health effects of the selected berry fruits constituents.

During the past decade, it has become increasingly clear that oxidative stress and inflammation are key features in a number of chronic diseases. The evidence strongly suggests that the reactive oxidant species (ROS) and free radicals are part of normal metabolism; radicals are generated and produced in an extensive range of physiological processes from normal metabolic activity and lifestyle exposures [106-108]. They are very reactive, can cause oxidative damage to the molecules in a cell, and have negative impacts on the cellular metabolism. Oxidative stress is an imbalance between the production of ROS and antioxidant defense, and may lead to oxidative damage. This biological condition may result from insufficiency of antioxidant defense mechanisms, intense production of ROS, and excessive activation of ROS systems, which are implicated in aging and in the pathology of many chronic disorders, including cancer, cardiovascular diseases, inflammation, diabetes, Parkinson´s and Alzheimer´s disease and other pathologies [109,110].

Antioxidant Properties

Dietary antioxidants can play an important role in mitigating the damaging effects of ROS on cellular macromolecules, and thereby reducing chronic disease risk [111-113]. The indicated properties of fruit and vegetable compounds determine their health-promoting properties [10]. Overall, phenolic compounds found in plant foods have multiple paths for benefiting human health, most notably through their actions as antioxidants and modifying cellular events. Their specific actions are likely to be dependent on the composition and time course of compound/metabolites appearing in plasma [114-117].

The antioxidant capacity (AOC) has been proposed as an indicator of the presence of beneficial bioactive compounds in foodstuffs and therefore, their healthfulness [118]. However, variability in the measurements between foodstuff samples and quantification methods makes the compilation of a phytochemical index, in a standardized way, very difficult. Several research groups have published lists of AOC values of numerous foods using their own food sources and methodologies [68,119-122]. The antioxidant activity of bioactive constituents of berries fruits has been assessed using *in vitro* assays by measuring the ability to reduce and trap free radicals; their potential as an antioxidant is usually measured by comparison with a reference substance, commonly Trolox (trade name of 6-hydroxy-2,5,7,8-tetramethylchroman-2-carboxylic acid, a water-soluble derivative of vitamin E) [5].

There is considerable *in vitro* evidence showing that berry phenolics are powerful antioxidants. When results are compared, it is evident that berry fruits are consistently ranked among the top sources of total phenolics and AOC, containing levels up to four times greater than other fruits, 10 times greater than vegetables, and 40 times greater than cereals. Berry phenolics are also potent antioxidants toward oxidation of bulk lipids [121,123]. Raspberries have been repeatedly ranked within the top 10 commonly consumed foods tested for their AOC values [119,121].

Berry fruits owe their antioxidant properties mainly to phenolic compounds, including phenolic acids, tannins, stilbenes and flavonoids which are represented by anthocyanins, flavonols and flavanols. The antioxidant effect of berry phenolics is strongly dependent on the choice of berry raw material; also the antioxidant activity differs between phenolic constituents (anthocyanins, ellagitannins, and proanthocyanidins).

Table 4. Antioxidant capacity in berry fruits

Species	ORAC[a] μmol/g fw	FRAP[b] μmol/g fw	ABTS[c] μmol/g fw	DPPH[d] μmol/g fw	References
Bilberry (*Vaccinium myrtillus*)	45	73	–	–	[24,52]
Blackberry (*Rubus fruticosus*)	13 – 56	88	20	36	[10,24,26,124]
Blueberry (*Vaccinium corymbosum*)	19 – 97	19 – 121	–	–	[24,55]
Chokeberry (*Aronia melanocarpa*)	160	–	–	–	[55]
Cranberry (*Vaccinium macrocarpon*)	19	–	–	–	[55]
Grapes (*Vitis vinifera* L.)	17	–	–	4	[18,56]
Raspberry (*Rubus idaeus*)	8 – 77	23	–	25	[26,57,58]
Strawberry (*Fragaria x ananassa*)	21–24	25--33	12	7	[26,56,58]

aORAC: Oxygen Radical Absorbance Capacity; bFRAP: Ferric Reducing Ability of Plasma; cABTS: 2,2'-Azinobis (3-ethylbenzothiazoline-6-sulfonic acid); dDPPH: 2,2-Diphenyl-1-picrylhydrazil; Units: µol equivalent trolox/mL; fw: fresh weight.

On the other hand, the antioxidant activity is determined by the species, variety, cultivation, region, weather conditions, ripeness, harvesting time, storage time and conditions. Chokeberry, bilberry, blueberry and strawberry contain large amounts of phenolics and are marked by particularly high antioxidant capacity (Table 4) [29,30,49-51,54,55,123]. On the other hand, wild berries have significantly higher antioxidant activities than domestic berries and also a higher content of phenolics (except for cranberry) [50,51,115].

Disease Prevention

Epidemiological studies have proposed a relationship between high flavonoid consumption and decreased risk of cancer, cardiovascular disease, and other age-related diseases. Thus, enhancing flavonoid biosynthesis in crops may result in foods with benefits to human health [36]. The phenolic compounds in the diet have positive effects within the gastrointestinal tract; some of them are binding of iron, scavenging reactive nitrogen, chlorine, and oxygen species, and inhibition of cyclooxygenases and lipoxygenases. Phenolic compounds have been also suggested to prevent the adverse affects of fungal toxins (mycotoxins) in human health and to serve in their detoxification [125].

There is substantial evidence that flavonoids, especially quercetin, reduce the risk of lung cancer; but also protect against coronary heart disease and atherosclerosis, as well as inflammation. Resveratrol has been shown to have cancer chemopreventive activity in the three major stages of carcinogenesis: promotion, initiation, and progression [95]. The anti-carcinogenic effects of resveratrol have been tested *in vitro* and *in vivo* for different researches and with diverse methods. On the other hand, resveratrol has been also reported to offer protection against cardiovascular diseases [5,16,34]. Ellagitannins are dietary polyphenols containing ellagic acid subunits that are thought to act as cancer chemo-preventive agents. Proanthocyanidins and tannin-like compounds are complex flavonoid polymers, and may have properties that contribute to health benefits in humans. As reducing agents, they may participate in prevention of cancers of the digestive tract and inner organs; they may also protect low density lipids (LDLs) against oxidation and inhibit platelet aggregation; which would act as a preventative of cardiovascular diseases [97].

On the other hand, obesity is recognized as a major health issue in the United States and in many other countries. Diet is one of the most important components of a multitude of complex factors that can affect this problem and health. Prior *et al.* [52] feeding mice with isolated anthocyanins from blueberry and strawberry found decreased weight gain and body fat, although the differences were not always statistically significant. However, feeding of the whole berry appears to have a negative effect in terms of increasing adiposity.

Anti-Inflammatory

Inflammation is a normal protective response induced by tissue injury or infection to combat foreign invaders in the body. Chronic inflammation is associated with several human pathologies and causes the up-regulation of several pro-inflammatory proteins in affected tissues. In this process there are mediators which somehow may regulate cellular adhesion molecules in inflamed tissues [126]. Among numerous pro- inflammatory enzymes, inducible nitric oxide synthase (iNOS) and cyclooxygenase 2 (COX-2) produce nitric oxide (NO) and prostaglandin E2 (PGE2) during the inflammation process (127). Cuevas-Rodríguez *et al.* [50] analyzed total polyphenolic compounds, total anthocyanins and total proanthocyanidin of four wild blackberry, one domesticated noncommercial breeding line, and one commercial cultivar (Tupy) to inhibit the inflammatory process. Nitric oxide (NO) and prostaglandin E2 (PGE2) production, inducible nitric oxide synthase (iNOS) and cyclooxygenase-2 (COX-2) expression were evaluated and the authors reported that the antioxidant capacity was significantly correlated with NO inhibition. The combined results from this study suggest that dietary consumption of blackberries may reduce the oxidative stress generated by NO and the expression of pro-inflammatory proteins such as COX-2 and iNOS, and the protection against oxidation-inflammation-related diseases. In addition, given the particularly strong bioactivities of compounds found in wild genotypes of Mexican blackberries, they concluded that these genotypes may be useful in plant-breeding programs designed to obtain new varieties with enhanced nutraceutical potential [50,51].

On the other hand, bioactive compounds may act as inflammation modulator agents, for example resveratrol in berries has shown very good anti-inflammatory effects; and anthocyanins have also shown potent anti-inflammatory activities [128-130].

Anticarcinogenic and Antimutagenic Activity

Anticarcinogenic and antimutagenic activity of some compounds in vegetables and fruits are effective to inhibit tumor initiation for influencing carcinogen metabolism. Phenolics and carotenoids can modulate some biochemical stages in carcinogenesis and cell signaling pathways to inhibit cancer progression [3,126,131,132]. Protective effects of polyphenolics against cancer extend beyond their antioxidant roles; many groups have been investigating the antitumor properties of phytochemicals and phytochemical-rich foods. Phenolics maybe blocking agents at the initiation stage of tumorogenesis and influence the metabolism of procarcinogens to stimulate the detoxification of carcinogens to their secretion from the body [2,131]. Cancer chemopreventive agents can act at different stages of the disease process by inhibiting formation of carcinogens, blocking initiation of carcinogenesis, or suppressing progression and proliferation of tumors [133].

The resveratrol in berries is a promising and potential chemopreventive. Chemopreventive action of resveratrol has been corroborated by its ability to block the activation of various carcinogens and also to stimulate detoxification, to prevent oxidative damage of DNA, to reduce inflammatory responses, and to block angiogenic and metastatic processes for tumor progression [85,89,128]. Anthocyanins possess also chemopreventive properties. Some reports demonstrate that flavonoids and anthocyanins inhibit the proliferation of human hepatocellular liver carcinoma cells (HepG2) and inhibited also esophageal tumors induced in rodent [134,135].

Seeram *et al.* [101] reported antiproliferative and pro-apoptotic effects of some berry extracts. When they increased berry extracts concentrations the inhibition of cell proliferation was increased too; the black raspberry showed the highest value. On the other hand, Vattem *et al.* [136] found antimutagenic activity in cranberry.

Cardioprotection

Phenolic compounds in berries have important role in cardioprotection. Numerous studies *in vitro* demonstrated that phenolic compounds can inhibit oxidation of LDL (low density lipoproteins), and oxidized LDL is the main constituent of atherogenic plaques, which are the basis of cardiovascular disorder [2,124]. Also, the anthocyanins have effects on cholesterol distribution, protect endothelial cells from inflammatory signals and induce relaxation in coronary arteries [137,138].

Anti-Ageing and Degenerative Diseases

Ageing process results in a various lifestyle diseases, mainly cardiovascular diseases and cancer, as well as other disorders, such as rheumatoid arthritis, lung diseases, cataract, Parkinson's or Alzheimer's disease [10,130]. The polyphenolics in fruits and vegetables have been shown to retard and even reverse age-related decrements in motor and cognitive performance. These effects may be the result of the polyphenols increasing antioxidant and/or anti-inflammatory levels, or by direct effects on signaling in the brain. Increased dietary intake of berry fruit has a positive and profound impact on human health, performance, and disease [139,140]. Also the efficacy of antioxidants, such as phenolics, carotenoids, vitamin C and vitamin E may reduce the deleterious effects of brain ageing. Blueberries, cranberries and strawberries have shown notorious actions in reversing the behavioral deficits [141-143].

Resveratrol has been identified to prolong the lifetime in certain model systems for ageing; this compound may alter chromatin structure, transcription and prevent age related cardiac dysfunction in mice [94]. Flavonoids (including anthocyanins) and other polyphenols can have effects in cell signaling and decrease oxidative damage, and also might act directly on cognition. These effects may contribute to the prevention of age-related and pathological degenerative processes in the brain [144]. On the other hand, anthocyanins in berries play beneficial roles in reversing age related cognitive impairment and protect against neurodegenerative disorders. Milbury and Kalt [145] reported that the plausible mechanism may be by modulation of signal transduction processes and/or gene expression in brain tissue, rather than by direct antioxidant radical quenching.

Antidiabetic

Anthocyanins and aglycones may have beneficial effects on diabetes, because they interfere with glucose absorption, inhibit active transport and they may have a protective effect on pancreatic cells. Simultaneous and daily administration to rats of anthocyanins and streptozotocin (diabetogenic compound with betacytotoxic effects) decrease glucose concentration in urine and serum. On the other hand, anthocyanins stimulate insulin secretion of rodent pancreatic beta-cells; the most potent stimulators are cyanidin, delphinidin and pelargonidin. Moreover, anthocyanins can inhibit α-glucosidase activity and may reduce blood glucose levels after starch-rich meals [66,74].

Other Biological Effects of Selected Constituents of Berries

Another effect of bioactive constituents in berry fruits is the antimicrobial activity. For example, they are useful for prevention of urinary tract infections; the proanthocyanidins can inhibit the adhesion of *E. coli* in the urinary tract [146,147]. Also some bioactive constituents in berries help to inhibit formation of biofilms (dental plaques) and adhesion of *streptococcus* and show anti-caries properties [148]. Berries flavonoids are very interesting for bone health and prevention of osteoporosis. It has been reported the effect of genistein and diadzein, also quercetin and kaempferol aglycones to suppress osteoclastic bone resorption in tissue culture systems and apoptosis in a rabbit bone osteoclast model [149-152]. Anthocyanins present protective gastric effects; this group of compounds prevents or lowers the inflammatory process involved in gastric injury and has been shown that cyanidin protects gastric mucosa from the damage caused by aspirin [74,153].

Berries

Blackberries

In blackberries (*Rubus fruticosus*, *R. ursinus* and *R. argutus*) 14 phenolic acids were found, the major being *p*-coumaric acid [25,59,75]. The major anthocyanins in blackberries are derivatives of cyaniding and the total of anthocyanins increased considerably during ripening; however, total phenolics did not show a marked change with maturity; but antioxidant activities also increased with ripening [34,43]. Interestingly, the proportions of anthocyanins varied greatly among cultivars, but the qualitative composition of polyphenolics is similar for all cultivars, even when quantitatively may be very different [43]. Cuevas-Rodríguez *et al.* [50] concluded that the four Mexican wild blackberries analyzed exhibited high polyphenolic concentrations; however, they reported considerably variation in bioactive polyphenolic content in different blackberry genotypes. Thus, the wild genotypes of Mexican blackberries are rich sources of polyphenolics compounds and can be used as a plant source for breeding programs to develop new super Mexican cultivars/varieties with elevated polyphenolic content with nutraceutical potential because of their antioxidant and anti-inflammatory properties [50,51]. Eleven ellagitannins were identified in the blackberry flesh, seeds, and torus; there are also multiple isomers of most ellagitannins. However, most were present only in the seeds with only a few present in all three regions of the fruit [154].

Blackberries are a rich source of polyphenolics which may contribute to reducing the risk of chronic diseases; they are usually consumed frozen or in thermally processed forms after storage. Processing usually resulted of losses in polyphenols, and in consequence also resulted in losses of antioxidant capacity [155]. Shukitt-Hale *et al.* [140] concluded that blackberries have positive effects on age-related changes in motor and spatial working memory performance. This berry can strengthen the brain against the ravages of time, could retard or prevent the development of age related neurodegenerative diseases and can reduce oxidative stress and inflammation superimposed upon a stress-vulnerable aging brain.

Blueberries

According to Ayaz *et al.* [156] the wild blueberry *(Vaccinium corymbosum)* growing in Turkey presented mainly an ester of caffeic acid and of quinic acid (chlorogenic acid); but in wild blueberry grown in Northeastern Poland were characterized 17 phenolic acids, the most common was vanillic acid; however other studies only identified five phenolic acids (caffeic, gallic, ferulic, ellagic and *p*-coumaric) in *V. ashei* and *V. corymbosum* [25,59,61,75]. The major components in blueberries are malvidin-3-O-arabinoside and the 3-O-galactosides of cyanidin, delphinidin, petunidin and malvidin, with many minor anthocyanins also being present [34,157].

Blueberry has high antioxidant activity among fresh fruits and genetic differences have been demonstrated in several studies [18,52,158,159]. Connor *et al.* [23] reported that cultivar differences for antioxidant activity exist in ripe blueberry fruit at harvest and during cold storage, and antioxidant activity correlated with total phenolic content and especially with anthocyanin content. Howard *et al.* [160] made a jam with fresh blueberries and stored for six months at 4 and 25 °C. Marked losses of anthocyanins and procyanidins occurred over six months of storage at 25 °C. Jams stored at 4 °C retained higher levels of anthocyanins, procyanidins, and antioxidant properties. The authors concluded that blueberry jams should be refrigerated to retain polyphenolics and antioxidant capacity.

Lacueva *et al.* [161] reported that blueberry supplementation and cognition are positively correlated with the total number of anthocyanin compounds found in the different brain regions; anthocyanins enhanced cognitive behavioral performance and have important benefits on the progression of ageing and neurodegenerative disease. Joseph *et al.* [162] found that blueberry is effective in reversing age-related deficits and Alzheimer's disease in rodents. Various studies have demonstrated that dietary supplementation with blueberry polyphenolics may have beneficial actions on motor and cognitive function, and suggested that blueberry supplementation enhanced several signaling pathways which have been widely shown to be important in memory formation [92,144,162]. Krikorian *et al.* [84] indicated that wild blueberry juice in the daily diet for 12 weeks improved memory function in older adults with early memory decline; they also found diminished depressive symptoms and reduced fasting glucose levels. Also anthocyanin extracts of wild and cultivated blueberries enhanced eye health. Generally, the daily dose recommended is 25 mg of anthocyanins, which is equivalent to less than a handful of blueberries [123].

Blueberries have favorable effects on metabolic syndrome (characterized by abdominal adiposity, dyslipidemia or high triglycerides and low HDL cholesterol, hypertension, impaired glucose tolerance, elevated oxidative stress, inflammation, and atherosclerotic cardiovascular disease) and diabetes type 2 in obese animals [52,159]. However, Basu *et al.* [19] reported that blueberry supplementation for eight week did not affect fasting serum glucose, insulin, lipid profiles, and body weight or waist circumference; but significantly decreased systolic and diastolic blood pressures. This is the first report that blueberries may have antihypertensive effects in people with metabolic syndrome and the authors also suggested a cardio-protective role.

Cranberries

Cranberries (*Vaccinium, macrocarpon, V. microcarpum, V. erythrocarpum, V. oxycocco*) are known for their elevated concentration of anthocyanins and significant content of flavonols, flavan-3-ols, tannins (ellagitannins and proanthocyanidins), and phenolic acid derivatives. The major anthocyanins are galactosides and arabinosides of cyanidin and peonidin [34,163,164]. However, a large variety of bioactive compounds are found in cranberries, like flavonols (quercetin 3-galactoside), the flavan-3-ols (catechin and epicatechin), other anthocyanins (cyaniding 3-galactoside, cyanidin 3-arabinoside, peonidin 3-galactoside, and peonidin 3-arabinoside), the tannins (ellagitannins and proanthocyanidins), and the phenolic acid derivatives (ferulic acid, *p*-coumaric acid, coumaroylglucose, feruloylglucose, caffeoylglucose, chlorogenic acid, ellagic acid, and *p*hydroxybenzoic acids) [61,163-168].

The data strongly suggest that cranberry consumption could help protect against cardiovascular diseases, prevention of urinary tract infections, clearance of stomach pathogens, disruption of oral pathogen virulence and biofilm formation, depression of viral infectivity in vitro, dental health, *Helicobacter pylori*-induced stomach ulcers, inhibition of Alzheimer's disease, promotion of cardiovascular health, prevention and inhibition of cancer, and modulation of inflammatory responses [13,101,163,165,167,169]. Also extract of cranberry proanthocyanidin has potent effects on cell cycle regulation, cell viability, cell proliferation and apoptosis of esophageal adenocarcinoma cells [170].

As a complex mixture of phytochemicals, cranberry induces their biological effects by a multitude of molecular mechanisms, sometimes competing and sometimes additive or synergistic. These mechanisms may be divided into the following three categories: pathogen interactions, antioxidant mechanisms and effects on signal transduction, and protein expression and activity [167].

The antioxidant capacity of cranberry is affected by cultivars and storage temperatures. Wang and Stretch [54] reported that antioxidant values, anthocyanins and total phenolics contents increased during storage; the highest increases occurred at 15 °C storage; but at 20 °C had lower values than those stored at 15 °C. Also the authors reported a positive relationship between antioxidant values and anthocyanin or phenolic content in all ten cranberry cultivars at different storage temperatures.

Raspberries

Red raspberries (*Rubus idaeus*) contain essential minerals, vitamins, fatty acids and dietary fiber, as well as a wide range of polyphenolic phytochemicals and low calories. Polyphenols primarily are anthocyanins and hydrolysable tannins. They are a particularly rich source of cyanidin glycosides and have elevated ellagitannin content [39]. Raspberries have attractive color and great flavor. Red raspberries have economical importance and widely consumed fresh, frozen, or in processed forms, such as jellies, jams, and juices, whereas black raspberries (*R. occidentalis*) are less commonly grown and consumed. On the other hand, raspberries are among the fruits containing the highest antioxidant levels; freshly picked commercial and frozen contain similar levels of phytochemicals and antioxidants per serving. It is the cultivar and growing conditions that mainly affect the phytochemical content of the fruit [39,171]. Beekwilder *et al.* [171] have shown that the antioxidant content of raspberry fruits is determined by a diverse range of components, which provide unequal contributions to the total antioxidant activity; furthermore, during development and ripening, significant shifts occur for the contributions of the different classes of compounds, which cannot be detected by a general determination of total antioxidant activity. The antioxidant activity of the raspberry is directly related to the total amount of phenolics and flavonoids found; however, no relationship is found between antiproliferative activity and total amount of phenolics/flavonoids found [134].

The dominant antioxidants could be classified as anthocyanins, ellagitannins, and proanthocyanidin-like tannins; however, the antioxidant detection system clearly indicates that the ellagitannins make major contributions to the total antioxidant activity [171]. The ellagitannin content varies amply among varieties; this is an important issue for breeding programs [70,80,171]. The mainly anthocyanins are derivatives of cyanidins, and contain ten or more anthocyanins in the form of cyanidin and pelargonidin-3-*O*-sugar conjugates; also contain quercetin-3-glucuronide, kaempferol-3-glucuronide and the mayor flavan-3-ol is (+)-catechin [34,70].

The phenolic profile of red raspberries contributes to the antioxidant activity; it appears to beneficially modulate enzyme activity, cellular pathways, and gene expression as well; and reduces oxidized-LDL, antiatherosclerotic, anti-inflammatory activities, and may provide protection against cardiovascular diseases [39,85,87,100,171,172]. Many studies *in vitro* have demonstrated raspberry phytochemicals' ability to reduce cancer cell growth and to be effective in reducing vascular endothelial growth factor (VEGF) expression, a promoter of angiogenesis, critical step for tumor metastasis [13,173]. There is a lot of evidence of the protective role of red raspberry phytochemicals against cancers of the gastrointestinal tract. However, there is little evidence for their protection against other cancers. Even though these compounds are poorly absorbed, water-soluble, and quickly excreted, further research on their tissue accumulation may alter this perspective [174-176]. Additionally, raspberry phytochemicals have shown potential to improve glucose control in diabetics [177].

Strawberries

Strawberries (*Fragaria × ananassa*) are an important source of vitamin C and bioactive compounds with physiological effects in the human body and they are rich in a variety of phytochemicals that have been shown to be bioactive. The phenolic profile of strawberries from diverse origins has been studied and varies with the cultivar, growing conditions, degree of ripeness, and handling after harvest [14,15,35,178]. Tulipani *et al.* [178] reported the characterization of phytochemical and antioxidant profiles of nine different genotypes of strawberry; they measured the total flavonoid, anthocyanin, vitamin C, and folate contents; and also the cultivar effects on the total antioxidant capacities. This study showed the important role played by the genetic background on the chemical and antioxidant profiles of strawberry fruits, because significant differences were found between genotypes. Buendía *et al.* [179] reported 15 phenolic compounds in cultivars grown in Spain. They can be classified into six groups: ellagitannins, ellagic acid conjugates, hydroxycinnamic acids (pcoumaric and ferulic acid derivatives), flavonols (quercetin and kaempferol conjugates), proanthocyanidins (flavan-3-ols (+)-catechin) and anthocyanins (pelargonidin and cyaniding derivatives). Very simple anthocyanin profiles are found in strawberries; contain predominant glucoside of pelargonidin and cyanidin [34,79]. However, the ellagic acid is an important phenolic compound but proanthocyanidins are the main strawberry phenolic compounds [61,71,179]. Zhang et al. [20] reported ten phenolic compounds [cyanidin-3-glucoside, pelargonidin, pelargonidin-3-glucoside, pelargonidin-3-rutinoside, kaempferol, quercetin, kaempferol-3-(6′-coumaroyl-glucoside), 3,4,5-trihydroxyphenyl-acrylic acid, glucose ester of (*E*)-*p*-coumaric acid, and ellagic acid in strawberries.

The total phenolic content of 15 strawberry cultivars showed quantitative and qualitative differences among cultivars; all cultivars were grown under the same agronomic conditions and harvested at the same time to avoid environmental and agronomic effects on phenolic composition; this opens the opportunity for selecting cultivars with outstanding phenolic profiles [179]. These differences could be explained by the various extraction solvents and conditions used or because during maturation the amount of phenolic compounds changed significantly and the fruits analyzed had different ripening state or because of their genetic background [42,179]. Since strawberries are rich in phenolic compounds, such as anthocyanin, catechin and ellagic acid, their potential contribution to health is in effect very important. Total antioxidant capacity was determined using three different methods, and the results demonstrated that the consumption of strawberries could increase the antioxidant capacity of serum in humans. Antioxidant power of the phenolic compounds in strawberries has the potential to lower the risk of heart disease. Studies of the individual components have demonstrated inhibition of LDL oxidation and lipid peroxidation, and suppression of inflammation. The antioxidant activity of strawberries also has the potential to provide benefits to the aging brain. Zhang *et al.* [20] reported that cyanidin-3-glucoside, pelargonidin and pelargonidin-3-rutinoside are the most potent antioxidants in strawberries.

Many studies of the individual compounds have demonstrated anticancer activity, blocking initiation of carcinogenesis, and suppressing progression and proliferation of tumors. For ellagic acid and quercetin, there is a huge body of literature on this topic. In addition to the decrease in risk for cancer and heart disease, the phenolics in strawberries have effects on the immune system that may be important in the prevention of a variety of conditions (35, 180).

Other Berries

Burns-Kraft *et al.* [33] evaluated four wild berry species; serviceberry (*Amelanchier alnifolia*), cranberry (*Viburnum trilobum*), chokecherry (*Prunus virginiana*) and buffaloberry (*Shepherdia argentea*). Their results demonstrated that these berries, traditionally consumed by tribal cultures, contain a rich array of phytochemicals that have the capacity to promote health. The range of phytochemicals among the different species implies that the traditional tribal diet consisted of a rich array of bioactive compounds that may have promoted health and provided protection from chronic diseases by a range of potential mechanisms. Phenolic acids, anthocyanins, and proanthocyanidins were hypoglycemic agents, and also showed the ability to modulate lipid metabolism and energy expenditure in a manner consistent with improving metabolic syndrome [33].

Chokeberry fruit and its products supplement the treatment of hypertension, atherosclerosis and gastrointestinal tract disorders. The bioactive compounds found in chokeberry strengthen blood vessel walls and improve their elasticity and improves peripheral circulation of the blood and boosts the body's resistance to infections [181]. The compounds found in bilberry also have a beneficial impact on the circulatory system. Bilberry anthocyanins improve the elasticity and permeability of the capillary vessels of the eyeball, thus improving microcirculation of the blood and vision at dusk and at night. Owing to those properties, the anthocyanins of bilberry are applied in the production of ophthalmic preparations [10,182].

Solanum indicum L., also known as "bitter berries", is cultivated in many parts of Africa and the Arabian Peninsula for culinary purposes and also is used as an herbal remedy for several diseases such as diarrhea, malaria and prostate diseases. This type of berry should be consumed at full ripeness because there is the time in which putatively bioactive molecules are in more concentration. Considering its high content of antioxidants the bitter berries might be considered as an interesting food to improve the antioxidant status of people living in the sub-Saharan Africa [183].

Aristotelia chilensis belongs to the Elaeocarpaceae family, is commonly known as "maqui" and grows in the temperate forests of central to southern Chile and western Argentina. *V. floribundum* commonly known as "mortin" is a deciduous, spreading shrub that belongs to the family Ericaceae. *A. chilensis* and *V. floribundum* contain phytochemicals that limit adipogenesis and lipid accumulation in fat cells and inflammatory pathways in macrophages *in vitro*. The potency of these extracts to reduce inflammation *in vitro* depends on their phytochemical composition [184].

Research Challenges

Plant foods, but especially fruits and vegetables, have been identified in epidemiological research as the key components of dietary patterns with the capability to reduce risk for the development of chronic degenerative diseases such as diabetes of type II, coronary heart diseases, cancers and degenerative processes associated with aging. Bioactive compounds that elicit physiologic responses to influence or modulate processes of metabolism, oxidative stress and inflammation, which promote health and reduce diseases risks are nowadays of the most importance. Fruits rich in simple and complex phenolic constituents have been found to have a unique role in disease risk reduction through different mechanisms to mitigate oxidative stressors that contribute to diseases. The inverse relationship between fruit and vegetable intake and risk of cardiovascular and neurodegenerarive diseases, cancers, diabetes or osteoporosis has been mostly ascribed to phenolics.

Research carried out in the past decade has demonstrated the important role played by fruit berries to increase the antioxidant capacity of the blood because they are a rich source of phytochemicals, in particular different phenolic compounds and vitamin C. Dietary antioxidants are a key player in mitigating the damaging effects of reactive oxygen species on macromolecules such as DNA, proteins and lipids thereby reducing chronic disease risks. Various investigations have also shown that concentrations of phytochemicals in berries is influenced by several factors including cultivar genetics, environmental conditions, degree of ripeness, and fruit processing and storage conditions. It has been found that some wild berry cultivars contain remarkable quantities of some phenolic constituents. Therefore, these genetic materials may be well used to develop new crops with remarkable amounts of specific phytochemicals.

In spite that great research advances have been made over the last years, several key epidemiological studies are pending such as addressing the relationship between consumption of berries phytochemicals and the incidence of chronic diseases in humans; these investigations should be carried out in medium to long-term periods of time.

Human studies are also necessary to understand the interactions between berry phenolics and colon microflora. It is now known that more than one thousand different types of bacteria are found in the colon which weigh about 1.5 kg in each human being, and some of them have been never isolated and identified; thus, it is a challenge the understanding of how the colon environment and how the microbiota could be modified, and their corresponding reaction, by berry phytochemicals absorption. It is also a challenge performing human studies to establish optimum intake levels of berries of well-known composition related to safety, and disease prevention.

It is now expected that research in the postgenomic era will be able to provide information on the role of the diet, nutrition, health and diseases susceptibility and risks for each individual. Researches in different laboratories of the world on nutrigenomics (effects of nutrients on the genome, proteome and metabolome) and nutrigenetics (genetic interactions between diet and disease) are nowadays receiving special attention.

Ingestion of berry phytochemicals and their biological effects at cellular and tissue levels will be more efficiently assessed by using the new molecular tools for a better understanding of their health benefits; within this same strategy, studies on gene – nutrient interactions should lead to the prevention of chronic human diseases. In view of the solid scientific progress achieved in the past decades of the last century, the years ahead should most likely give the answers to these challenges and will provide as a result a better quality of life.

Acknowledgments

We recognize partial financial support on berries studies from Consejo Nacional de Ciencia y Tecnología – México.

Reference

[1] Yao, L.H.; Jiang, Y.M.; Shi, J.; Tomás-Barberán, F.A; Datta, N.; Singanusong, R.; Chen, S.S. Flavonoids in food and their health benefits. *Plant Foods for Human Nutrition*, 2004, *59*, 113-122.

[2] Scalbert, A.; Manach, C.; Morand, C.; Rémésy, C.; Jiménez, L. Dietary polyphenols and the prevention of diseases. *Critical Reviews in Food Science and Nutrition*, 2005, *45*, 287-306.

[3] Santos-Cervantes, M.E.; Ibarra-Zazueta, M.E.; Loarca-Piña, G.; Paredes-López, O.; Delgado-Vargas, F. Antioxidant and antimutagenic activities of *Randia echinocarpa* fruit. *Plant Foods for Human Nutrition*, 2007, *62*, 71-77.

[4] Yin, X.; Quan, J.; Kanazawa, T. Banana prevents plasma oxidative stress in healthy individuals. *Plant Foods for Human Nutrition*, 2008, *63*, 71-76.

[5] Paredes-López, O.; Cervantes-Ceja, M.; Vigna-Pérez, M.; Hernández-Pérez, T. Berries: Improving human health and healthy aging, and promoting quality life- A Review. *Plant Foods for Human Nutrition*, 2010, *65*, 299-308.

[6] Knekt, P.; Kumpulainen, J.; Jarvinen, R.; Rissanen, H.; Heliövaara, M.; Reunanen, A; Hakulinen, A.; Aromaa, A. Flavonoid intake and risk of chronic diseases. *The American Journal Clinical Nutrition*, 2002, *76*, 560-568.

[7] Kris-Etherton, P.M.; Lefevre, M.; Beecher, G.R.; Gross, M.D.; Keen, C.L.; Etherton, T.D. Bioactive compounds in nutrition and health-research methodologies for establishing biological function: the antioxidant and anti-inflammatory effects of flavonoids on atherosclerosis. *Annual Review of Nutrition*, 2004, *24*, 511-538.

[8] Mennen, L.I.; Sapinho, D.; de Bree, A.; Arnault, N.; Bertrais, S.; Galan, P.; Hercberg, S. Consumption of foods rich in flavanoids to a decreased cardiovacular risk in apparently healthy French woman. *American Society of Nutrition Science*, 2004, *134*, 923-926.

[9] Most, M.M. Estimated phytochemical content of the dietary approaches to stop hypertension (DASH) diet is higher than in the control study diet. *Journal of American Dietetic Association*, 2004, *104*, 1725-1727.

[10] Szajdek, A.; Borowska, E.J. Bioactive compounds and health-promoting properties of berry fruits: A review. *Plant Foods for Human Nutrition*, 2008, *63*, 147-156.

[11] Sampson, L.; Rimm, E.; Hollman, P.C.M.; de Vries, J.H.M.; Katan, M.B. Flavonol and flavone intakes in US health professionals. *Journal of the American Dietetic Association*, 2002, *102*, 1414-1420.

[12] Pérez-Jiménez, J.; Neveu, V.; Vos, F.; Scalbert, A. Systematic analysis of the content of 502 polyphenols in 452 foods and beverages: an application of the phenol-explorer database. *Journal of Agricultural and Food Chemistry*, 2010, *58*, 4959-4969.

[13] Liu, Z.; Schwimer, J.; Liu, D.; Greenway, F.L.; Anthony, C.T.; Woltering, E.A. Black raspberry extract and fractions contain angiogenesis inhibitors. *Journal of Agricultural and Food Chemistry*, 2005, *53*, 3909-3915.

[14] Seeram, N.P. Berry fruits: Compositional elements, biochemical activities, and the impact of their intake on human health, performance, and disease. *Journal of Agricultural and Food Chemistry*, 2008, *56*, 627-629.

[15] Seeram, N.P. Berry fruits for cancer prevention: Current status and future prospects. *Journal of Agricultural and Food Chemistry*, 2008, *56*, 630-635.

[16] Seeram, N.P. Recent trends and advances in berry health benefits research. *Journal of Agricultural and Food Chemistry*, 2010, *58*, 3869-3870.

[17] Ben-Amotz, A.; Levy, Y. Bioavailability of a natural isomer mixture compared with synthetic all-trans beta-carotene in human serum. *The American Journal Clinical Nutrition*, 1996, *63*, 729-734.

[18] Wang, H.; Cao, G.; Prior, R.L. Total antioxidant capacity of fruits. *Journal of Agricultural and Food Chemistry*, 1996, *44*, 701-705.

[19] Basu, A.; Du, M.; Leyva, M.J.; Sánchez, K.; Betts, N.M.; Wu, M.; Aston, C.E.; Lyons, T.J. Blueberries decrease cardiovascular risk factors in obese men and women with metabolic syndrome. *Journal of Nutrition*, 2010, *140*, 1582-1587.

[20] Zhang, P.; Seeram, N.; Lee, R.; Feng, L.; Heber, D. Isolation and identification of strawberry phenolics with antioxidant and human cancer cell antiproliferative properties. *Journal of Agricultural and Food Chemistry*, 2008, *56*, 670–675

[21] Häkkinen, S.H.; Törrönen, A.R. Content of flavonols and selected phenolic acids in strawberries and Vaccinium species: Influence of cultivar, cultivation site and technique. *Food Research International*, 2000, *33*, 517-524.

[22] Kähkönen, M.P.; Hopia, A.I.; Heinonen, M. Berry phenolics and their antioxidant activity. *Journal of Agricultural and Food Chemistry,* 2001, *49*, 4076-4082.

[23] Connor, A.M.; Luby, J.J.; Hancock, J.F.; Berkheimer, S. Hanson, EJ. Changes in fruit antioxidant activity among blueberry cultivars during cold-temperature storage. *Journal of Agricultural and Food Chemistry,* 2002, *50*, 893-898.

[24] Moyer, R.A.; Hummer, K.E.; Finn, C.E.; Frei, B.; Wrolstad, R.E. Anthocyanins, phenolics, and antioxidant capacity in diverse small fruits: *Vaccinium, Rubus*, and *Ribes*. *Journal of Agricultural and Food Chemistry*, 2002, *50*, 519-525.

[25] Sellappan, S.; Akoh, C.C.; Krewer, G. Phenolic compounds and antioxidant capacity of Georgia-grown blueberries and blackberries. *Journal of Agricultural and Food Chemistry*, 2002, *50*, 2432-2438.

[26] Wang, S.Y.; Lin, H.S. Antioxidant activity in fruits and leaves of blackberry, raspberry, and strawberry varies with cultivar and developmental stage. *Journal of Agricultural and Food Chemistry*, 2000, *48*, 140-146.

[27] Borowska, J.; Szajdek, A. Antioxidant activity of berry fruits and beverages. *Polish Journal of Natural Science*, 2003, *14*, 521-528.

[28] Hakala, M.; Lapveteläinen, A.; Huopalahti, R.; Kallio, H.; Tahvonen, R. Effects of varieties and cultivation conditions on the composition of strawberries. *Journal of Food Composition and Analysis*, 2003, *16*, 67-80.

[29] Benvenuti, S.; Pellati, F.; Melegari, M.; Bertelli, D. Polyphenols, anthocyanins, ascorbic acid, and radical scavenging activity of *Rubus*, *Ribes* and *Aronia*. *Journal of Food Science*, 2004, *69*, 64-69.

[30] Skupień, K.; Oszmiański, J. Comparison of six cultivars of strawberries (*Fragaria ananassa* Duch.) grown in northwest Poland *European Food Research and Technology*, 2004, *219*, 66-70.

[31] Taruscio, T.G.; Barney, D.L.; Exon, J. Content and profile of flavonoid and phenolic acid compounds in conjunction with the antioxidant capacity for a variety of northwest Vaccinium berries. *Journal of Agricultural and Food Chemistry*, 2004, *52*, 3169-3176.

[32] Lila, M.A. The nature-versus-nurture debate on bioactive phytochemicals: The genome versus terroir. *Journal of the Science and Food Agriculture*, 2006, *86*, 2510-2515.

[33] Burns-Kraft, T.; Dey, M.; Rogers, R.; Ribnicky, D.; Gipp, D.; Cefalu, W.; Raskin, O.; Lila, M.A. Phytochemical composition and metabolic performance-enhancing activity of dietary berries traditionally used by native North Americans. *Journal of Agricultural and Food Chemistry*, 2008, *56*, 654-660.

[34] Del Río, D.; Borges, G.; Crozier, A. Berry flavonoids and phenolics: Bioavailability and evidence of protective effects. *British Journal of Nutrition*, 2010, *104*, S67-S90.

[35] Hannum, S.M. Potential impact of strawberries on human health: a review of the science. *Critical Reviews in Food Science and Nutrition*, 2004, *44*, 1-17.

[36] Vermerris, W.; Nicholson, R. *Phenolic Compound Biochemistry*. Springer Science+Business Media B.VI; 2008.

[37] Cohen, S.D.; Kennedy, A. Plant metabolism and the environment: Implications for managing phenolics. *Critical Reviews in Food Science and Nutrition*, 2010, *50*, 620-643.

[38] Rice-Evans, C.A.; Miller, N.J.; Paganga, G. Structure–antioxidant activity relationships of flavonoids and phenolic acids. *Free Radical Biology & Medicine*, 1996, *20*, 933-956.

[39] Rao, A.V.; Snyder, D.M. Raspberries and human health: A review. *Journal of Agricultural and Food Chemistry*, 2010, *58*, 3871-3883.

[40] Espín, J.C.; Tomás-Barberan, F.A. Phenolic compounds and related enzymes as determinants of fruits and vegetables quality. *Journal of the Science of Food and Agriculture*, 2001, *81*, 853–876.

[41] Delgado-Vargas, F.; Jiménez-Aparicio, A.; Paredes-López, O. Natural pigments: Carotenoids, anthocyanins and betalains - Characteristics, biosynthesis, processing and stability. *Critical Reviews in Food Science and Nutrition*, 2000, *40*, 173-289.

[42] Kosar, M.; Kafkas, E.; Paydas, S.; Baser, K.H.C. Phenolic composition of strawberry genotypes at different maturation stages. *Journal of Agricultural and Food Chemistry*, 2004, *52*, 1586-1589.

[43] Siriwoharn, T.; Wrolstad, R.E.; Finn, C.E.; Pereira, C. Influence of cultivar, maturity, and sampling on blackberry (*Rubus* L. hybrids) anthocyanins, polyphenolics, and

antioxidant properties. *Journal of Agricultural and Food Chemistry*, 2004, *52*, 8021-8030.

[44] Reyes-Carmona, J.; Yousef, G.G.; Martínez-Peniche, R.A.; Lila, M.A. Antioxidant capacity of fruit extracts of blackberry (*Rubus* sp.) produced in different climatic regions. *Journal of Food Science*, 2005, *70*, S497-S503.

[45] Scalzo, J.; Politi, A.; Pellegrini, N.; Mezzetti, B.; Battino, M. Plant genotype affects total antioxidant capacity and phenolic contents in fruit. *Nutrition*, 2005, *21*, 207-213.

[46] Koca, I.; Karadeniz, B. Antioxidant properties of blackberry and blueberry fruits grown in the black sea region of Turkey. *Scientia Horticulturae*, 2009, *121*, 447-450.

[47] Kellogg, J.; Wang, J.; Flint, C; Ribnicky, D.; Kuhn, P.; González de Mejia, E.; Raskin, I; Lila, M.A. Alaskan wild berry resources and human health under the cloud of climate change. *Journal of Agricultural and Food Chemistry*, 2010, *58*, 3884-3900.

[48] Kalt, W.; Forney, C.F.; Martin, A.; Prior, R.L. Antioxidant capacity, vitamin C, phenolics, and anthocyanins after fresh storage of small fruits. *Journal of Agricultural and Food Chemistry*, 1999, *47*, 4638-4644.

[49] Deighton, N.; Brennan, R.; Finn, C.; Davies, H.V. Antioxidant properties of domesticated and wild Rubus species. *Journal of the Science of Food and Agriculture*, 2000, *80*, 1307-1313.

[50] Cuevas-Rodríguez, E.; Yousef, G.; García-Saucedo, P.; López-Medina, J.; Paredes-López, O.; Lila, M.A. Characterization of anthocyanins and proanthocyanidins in wild and domesticated Mexican blackberries (*Rubus* spp.). *Journal of Agricultural and Food Chemistry*, 2010, *58*, 7458-7464.

[51] Cuevas-Rodríguez, E.; Día, V.; Yousef, G.; García-Saucedo, P.; López-Medina, J.; Paredes-López, O.; González de Mejía, E.; Lila, M.A. Inhibition of pro-inflammatory responses and antioxidant 2 capacity of Mexican blackberry (*Rubus* spp.) extracts. *Journal of Agricultural and Food Chemistry*, 2010, *58*, 9542-9548.

[52] Prior, R.L.; Cao, G.; Martin, A.; Sofic, E.; McEwen, J.; O'Brien, C.; Lischner, N.; Ehlenfeldt, M.; Kalt, W.; Krewer, G.; Mainland, C.M. Antioxidant capacity as influenced by total phenolic and anthocyanin content, maturity, and variety of *Vaccinium* species. *Journal of Agricultural and Food Chemistry*, 1998, *46*, 2686-2693.

[53] Heinonen, I.M.; Meyer, A.S.; Frankel, E.N. Antioxidant activity of berry phenolics on human low-density lipoprotein and liposome oxidation. *Journal of Agricultural and Food Chemistry*, 1998, *46*, 4107-4112.

[54] Wang, S.Y.; Stretch, A.W. Antioxidant capacity in cranberry is influenced by cultivar and storage temperature. *Journal of Agricultural and Food Chemistry*, 2001, *49*, 969-974.

[55] Zheng, W.; Wang, S.Y. Oxygen radical absorbing capacity of phenolics in blueberries, cranberries, chokeberries and lingonberries. *Journal of Agricultural and Food Chemistry*, 2003, *51*, 502-509.

[56] Kevers, C.; Falkowski, M.; Tabart., J; Defraigne, J.O.; Dommes, J.; Pincemail, J. Evolution of antioxidant capacity during storage of selected fruits and vegetables. *Journal of Agricultural and Food Chemistry*, 2007, *55*, 8596-8603.

[57] Wada, L.; Ou, B. Antioxidant activity and phenolic content of Oregon caneberries. *Journal of Agricultural and Food Chemistry*, 2002, *50*, 3495-3500.

[58] Proteggentea, A.R.; Pannalaa, A.S.; Pagangaa, G.; Burenb, L.; Wagnera, E.; Wisemanb, S.; van de Putb, F.; Dacombec, C.; Rice-Evans, C.A. The antioxidant activity of regularly consumed fruit and vegetables reflects their phenolic and vitamin C composition. *Free Radical Research*, 2002, *36*, 217-233.

[59] Zadernowski, R.; Naczk, M.; Nesterowicz, J. Phenolic acid profiles in some small berries. *Journal of Agricultural and Food Chemistry*, 2005, *53*, 2118-2124.

[60] Tomás-Barberán, F.A.; Clifford, M.N. Dietary hidroxybenzoic acid derivates-nature, occurrence and dietary burden. *Journal of the Science of Food and Agriculture*, 2000, *80*, 1024-1032.

[61] Mattila, P.; Hellstrón, J.; Torronen, R. Phenolic acids in berries, fruits, and beverages. *Journal of Agricultural and Food Chemistry*, 2006, *54*, 7193-7199

[62] Lafay, S.; Izquierdo, G.A. Bioavailability of phenolic acids. *Phytochemistry Reviews*, 2008, *7*, 301-311.

[63] Burton-Freeman, B. Postprandial metabolic events and fruit-derived phenolics: A review. *British Journal of Nutrition*, 2010, *104*, S1-S14.

[64] Pimiä, P.R.; Nohynek, L; Alakomi, H.L.; Caldentey, O.K.M. The action of berry phenolics against human intestinal pathogens. *BioFactors*, 2005, *23*, 243-251.

[65] Andersen, M.O.; Markham; R.K. *Flavonoids: chemistry, biochemistry and applications*. CRC Press; 2006; pp 219-225.

[66] Han, X.; Shen, T.; Lou, H. Dietary polyphenols and their biological significance. *International Journal of Molecular Science*, 2007, *8*, 950-988.

[67] Gu, L.; Kelm, M.A.; Hammerstone, J.F.; Beecher, G.; Holden, J.; Haytowitz, D.; Prior R.L. Concentrations of proanthocyanidins in common foods and estimations of normal consumption. *Journal of Nutrition*, 2004, *134*, 613-617.

[68] Wu. X.; Gu, L.; Beecher, G.R.; Holden, J.M.; Haytowitz, D.B.; Gebhardt, S.E.; Prior, R.L. Characterization of anthocyanins and proanthocyanidins in some cultivars of Ribes, Aronia, and Sambucus and their antioxidant capacity. *Journal of Agricultural and Food Chemistry*, 2004, *52*, 7846-7856.

[69] Häkkinen, S.H.; Karenlampi. S.K.; Heinonen. M.; Mykkanen, H.M.; Torronen, R. Content of the flavonols quercetin, myricetin, and kaempferol in edible berries *Journal of Agricultural and Food Chemistry*. 1999, *47*, 2274-2279.

[70] Maatta-Riihinen, K.R.; Kamal-Eldin, A.; Tarranen, A.R. Identification and quantification of phenolic compounds in berries of *Fragaria* and *Rubus* species (family Rosaceae). *Journal of Agricultural and Food Chemistry*, 2004, *52*, 6178-6187.

[71] http://en.wikipedia.org/wiki/Phenolic_compounds_in_wine

[72] Clifford, M.N. Review. Anthocyanins-nature, occurrence and dietary burden. *Journal of the Science of Food and Agriculture*, 2000, *80*, 1063-1072.

[73] Gould, K.; Davies, K.; Winefield, C. *Anthocyanins: Biosynthesis, functions and applications*. Springer, Science, 2008.

[74] Pascual-Teresa, S.; Sánchez-Ballesta, M.T. Anthocyanins: From plant to health. *Phytochemistry Reviews*, 2008, *7*, 281-299.

[75] Häkkinen, S.H.; Kärenlampi, S.O.; Mykkänen, H.M.; Heinonen, I.M.; Törrönen, A.R. Ellagic acid content in berries: influence of domestic processing and storage. *European Food Research and Technology*, 2001, *212*, 75-80.

[76] Yilmaz, Y.; Toledo, R.T. Major flavonoids in grape seeds and skin: antioxidant capacity of catechin, epicatechin and gallic acid. *Journal of Agricultural and Food Chemistry*, 2004, *52*, 255-260.
[77] Pawlowska, M.A.; Olesker, W.; Braca, A. Quali-quantitative analyses of flavonoids of *Morus nigra* L. and *Morus alba* L. (Moraceae) fruits. *Journal of Agricultural and Food Chemistry*, 2008, *56*, 3377-3380.
[78] Koponen, J.M.; Happonen A.M.; Mattila, P.H.; Törrönen, R. Contents of anthocyanins and ellagitannins in selected foods consumed in Finland. *Journal of Agricultural and Food Chemistry*, 2007, *55*, 1612-1619.
[79] Wu, X.; Beecher, G.; Holden, J.M.; Haytowitz, B.D.; Gebhardt, E.S.; Prior, L.R. Concentrations of anthocyanins in common foods in the United States and estimation of normal consumption. *Journal of Agricultural and Food Chemistry*, 2006, *54*, 4069-4075.
[80] Anttonen, M.J.; Karjalainen, R.O. Environmental and genetic variation of phenolic compounds in red raspberry. *Journal Food Composition and Analysis*, 2005, *18*, 759-769.
[81] Castaneda-Ovando, A.; Pacheco-Hernández, M.D.; Paez-Hernández, M.E.; Rodríguez, J.A.; Galan-Vidal, C.A. Chemical studies of anthocyanins: A review. *Food Chemistry*, 2009, *113*, 859-871.
[82] Puupponen-Pimiä, R.; Nohynek, L.; Alakomi, H.-L.; Oksman-Caldentey, K.-M. Bioactive berry compounds-novel tools against human pathogens. *Applied Microbiology and Biotechnology*, 2005, *67*, 8-18.
[83] Mazza, G. Anthocyanins and heart health. *Annali dellIstituto Superiore di Sanita*, 2007, *43*, 369-374.
[84] Krikorian, R.; Shidler, M.; Nash, T.; Kalt, W.; Vinqvist-Tymchuk, M.; Shukitt-Hale, B.; Joseph, J. Blueberry supplementation improves memory in older adults. *Journal of Agricultural and Food Chemistry*, 2010, *58*, 3996-4000.
[85] Kundu, K.J.; Surh, J.Y. Cancer chemopreventive and therapeutic potential of resveratrol: Mechanism perspectives. *Cancer Letter*, 2008, *269*, 243-261.
[86] Wang, J.; Mazza, G. Effects of anthocyanins and other phenolic compounds on the production of tumor necrosis factor R in LPS/IFN-γ-activated RAW 264.7 macrophages. *Journal of Agricultural and Food Chemistry*, 2002, *50*, 4183-4189.
[87] Wang, J.; Mazza, G. Inhibitory effects of anthocyanins and other phenolic compounds on nitric oxide production in LPS/IFN-γ-activated RAW 264.7 macrophages. *Journal of Agricultural and Food Chemistry*, 2002, *50*, 850-857.
[88] Lyons, M.; Yu, C.; Tomas, R.B.; Cho, S.Y; Reiboldt, W.; Lee, J.; van Breemen, R.B. Resveratrol in raw and baked blueberries and bilberries. *Journal of Agricultural and Food Chemistry*, 2003, *57*, 5867-5870.
[89] Rimando, M.A.; Kalt, W.; Magee, B.J.; Dewey, J; Ballington, R.J. Resveratrol, pterostilbene and piceatannol in *Vaccinium* berries. *Journal of Agricultural and Food Chemistry*, 2004, *52*, 4713-4719.
[90] Potter, G.A.; Paterson, L.H.; Wanogho, E.; Perry, P.J.; Butler, P.C.; Ijaz, T.; Ruparelia, K.C.; Lamb, J.H.; Farmer, P.B.; Stanley, L.A.; Burke, M.D. The cancer

chemopreventive agent resveratrol is converted to the anticancer agent piceatannol by the cytrochrome P450 enzyme CYPIBI. *British Journal of Cancer*, 2002, *86*, 774-778.

[91] Aggarwal, B.B.; Shishodia, S. *Resveratrol in Health and Diseases*. CRC Press; 2006.

[92] Joseph, J.A.; Fisher D.R.; Cheng, V.; Rimando, A.M.; Hale, S.B. Cellular and behavioral effects of stilbene resveratrol analogues: Implications for reducing the deleterious effects of aging. *Journal of Agricultural and Food Chemistry*, 2008, *56*, 10544-10551.

[93] Mizuno, C.S.; Schrader, K.K.; Rimando, A.M. Alguicidal activity of stilbene analogues. *Journal of Agricultural and Food Chemistry*, 2008, *56*, 9140-9145.

[94] Shakibaei, M.; Harikumar, B.K.; Aggarwal, B.B. Resveratrol addiction: To die or not to die. *Molecular Nutrition & Food Research*, 2009, *53*, 115-128

[95] Jang, M.; Cai, L.; Udeani, G.O.; Slowing, K.V.; Thomas, C.F.; Beecher, C.W.W.; Fong, H.S.; Farnsworth, N.R.; Kinghorn, A.D.; Mehta, R.G.; Moon, R.C.; Pezzuto, J.M. Cancer chemopreventive activity of resveratrol, a natural product derived from grapes. *Science,* 1997, *275*, 218-220.

[96] Khanbabaee, K.; Ree, V. Tannins: Classification and definition. *Natural Product Reports Articles*, 2001, *18*, 641-649.

[97] Santos-Buelga, C.; Scalbert, A. Review. Proanthocyanidins and tannin-like compounds-nature, occurrence, dietary intake and effects on nutrition and health. *Journal of the Science of Food and Agriculture*, 2000, *80*, 1094-1117.

[98] Dewick, P.M. *Medicinal Natural Products: A Biosynthetic Approach*. John Wiley & Sons, Ltd., 2002.

[99] Quideau, S. *Chemistry and biology of ellagitannins: An underestimated class of bioactive plant polyphenols*. Singapore: World Scientific Publishing, 2009.

[100] Mullen, W.; McGinn, J.; Lean, M.E.J.; MacLean, M.R.; Gardner, P.; Duthie, G.G.; Yokota, T.; Crozier, A. Ellagitannins, flavonoids, and other phenolics in red raspberries and their contribution to antioxidant capacity and vasorelaxation properties. *Journal of Agricultural and Food Chemistry*, 2002, *50*, 5191-5196.

[101] Seeram, N.P.; Adams, L.; Zhang, Y.; Lee, R.; Sand, D.; Scheuller, H.; Heber. D. Blackberry, black raspberry, blueberry, cranberry, red raspberry, and strawberry extracts inhibit growth and stimulate apoptosis of human cancer cells *in vitro*. *Journal of Agricultural and Food Chemistry*, 2006, *54*, 9329-9339.

[102] Bakkalbasi, E.; Montes, O.; Artik, N. Food ellagitannins-occurrence, effects of processing and storage. *Critical Reviews in Food Science and Nutrition*, 2009, *49*, 283-298.

[103] Amakura, Y.; Okada, M.; Tsuji, S.; Tonogai, Y. High performance liquid chromatographic determination with photo diode array detection of ellagic acid in fresh and processed fruits. *Journal of Chromatography*, 2000, *896*, 87-93.

[104] Oszmiański, J.; Wojdylo, A. *Aronia melanocarpa* phenolics and their antioxidant activity. *European Food Research and Technology*, 2005, *221*, 809-813.

[105] Wang, L.; Hecht, S.; Carmella, S.; Seguin, C.; Rocha, C.; Yu, N.; Stoner, K.; Chiu, S.; Stoner, G. Berry ellagitannins may not be sufficient for prevention of tumors in the rodent esophagus. *Journal of Agricultural and Food Chemistry*, 2010, *58*, 3992-3995.

[106] Simonian, N.A.; Coyle, J.T. Oxidative stress in neurodegenerative diseases. *Annual Review of Pharmacology and Toxicology*, 1996, *36*, 83-106.

[107] Bokov, A.; Chaudhurie, A.; Richardson, A. The role of oxidative damage and stress in aging. *Mechanisms of Ageing and Development*, 2004, *125*, 811-826.

[108] Madamanchi, N.R.; Vendrov, A.; Runge, M.S. Oxidative stress and vascular disease. *Arteriosclerosis Thrombosis and Vascular Biology*, 2005, *25*, 29-38.

[109] Ames, B.N.; Gold, L.S. Too many rodent carcinogens: mitogenesis increases mutagenesis. *Science,* 1991, *249*, 970-971.

[110] Winterbourn, C.C. Reconciling the chemistry and biology of reactive oxygen species. *Nature Chemical Biology*, 2008, *4*, 278-286.

[111] Rice-Evans, C.A.; Miller, N.J; Bolwell, P.G.; Bramley, P.M.; Pridham, J.B. The relative antioxidant activities of plant-derived polyphenolic flavonoids. *Free Radical Research*, 1995, *22*, 375-383.

[112] Harborne, J.B.; Williams, C.A. Advances in flavonoid research since 1992. *Phytochem*, 2000, *5*, 481-504.

[113] Heim, K.E.; Tagliaferro, A.R.; Bobilya, D.J. Flavonoid antioxidants: chemistry, metabolism and structure–activity relationships. *Journal of Nutritional Biochemistry*, 2002, *13*, 572-584.

[114] Hollman, P.C.; van Trijp, J.M.; Buysman, M.N.; Martijn, S.G.; Marcel, J.B; de Vries, J.H.M.; Katan, M.B. Relative bioavailability of the antioxidant flavonoid quercetina from various foods in man. *FEBS Letter*, 1997, *418*, 152-156.

[115] Ehala, S.; Vaher, M.; Kaljurand, M. Characterization of phenolic profiles of northern european berries by capillary electrophoresis and determination of their antioxidant activity. *Journal of Agricultural and Food Chemistry*, 2005, *53*, 6484-6490.

[116] Manach, C.; Williamson, G.; Morand, C.; Scalbert, A.; Rémésy, C. Bioavailability and bioefficacy of polyphenols in humans. I. Review of 97 bioavailability studies. *The American Journal Clinical Nutrition*, 2005, *81*, 230S-242S.

[117] Crozier, A.; Jaganath, I.B.; Clifford, M.N. Dietary phenolics: chemistry, bioavailability and effects on health. *Natural Product Reports Articles*, 2009, *26*, 1001-1043.

[118] McCarty, M.F. Optimizing endothelial nitric oxide activity may slow endothelial aging. *Medical Hypotheses*, 2004, *63*, 719-723.

[119] Pellegrini, N.; Serafini, M.; Colombi, B.; Del Rio, D.; Salvatore, S.; Bianchi, M.; Brighenti, F. Total antioxidant capacity of plant foods, beverages and oils consumed in Italy assessed by three different *in vitro* assays. *Journal of Nutrition*, 2003, *133*, 2812-2819.

[120] Beer, C.; Myers, R.A.; Sorenson, J.H.; Bucci, L.R. Comprehensive comparison of the antioxidant activity of fruits and vegetables based on typical serving sizes from common methods. *Current Topics in Nutraceutical Research*, 2004, *2*, 227-250.

[121] Halvorsen, B.L.; Holte, K.; Myhrstad, M.C.W.; Barikmo, I.; Hvattum, E.; Remberg, S.F.; Wold, A.B.; Haffner, K.; Bauger, A.H.; Andersen, L.F.; Moskaug, O.; Jacobs, D.R.; Blomhoff, R. A systematic screening of total antioxidants in dietary plants. *Journal of Nutrition*, 2002, *132*, 461-471.

[122] Halvorsen, B.L.; Carlsen, M.H.; Phillips, K.M.; Boehn, S.K.; Holte, K.; Jacobs, D.R.; Blomhoff, R. Content of redox-active compounds (ie., antioxidants) in foods consumed in the United States. *The American Journal Clinical Nutrition*, 2006, *84*, 95-135.

[123] Heinonen, M. Antioxidant activity and antimicrobial effect of berry phenolics – a Finnish perspective. *Molecular Nutrition & Food Research*, 2007, *51*, 684-691.

[124] Ozgen, M.; Reese, N.R.; Tulio, Z.A.; Scherens, J.C.; Miller, R. (ABST) Method to measure antioxidant capacity of selected small fruits and comparison to ferric reducing antioxidant power (FRAP) and 2,2′-diphenyl-1-picrylhydrazyl(DPPH) methods. *Journal of Agricultural and Food Chemistry*, 2006, *54*, 1151-1157.

[125] Beekrum, S.; Govinden, R.; Padayachee, T.; Odhav, B. Naturally occurring phenols: a detoxification strategy for fumonisin B-1. *Food Additives & Contaminants*, 2003, *20*, 490-493.

[126] Stevenson, D.E.; Huso, R.D. Review. Polyphenolic phytochemicals - just antioxidants or much more? *Cellular and Molecular Life Science*, 2007, *64*, 2900-2916.

[127] Shin, K.; Kim, I.; Park, Y.; Ha, J.; Choi, J.; Park, H.; Lee, Y.S.; Lee, K. Anti-inflammatory effect of caffeic acidmethyl ester and itsmode of action through the inhibition of prostaglandin E2, nitric oxide and tumor necrosis factor-R production. *Biochemical Pharmacology*, 2004, *68*, 2327-2336.

[128] Bhat, P.K.L.; Kosmeder, J.W.; Pezzuto, J.M. Biological effects of resveratrol. *Antioxidant & Redox Signal*, 2001, *3*, 1041-1064.

[129] Pergola, C.; Rossi, A.; Dugo, P.; Cuzzocrea, S.; Sautebin, L. Inhibition of nitric oxide biosynthesis by anthocyanin fraction of blackberry extract. *Nitric Oxide*, 2006, *15*, 30-39.

[130] Hale, S.B.; Lau, C.F.; Joseph, A.J. Berry fruit supplementation and the aging brain. *Journal of Agricultural and Food Chemistry*, 2008, *56*, 636-641.

[131] Surh, Y.J. Cancer chemoprevention with dietary phytochyemicals. Rev. *Nature*, 2003, *3*, 768-780.

[132] Coulder, I.D.; Hardy, M.L.; Morton, S.C.; Hilton, L.G.; Tu, W.; Valentine, D.; Shelelle, P.G. Antioxidants vitamin C and vitamin E for the prevention and treatment of cancer. *Journal of General Internal Medicine*, 2006, *21*, 735-744.

[133] Hannum, S. M. Potential impact of strawberries on human health: A review of the Science. *Critical Reviews in Food Science and Nutrition*, 2004, *44*, 1-17.

[134] Liu, M.; Li, X.Q.; Weber, C.; Lee, C.Y.; Brown, J.; Liu, R.H. Antioxidant and antiproliferative activities of raspberries. *Journal of Agricultural and Food Chemistry*, 2002, *50*, 2926-2930.

[135] Stoner, G.D.; Wang, L.S.; Zirki, N.; Chen, T.; Hecht, S.S.; Huang, C.; Sardo, C.; Lechner, J.F. Cancer prevention with freeze-dried berries and berry components. *Cancer Biology*, 2007, *17*, 403-410.

[136] Vattem, D.A.; Jang, H.D.; Levin, R.; Shetty, K. Synergism of cranberry phenolics with ellagic acid and rosmarinic acid for antimutagenic and DNA protection functions. *Journal of Food Biochemistry*, 2006, *30*, 96-116.

[137] Bell, D.R.; Gochenaur, K. Direct vasoactive and vasoprotective propierties of anthocyanins-rich extracts. *Journal of Applied Physics*, 2006, *100*, 1164-1170.

[138] Xia, M.; Lin, W.; Zhu, H. Anthocynin prevents CD-40- activated proinflammatory signaling in endothelial cells by regulation cholesterol distribution. *Arteriosclerosis Thrombosis and Vascular Biology*, 2007, *27*, 519-1749.

[139] Shukitt-Hale, B.; Lau, F.C.; Joseph, J.A. Berry fruit supplementation and the aging brain. *Journal of Agricultural and Food Chemistry*, 2008, *56*, 636-641.

[140] Shukitt-Hale, B.; Cheng, V.; Joseph, J.A. Effects of blackberries on motor and cognitive function in aged rats. *Nutritional Neuroscience*, 2009, *12*, 135-140.

[141] Deschamps, V.; Barberger-Gateau, P.; Peuchant, E.; Orgogozo, J.M. Nutritional factors in cerebral aging and dementia: Epidemiological arguments for a role of oxidative stress. *Neuroepidemilogy*, 2001, *20*, 7-15.

[142] Hale, S.B.; Galli, R.; Meterko, V.; Carey, A.; Beilinski, D.; Mcghie, T.; Joseph, J. Dietary supplementation with fruit polyphenolics ameliorates age-related deficits in behavior and neuronal markers of inflammation and oxidative stress. *Age*, 2005, *27*, 49-57.

[143] Hale, S.B.; Cheng, V.; Beilinski, D.; Carey, A.; Lau, F.; Seeram, N.; Heber, D.; Joseph, J.A. Differential brain regional specificity to blueberry and strawberry polyphenolis in improved motor and cognitive function in aged rats. *Society of Neuroscience Abstracts*, 2006, *32*, 81-15.

[144] Barros, D.; Amaral, O.B.; Geracitano, I.I.; Bassols Raseira, L.; Teresinha Henriques, A.; Ramírez, M.R. Behavioral and genoprotective effects of *Vaccinium* berries intake in mice. *Pharmacology, Biochemistry and Behavior*, 2006, *84*, 229-234.

[145] Milbury, P.; Kalt, E. Xenobiotic metabolism and berry flavonoid transport across the blood-brain barrier. *Journal of Agricultural and Food Chemistry*, 2010, *58*, 3950-3956.

[146] Howell, A.B.; Reed, J.D.; Krueger, C.G.; Winterbottom, R.; Cunningham, D.; Leahy, M. A type cranberry proanthicyanidins and uropathigenic bacterial antiadhesion activity. *Phytochemistry*, 2005, *66*, 2281-2291.

[147] Nohynek, J.L.; Alakomi, L.H.; Kahkonen, P.M.; Heinonen, M.; Helander, M.; Clanderntey, O.K.; Pimia, P.R. Berry phenolics: Antimicrobial properties and mechanisms of action against severe human pathogens. *Nutrition and Cancer*, 2006, *54*, 18-32.

[148] Bodet, C.; Grenier, D.; Chandad, F.; Ofek, I; Steinberg, D. Potential oral health benefits of cranberry. *Critical Reviews in Food Science and Nutrition*, 2008, *48*, 672-680.

[149] Gao, Y.H.; Yamaguchi, M. Suppressive effect of genistein on rat bone osteoclasts: Involvement of protein kinase inhibition and protein tyrosine phosphatase activation. *Journal of Molecular Medicine*, 2000, *5*, 261-267.

[150] Okamoto, F.; Okabe, K.; Kajiya, H. Genistein, a soybean isoflavone, inhibits inward rectifier K(+) channels in rat osteoclast. *Japanese Journal of Physiology*, 2001, *51*, 501-509.

[151] Rassi, C.M.; Kasum, C.M. Dietary flavonoids: Bioavailability, metabolic effects, and safety. *Annual Review of Nutrition*, 2002, *22*, 19-34.

[152] Habauzit, V.; Horcajada, M.N. Phenolics phytochemicals and bone. *Phytochem Rev*, 2008, *7*, 313-344.

[153] Galvano, F.; La Fauci, L.; Lazzarino, G. Cyanidins: Metabolism and biological properties. *Journal of Nutritional Biochemistry*, 2004, *15*, 2-11.

[154] Hager, T.J.; Howard, L.R.; Liyanage, R.; Lay, J.; Prior; R.L. Ellagitannin composition of blackberry as determined by HPLC-ESI-MS and MALDI-TOF-MS. *Journal of Agricultural and Food Chemistry*, 2008, *56*, 661-669.

[155] Hager, T.J.; Howard, L.R.; Prior, R.L. Processing and storage effects on monomeric anthocyanins, percent polymeric color, and antioxidant capacity of processed blackberry products. *Journal of Agricultural and Food Chemistry*, 2008, *56*, 689-695.

[156] Ayaz, F.A.; Ayaz, H.S.; Gruz, J.; Novak, O.; Strnad, M. Separation, characterization and quantitation of phenolic acids in a little-known blueberry *(Vaccinium arctostaphylos L.)* fruit by HPLC-MS. *Journal of Agricultural and Food Chemistry* 2005, *53*, 8116-8122.

[157] Nicoue, E.M.; Savard, S.; Belkacemi, K. Anthocyanins in wild blueberries of Quebec: Extraction and identification. *Journal of Agricultural and Food Chemistry*, 2007, *55*, 5626-5635.

[158] Ehlenfeldt, M.K.; Prior, R.L. Oxygen radical absorbance capacity (ORAC) and phenolic and anthocyanin concentrations in fruit and leaf tissues of highbush blueberry. *Journal of Agricultural and Food Chemistry*, 2001, *49*, 2222-2227.

[159] Prior, R.L.; Wu, X.; Gu, L.; Hager, T.; Hager, A.; Howard, L.R. Whole berries versus berry anthocyanins: Interactions with dietary fat levels in the C57BL/6J mouse model of obesity. *Journal of Agricultural and Food Chemistry*, 2008, *56*, 647-653.

[160] Howard, L.; Castrodale, C.; Brownmiller, C.; Mauromoustakos, A. Jam processing and storage effects on blueberry polyphenolics and antioxidant capacity. *Journal of Agricultural and Food Chemistry*, 2010, *58*, 4022-4029.

[161] Lacueva, A.C.; Hale, S.B.; Galli, L.R.; Jáuregui, O.; Raventos, R.M.; Joseph, J.A. Anthocyanins in aged blueberry-fed rats are found centrally and may enhance memory. *Neuroscience and Nutrition*, 2005, *8*, 111-120.

[162] Joseph, J.A.; Denisova, N.A.; Arendash, G.; Gordon, M.; Diamond, D.; Hale, S.B.; Morgan, D. Blueberry supplementation enhances signaling and prevents behavioral deficits an Alzheimer disease. *Neuroscience and Nutrition*, 2003, *3*, 153-162.

[163] Côté, J.; Caillet, S.; Doyon, G.; Sylvain, J.F.; Lacroix, M. Analyzing cranberry bioactive compounds. *Critical Reviews in Food Science and Nutrition*, 2010, *50*, 872-888.

[164] Côté, J.; Caillet, S.; Doyon, G.; Sylvain, J.F.; Lacroix, M. Bioactive compounds in cranberries and their biological properties. *Critical Reviews in Food Science and Nutrition*, 2010, *50*, 666-679.

[165] Sun, J.; Liu, H.R. Cranberry phytochemical extracts induce cell cycle arrest and apoptosis in human MCF-7 breast cancer lines. *Cancer Letter*, 2005, *41*, 124-134.

[166] Zuo, Y.; Zhan, J. Separation, characterization, quantitation of benzoic and phenolic antioxidants in American cranberry fruit by GC-MS. *Journal of Agricultural and Food Chemistry*, 2002, *50*, 3789-3794.

[167] Pappas, E.; Schaich, K.M. Phytochemicals of cranberries and cranberry products: Characterization, potential health effects, and processing stability, *Critical Reviews in Food Science and Nutrition*, 2008, *49*, 741-781.

[168] White, B.; Howard, L.; Prior, R.L. Proximate and polyphenolic characterization of cranberry pomace. *Journal of Agricultural and Food Chemistry*, 2010, *58*, 4030-4036.

[169] White, B.; Howard, L.; Prior. R.L. Polyphenolic composition and antioxidant capacity of extruded cranberry pomace. *Journal of Agricultural and Food Chemistry*, 2010, *58*, 4037-4042.

[170] Kresty, L.; Howell, A.; Baird, M. Cranberry proanthocyanidins induce apoptosis and inhibit acid-induced proliferation of human esophageal adenocarcinoma cells. *Journal of Agricultural and Food Chemistry*, 2008, *56*, 676-680.

[171] Beekwilder, J.; Jonker, H.; Meesters, P.; Hall, R.D.; Van Der Meer, I.M.; De Vos, C.H.R. Antioxidants in raspberry: on-line analysis links antioxidant activity to a diversity of individual metabolites. *Journal of Agricultural and Food Chemistry*, 2005, *53*, 3313-3320.

[172] Serraino, I.; Dugo, L.; Dugo, P.; Mondello, L.; Mazzon, E.; Dugo, G.; Caputi, A.P.; Cuzzocrea, S. Protective effects of cyanidin-3-O-glucoside from blackberry extract against peroxynitrite-induced endothelial dysfunction and vascular failure. *Life Science*, 2003, *73*, 1097-1114.

[173] Huang, C.; Li, J.; Song, L.; Zhang, D.; Tong, Q.; Ding, M.; Bowman, L.; Aziz, R.; Stoner, G.D. Black raspberry extracts inhibit benzo(a)pyrene diol-epoxide-induced activator protein 1activation and VEGF transcription by targeting the phosphotidylinositol 3-kinase/Akt pathway. *Cancer Research*, 2006, *66*, 581-587.

[174] Chen, T.; Hwang, H.; Rose, M.E.; Nines, R.G.; Stoner, G.D. Chemopreventive properties of black raspberries in N-nitrosomethylbenzylamine-induced rat esophageal tumorigenesis:down-regulation of cyclooxygenase-2, inducible nitric oxide synthase. *Cancer Research*, 2006, *66*, 2853-2859.

[175] Chen, T.; Rose, M.E.; Hwang, H.; Nines, R.G.; Stoner, G.D. Black raspberries inhibit N-nitrosomethylbenzylamine (NMBA)-induced angiogenesis in rat esophagus parallel to the suppression of COX-2 and iNOS. *Carcinogenesis*, 2006, *27*, 2301-2307.

[176] Cooke, D.; Schwarz, M.; Boocock, D.; Winterhalter, P.; Steward, W.P.; Gescher, A.J.; Marczylo, T.H. Effect of cyanidin-3-glucoside and an anthocyanin mixture from bilberry on adenoma development in the ApcMin mouse model of intestinal carcinogenesis - relationship with tissue anthocyanin levels. *International Journal of Cancer*, 2006, *119*, 2213-2220.

[177] McDougall, G.J.; Stewart, D. The inhibitory effects of berry polyphenols on digestive enzymes. *Biofactors*, 2005, *23*, 189-195.

[178] Tulipani, S.; Mezzetti, B., Capocasa, F.; Bompadre, S.; Beekwilder, J.; de Vos, R.; Capanoglu, E.; Bovy, A.; Battino, M. Antioxidants, Phenolic compounds, and nutritional quality of different strawberry genotypes. *Journal of Agricultural and Food Chemistry*, 2008, *56*, 696-704.

[179] Buendía, B.; Gil, M.; Tudela, J.; Gady, A.L.; Medina, J.; Soria, C.; López, J.; Tomás-Barrera, F. HPLC-MS analysis of proanthocyanidin oligomers and other phenolics in 15 strawberry cultivars. *Journal of Agricultural and Food Chemistry*, 2010, *58*, 3916-3926.

[180] Cao, G.; Russell, R.M.; Lischner, N.; Prior R.L. Serum antioxidant capacity is increased by consumption of strawberries, spinach, red wine or vitamin C in elderly woman. *Journal of Nutrition*, 1998, *98*, 2383-2309.

[181] Ara, V. The black chokeberry: a healthy fruit that will soon be "on all tongues"? *Fruit Processing*, 2002, *12*, 500-506.

[182] Martín-Aragón, S.; Basabe, B.; Benedi, J.; Villar, A. Antioxidant action of *Vaccinium myrtillus* L. *Phytotherapy Research*, 1998, *12*, S104-S106.

[183] Dri, D.; Calani, L.; Mazzeo, T.; Scazzina, F.; Rinaldi, M.; Del Rio, D.; Pellegrini, N.; Brighenti, F. Effects of different maturity stages on antioxidant content of ivorian gnagnan (*Solanum indicum* L.) berries. *Molecules*, 2010, *15*, 7125-7138.

[184] Schreckinger, M.E.; Wang, J.; Yousef, G.; Lila M.A.; González de Mejia, E. Antioxidant Capacity and *in vitro* inhibition of adipogenesis and inflammation by phenolic extracts of *Vaccinium floribundum* and *Aristotelia chilensis Journal of Agricultural and Food Chemistry*, 2010, *58*, 8966-8976.

In: Berries: Properties, Consumption and Nutrition
Editor: Carlo Tuberoso

ISBN 978-1-61470-257-3

Chapter II

Resveratrol in Berries: A Review

Natividad Sebastià[1], José M. Soriano[1], Alegría Montoro[2], Pedro Pérez-Bermúdez,*[*3] and Isabel Gavidia[3]

[1]Department of Preventive Medicine, Faculty of Pharmacy,
University of Valencia, Burjassot, Spain
[2]Servicio de Protección Radiológica,
Hospital Universitario La Fe, Valencia, Spain
[3]Department of Plant Biology, Faculty of Pharmacy,
University of Valencia, Burjassot, Spain

Abstract

Resveratrol is a polyphenolic compound found in several plant tissues and organs which is mainly detected in berries. In plants resveratrol acts as a phytoalexin, that is, plant metabolites produced against pathogen attacks or certain environmental stress factors. This compound possesses diverse biochemical and physiological properties including anti-inflammatory and immunomodulatory activities plus a wide range of health benefits ranging from chemoprevention to cardioprotection. Furthermore, recent studies have suggested that resveratrol also possesses antiaging properties. The present review describes and compares the occurrence of resveratrol in berries including data on the origin of the samples analyzed, the incidence observed, and the range of concentrations reported. A brief description of resveratrol biosynthesis and its biotechnological implication is also included.

[*] Department of Plant Biology, Faculty of Pharmacy, University of Valencia, Av. Vicent Andrés Estellés s/n. 46100 Burjassot, Spain, E-mail: perezb@uv.es.

Introduction

Trans-Resveratrol (3,5,4'-trihydroxystilbene), a phytoalexin that belongs to the group of compounds known as stilbenes, was first discovered in white hellebore [1] and was isolated from grapes almost four decades later [2]. It occurs in both leaves and berries, and in other foods (nuts and cacao), and its production is known to increase in response to a microbial challenge or to some other exogenous stimuli including wounding, pathogen attack or ultraviolet radiation. Usually, resveratrol is the major stilbene in berries and takes two isomeric forms: *trans*- and *cis*-resveratrol.

In the past decade, stilbenoids have attracted much attention and a number of scientific papers has been published about their beneficial effects on health given their strong antioxidant activity. This activity has been reported in a number of studies which have demonstrated that resveratrol inhibits platelet aggregation and low-density lipoprotein oxidation [3] and that it acts as a cancer chemopreventive [4,5]. It is believed that *trans*-resveratrol is the compound primarily responsible for the "French Paradox", which refers to the French having lower incidences of cardiovascular disease despite consuming a diet high in saturated fats, thanks to their regular consumption of red wine.

Resveratrol is usually analyzed in berries by reversed-phase high-performance liquid chromatography (LC) with standard-bore columns. Most LC methods perform separation by gradient elution with spectrophotometric UV diode array detection (DAD) [6-8], fluorimetric [9], electrochemical [8] and mass spectrometry (MS) with an electrospray ionization (ESI) detector. Methods based on gas chromatography and gas chromatography-mass spectrometry (GC-MS) [10] have been proposed for resveratrol. However, derivatization is required prior to a GC analysis of this substance to enhance volatility, and this time-consuming procedure may result in some *trans* to *cis* isomerization of resveratrol [11]. Some applications have also involved the use of capillary electrophoresis for the determination of resveratrol in wine.

This chapter attempts to present a detailed account of the presence of resveratrol in berries and the main factors affecting its concentration in these fruits. An introductory description of the resveratrol biosynthetic pathway is also included.

Resveratrol Biosynthesis

In microorganisms and plants, but not animals, the shikimate pathway produces aromatic acids L-phenylalanine, L-tyrosine and L-tryptophan. L-phenylalanine is the main precursor of numerous distinct phenolic compounds (Figure 1).

The most usual first metabolic step in plants is catalyzed by the enzyme phenylalanine ammonia lyase (PAL) producing cinnamic acid, which is hydroxylated to coumaric acid with participation of a cytochrome P450. The coenzyme A ester of coumaric acid is the basic unit required for further chain extension with malonyl-CoA molecules; usually three molecules are sequentially added. A polyketide is formed as a result of the addition of six carbons. The metabolism of this compound is a divergent point for distinct metabolic routes in plants since the polyketide is a substrate of two different enzymes, chalcone synthase or stilbene synthase.

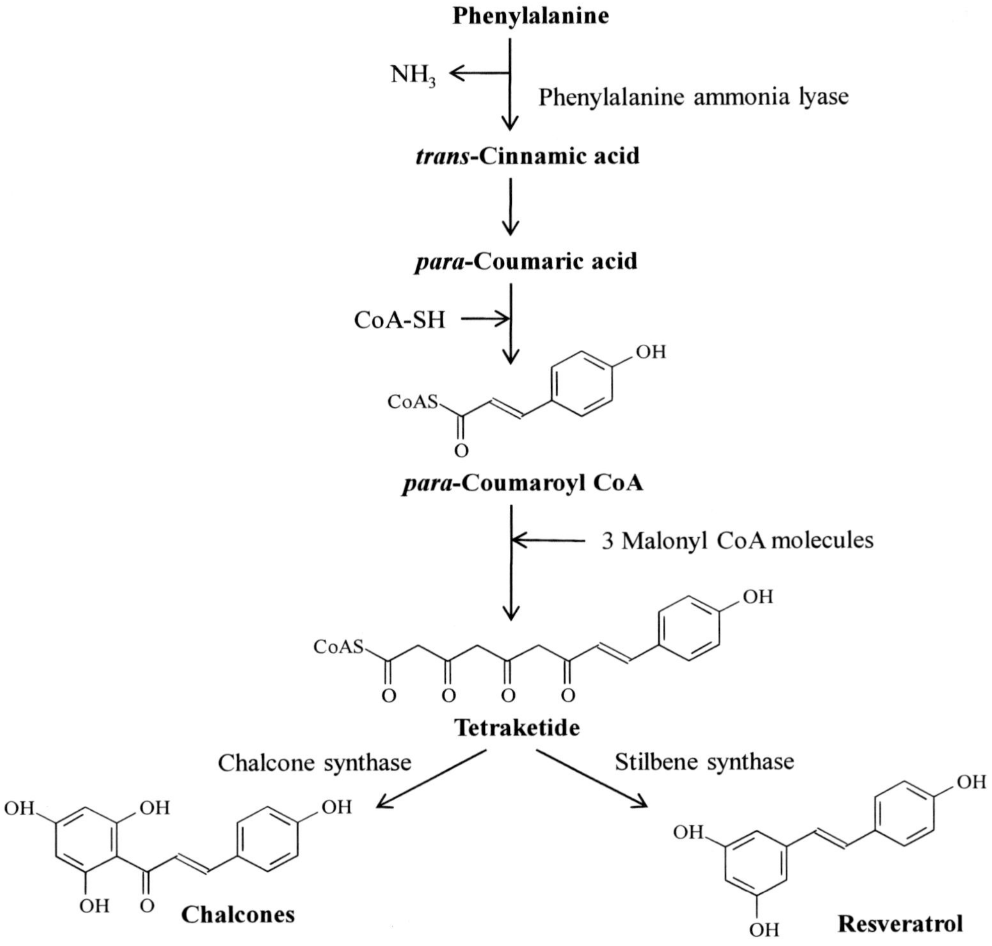

Figure 1. Steps and enzymes involved in the biosynthetic pathway of resveratrol.

Chalcone synthase is present in all plants and its activity leads to the production of chalcones, which are precursors of a wide range of phenolic compounds such as flavonoids and anthocyanins. In the other branch, the polyketide is folded by the stilbene synthase to produce the aromatic skeleton of the stilbene group, including *trans*- and *cis*-resveratrol, which can be further glycosylated to form piceids (Figure 1).

Most plants do not contain the enzyme required for resveratrol biosynthesis. Obviously, the stilbene synthase is the key enzyme for the genetically engineered production of resveratrol and stilbene derivatives.

Along these lines, the first data on cDNAs and genes for a stilbene synthase were obtained from peanuts and published by Schröder *et al.* [12]. Today there are many transgenic plants, as well as microorganisms, that synthesize ectopic resveratrol; for a recent review see Donnez *et al.* [13], who presented the state of the art of *trans*-resveratrol bioproduction by bacteria, yeasts and plant cells that determines the enhancement of the role of this compound in not only human health promotion, but also plant disease control.

Factors Affecting the Incidence and Concentration of Resveratrol in Berries

Resveratrol content of berries is low and extremely variable, and depends on numerous factors, as inferred from the numerous works carried out on resveratrol-producing plants, particularly on cultivars of *Vitis vinifera* and different species of the genus *Vaccinium*. Resveratrol production is firstly dependent on the type and variety of berry, and it is known that this metabolite accumulates differentially in skin, pulp or seeds. Although these intrinsic properties of berries are genetically determined, its final expression of resveratrol production throughout berry development is deeply altered by agricultural and environmental factors (management practices, soil, temperature, irrigation, pathogen attack, etc.) that affect the whole plant, or specifically berries. Moreover, the amount of resveratrol present in resveratrol-containing foods, berries or beverages, may be finally modulated in a greater or lesser extent by postharvesting practices in fruit processing, juice extraction, winemaking, etc.

The main factors affecting resveratrol concentration in berries, since their formation in the field until they are consumed in the human diet, are discussed below. The incidence and concentration range of resveratrol in several types of berries, besides the corresponding references, are shown in Table 1 (*Vitis vinifera* cultivars) and Table 2 (genus *Vaccinium*, *Morus* and *Fragaria*).

Intrinsic Properties of Berries

Grapevines are one of the most important plants due to the uses of their berries and products. In most grapevines, stilbenes mainly accumulate in berry skins, although these phenolic compounds are also found in much lower concentrations in seeds, pulp, grape stem and leaves. Nevertheless, Pastrana-Bonilla *et al.* [14] studied this variation in muscadine grapes (*V. rotundifolia*), which are indigenous to Southeast USA. These authors observed a different rank order of resveratrol (seeds >> skins > leaves >> pulp) since this phenolic compound in muscadine grape is, on average, five times more concentrated in seeds than in skins and 80 times higher than in pulp. Skins and seeds are discarded as waste during grape processing, for example in juice, wine or jelly production. This fact could prove an interesting fact because the nutraceutical industry may use seeds and skins as potential sources of resveratrol as these materials may provide an additional source of income for farmers or processors.

Resveratrol is the main stilbene in grapes, and red grapes and red wines are two of the major dietary sources of *trans*-resveratrol. Navarro *et al.* [15] analyzed resveratrol levels in the skins of four red grape berries used for winemaking (Bobal, Tempranillo, Cabernet Sauvignon and Crujidera), and concluded that the biosynthetic potential of these grapes to produce resveratrol largely depends on the grape variety (see Table 1), with a remarkably high content (245 $\mu g\ g^{-1}$ dw) found in Bobal berries. Similar results were reported for Californian table seedless grapes where *trans*-resveratrol content exhibited a ca. 20-fold variation between different clones, 0.16 μg/g in the Crimson cultivar *versus* 3.0 μg/g in the

Fantasia cultivar [16]. Romero-Pérez *et al.* [7] analyzed stilbene levels in the skins of three white grape berries and found that resveratrol content is also dependent on the cultivar (see Table 1).

Table 1. Incidence of resveratrol in grape samples

SOURCE	ORIGIN	INCIDENCE (positive samples/total samples)	RANGE	REFERENCE
Grape (*Vitis vinifera*)				
Grape extract				
Cv. Cabernet Sauvignon (red)	Oregon (USA)	(2/2)	2.45 µg/g dw	[25]
Cv. Cabernet Sauvignon (red)	Chile	(1/2)	0.5 µg/g fw	[54]
Cv. Concord (white grape concentrate)	Massachussets (USA)	(1/1)	1.16 µg/g	[55]
Cv. Concord (white grape extract)	Massachussets (USA)	(1/1)	0.43 µg/g fw	[55]
Cv. Concord (white grape powder)	Massachussets (USA)	(4/4)	0.53-2.70 µg/g dw	[55]
Cv. Crimson (red)	USA	-* (no data)	0.16 µg/g	[16]
Cv. Fantasia (red)	USA	-*	3.00 µg/g	[16]
Cv. Merlot (red)	Oregon (USA)	(2/2)	6.36 µg/g dw	[25]
Cv. Merlot (red)	Chile	(1/2)	0.5 µg/g fw	[54]
Cv. Muscadine (bronze)	Georgia (USA)	(12/15)	1 µg/g fw	[14]
Cv. Muscadine (purple)	Georgia (USA)	(12/15)	1 µg/g fw	[14]
Cv. Nebbiolo (red grape pulp)	Valtellina (Italy)	(4/4)	1 µg/g fw	[56]
Cv. Nero d'Avola (red grape pomace)	Siracusa (Italy)	(6/6)	6 µg/g dw	[11]
Cv. Pinot noir (red)	Oregon (USA)	(2/2)	5.75 µg/g dw	[25]
Cv. unknown (extract)	USA	-*	200 µg/g dw	[57]
Cv. unknown (extract)	Alicante (Spain)	-*	0.1 µg/g dw	[58]
Cv. unknown (table grape)	New Scotland (Canada)	(2/2)	6.47 µg/g dw	[25]
Red grape skins				
Cv. Bobal	Valencia (Spain)	(5/5)	245 µg/g dw	[15]
Cv. Bobal	Valencia (Spain)	(3/3)	80.03 µg/g	[59]
Cv. Cabernet Sauvignon	Valencia (Spain)	(5/5)	115 µg/g dw	[15]
Cv. Cabernet Sauvignon	Cataluña (Spain)	(13/13)	19.35-39.38 µg/g	[7]
Cv. Cariñena	Cataluña (Spain)	(13/13)	17.28-21.35 µg/g	[7]
Cv. Crujidera	Valencia (Spain)	(5/5)	120 µg/g dw	[15]
Cv. Merlot	Valencia (Spain)	(3/3)	21.5 µg/g	[59]
Cv. Merlot	Cataluña (Spain)	(13/13)	38.26 µg/g	[7]
Cv. Muscadine	Georgia (USA)	(27/30)	1-2 µg/g fw	[14]
Cv. Nebbiolo	Valtellina (Italy)	(4/4)	60 µg/g fw	[56]
Cv. Nero d'Avola	Siracusa (Italy)	(6/6)	27.5 µg/g dw	[11]
Cv. Tempranillo	Valencia (Spain)	(3/3)	174 µg/g	[59]
Cv. Tempranillo	Valencia (Spain)	(5/5)	32 µg/g dw	[15]
Cv. Tinto mozuelo	Valencia (Spain)	(3/3)	71.2 µg/g	[59]
Cv. unknown	USA	-*	50-100 µg/g fw	[4]
Cv. unknown	Alicante (Spain)	-*	0.15 µg/g dw	[58]
Cv. unknown	Turkey	-*	140-300 µg/g fw	[60]
White grape skins				
Cv. Macabeo	Cataluña (Spain)	(13/13)	47.6 µg/g	[7]
Cv. Palomino fino	Cádiz (Spain)	(25/25)	3.22 µg/g	[23]

Cv. Parellada	Cataluña (Spain)	(13/13)	11.04-16.59 μg/g	[7]
Cv. Xarel.lo	Cataluña (Spain)	(13/13)	18.13 μg/g	[7]

Numerous publications have reported that *trans*-resveratrol content in wines, transferred from skins to musts during maceration, differs according to the variety of grape used for winemaking (for a review, see Stervbo *et al.* [17]). Thus, Jeandet *et al.* [18] observed that the *trans*-resveratrol content of wines made with red grapes (var. Pinot noir) was around three times higher than in those made with white grapes (var. Chardonnay blanc) when vinted under the same conditions. In a comparison made among several grape juices varieties, Romero-Pérez *et al.* [19] observed that the highest levels of total resveratrol were found in the juices produced from Xarel.lo variety followed by those produced from cv. Parellada. These results are in agreement with those previously presented by the same authors [20] in white wines made from berries of the same varieties. In contrast to the prevalence of *trans*-resveratrol in red grapes, the highest concentrations of the stilbenes found in white grape juices were the piceid isomers, whereas *cis*-resveratrol could not be quantified or was not detected in any of the samples [21, 2]. Furthermore, it is important to note that significant differences can be found in resveratrol content between one vintage and another within the same grape variety [22, 23], and that much of the variance reported on resveratrol content in grape berries can also be explained by the age of the vines [24], the grape maturation stage [22] or the degree of infection by gray mold [18].

Regarding the berries from *Vaccinium* spp. several studies have taken it for granted that resveratrol is virtually always present in these woodland fruits, but in strongly variable concentrations.

Rimando *et al.* [25] analyzed the berries collected from different populations of *Vaccinium* located throughout US and Canadian territories to find that resveratrol concentrations ranged from 0.01 μg g^{-1} dw in Rabbiteye blueberry (*Vaccinium ashei* var. Reade) to 5.9 μg g^{-1} dw in Partridge berry (*Vaccinium vitis-idaea* var. Minor) (see Table 2). They also found that for each variety analyzed, resveratrol content varied not only among the different populations, but also within the berry samples collected from the same region.

As regards strawberry, Wang *et al.* [26] carried out a comparative study conducted with several cultivars. Both *cis*- and *trans*-resveratrol were detected in strawberry achenes (seeds) and pulp (receptacle tissue) although the stilbenoids were differentially distributed in the berry since was found to be higher in achenes than in fruit pulp: 1.64 μg g^{-1} dw and 0.83 μg g^{-1} dw, respectively. The obtained results demonstrate that resveratrol content in strawberry is also dependent on the variety analyzed since fruit from Ovation (B28), Mohawk, Earliglow and B35 had higher amounts of total resveratrol than the fruits of the other ten genotypes. Genotype Ovation (B28) contained the highest resveratrol quantity, whereas Latestar contained the least amount (see Table 2). Another berry that provides a large amount of resveratrol is mulberry (*Morus* spp.), as Song *et al.* [27] found that its concentrations range from 2.1 to 5.3 μg g^{-1} among the fruits of eight different species collected from several regions of China.

Agricultural and Environmental Factors

Soil. Soil significantly affects not only plant growth and development, but mineral and secondary metabolite accumulation in fruits. Along these lines, Bavaresco *et al.* [28] studied the interaction among soil type (neutral or calcareous), growth, stilbenoid accumulation and ochratoxin production in the grape cv. Merlot.

Table 2. Incidence of resveratrol in *Vaccinium* spp. berries, mulberry and strawberry

SOURCE	ORIGIN	INCIDENCE (positive samples / total samples)	RANGE	REFERENCE
Vaccinium spp.				
Bilberry (*V. myrtillus* L.)				
Bilberry	New Scotland (Canada)	(2/2)	0.77 µg/g dw	[25]
Bilberry extract	USA	-* (no data)	<100 µg/g dw	[57]
Heated bilberry	Poland	(3/3)	0.01 µg /g	[47]
Raw bilberry	Poland	(5/5)	0.02 µg /g	[47]
Blueberry cv. Elliot (*V. Elliotti* Cv. Chapman*)*				
Blueberry cv. Elliot	Mississippi (USA)	(2/2)	0.41-0.45 µg /g dw	[25]
Cranberry (*V. macrocarpon Ait*)				
Cranberry	Canada	(2/2)	0.9 µg/g dw	[25]
Deerberry (*V. stamineum* L.*)*				
Deerberry	North Carolina (USA)	(17/17)	0.05-0.5 µg /g dw	[25]
Highbush blueberry (*V.corymbosum* L.)				
Heated highbush blueberry	Michigan (USA)	(3/3)	0.02 µg /g	[47]
Highbush blueberry	Oregon (USA)	(4/4)	0.33-0.85 µg /g dw	[25]
Highbush blueberry	Southern United States	(3/3)	1.07 µg/g dw	[25]
Raw highbush blueberry	Michigan (USA)	(3/3)	0.03 µg /g	[47]
Lingonberry (*V. vitis-ideae* cv. *vitis-ideae*)				
Lingonberry	New Scotland (Canada)	(2/2)	0.59 µg/g dw	[25]
Lowbush blueberry (*V. angustifolium* cv. Aiton)				
Heated lowbush wild blueberry	New Scotland (Canada)	(3/3)	0.01 µg /g	[47]
Lowbush blueberry	New Scotland (Canada)	(3/3)	0.87 µg/g dw	[25]
Raw lowbush wild blueberry	New Scotland (Canada)	(3/3)	0.01 µg /g	[47]
Partridgeberry (*V. vitis-idaea* cv. Minor)				
Partridgeberry	New Scotland (Canada)	(2/2)	5.9 µg/g dw	[25]
Rabbiteye blueberry *(V. ashei* cv. Reade*)*				
Rabbiteye blueberry	USA	-*	1.69 µg/g dw	[25]
Rabbiteye blueberry	Mississippi (USA)	(3/3)	0.01-0.58 µg /g dw	[25]
Sparkleberry *(V. arboreum* cv. Marshall)				
Sparkleberry	Mississippi (USA)	(3/3)	0.12-0.52 µg /g dw	[25]
Mulberry (*Morus* spp.)				
Lyophilized mulberry	China	(13/41)	2.1-5.3 µg/g dw	[27]
Lyophilized mulberry fruit marc	China	(19/41)	1.0-6.8 µg /g dw	[27]
Strawberry (Fragaria × *ananassa* Duchesne)				
Cv. Allstar pulp	Maryland (USA)	(3/3)	0.83 µg/g dw	[26]

Cv. Allstar seeds	Maryland (USA)	(3/3)	1.64 μg/g dw	[26]
Cv. Ovation	Maryland (USA)	(3/3)	2.9-3.7 μg/g dw	[26]
Cv. Latestar	Maryland (USA)	(3/3)	0.7-1.6 μg/g dw	[26]
Cv. Honeoye	Maryland (USA)	(3/3)	1-1.4 μg/g dw	[26]
Cv. Earliglow	Maryland (USA)	(3/3)	0.8-1.5 μg/g dw	[26]
Cv. Kent	Maryland (USA)	(3/3)	0.7-1.1 μg/g dw	[26]

The authors reported that *trans*-resveratrol and viniferin berry concentrations are significantly affected by fungal infection and that the effect of soil type differs depending on the phenological phase of the berries: at veraison calcareous soil induces a higher level of both stilbenoids than neutral soil, whereas the exact opposite occurs during ripening. In control uninoculated berries, the lime stress condition of calcareous soil increases the level of stilbenes, especially at ripening.

Compost as a soil supplement can also enhance the level of total resveratrol content in fruits. Wang *et al.* [26] studied variations of resveratrol content in two strawberry cultivars (Allstar and Honeoye) in accordance with soil treatment. The fruits of the plants grown in 100% soil or 50% soil plus 50% sand presented low levels of resveratrol content. However in both cultivars, the fruit grown in 50% soil plus 50% compost or that grown in 100% compost had ca. 50% higher levels of resveratrol than fruits from plants grown without this supplement. Compost causes changes in soil's chemical and physical characteristics, increases beneficial microorganisms activity [29], and enhances nutrient availability and uptake [28, 29], thus resulting in high levels of antioxidants, including resveratrol, in strawberry fruits.

Temperature. In their study on strawberry plants, Wang *et al.* [26] employed two cultivars (Kent and Earliglow) to determine the effect of temperature on resveratrol production. They found the lowest resveratrol contents (ca. 0.7 - 0.8 μg g^{-1} dw) in the fruits collected from plants grown in cool day and night cycles (18/12 °C). They also observed that increasing the night temperature from 12 °C to 22 °C, and maintaining the day temperature constant at 25 °C, resulted in a significant increase in the resveratrol contents of the Kent and Earliglow fruits (1.0 – 1.3 μg g^{-1} dw). Finally, the highest day/night temperatures assayed (30/25 °C) yielded the fruits with the largest amount of resveratrol (1.1 - 1.5 μg g^{-1} dw).

In their work with white grapes of the Palomino fino cultivar, Palacios *et al.* [31] noted how lower temperatures (24-25 °C) than those expected in the growth area during grape maturation, combined with a high radiation level, lowers photosynthesis and the plant's general metabolism. All these factors lead to high total acidity and polyphenol values, including resveratrol, in juice. These authors concluded that situations of physiological stress caused by unfavorable climatic conditions increase resveratrol which is present mainly in its glycosylated forms.

CO_2 -enriched environment. Elevated carbon dioxide (plants grown in hill plasticultures *versus* plants grown in matted rows) affects resveratrol content in strawberry fruits since the berries collected had higher concentrations of total resveratrol when plants were grown in CO_2 -enriched environment. Two different conditions assayed that increase the CO_2 level (ambient + 300 μmol mol^{-1} CO_2 and ambient + 600 μmol mol^{-1} CO_2) resulted in increased resveratrol accumulation in strawberry fruits. Resveratrol concentration raised from 1.12 μg g^{-1} dw, determined in strawberries grown in ambient atmosphere, to 1.75 μg g^{-1} dw in those fruits grown in an environment enriched with 600 μmol mol^{-1} CO_2. An increase in resveratrol

in elevated CO_2-treated strawberries could help in quenching the excited state of active oxygen species and in reducing free radical activity [26].

Water stress. Roldán *et al.* [23] compared the effects of different factors on resveratrol production during two consecutive vintages of grapes cv. Palomino fino. They saw that a reduced level of precipitation from 600 mm, a suitable level for the maturation of this grape variety, to only 211 mm leads to a water stress situation. This scenario causes high resveratrol production in berries, mainly in the glycosylated form (piceids), that accumulates in skins and is stored for use as part of the plant's defense mechanism, whereas free isomers in juice spread.

Infection by fungi. As previously mentioned, much of the variance reported on resveratrol content in grape berries can be explained by the degree of fungal infections, more specifically by the gray mold caused by *Botrytis cinerea.* Jeandet *et al.* [18] put forward a hypothesis that the wines obtained from those grapes that had undergone a severe *Botrytis* infestation (80%) have poor resveratrol contents due to degradation by laccase enzymes, such as stilbene oxidase. This hypothesis is supported by the results of Roldán *et al.* [23], who observed that at more advanced infection stages, when *Botrytis* had accomplished its external development, a widespread decrease of the total resveratrol content in grape juice is observed at levels of the same order as the initial ones before infection.

Thus, resveratrol content in berries, and therefore in wine, seems to be the result of a balance between resveratrol synthesis by plant and resveratrol degradation by the pathogen. In fact one could expect an accumulation of resveratrol in the skin in response to infection by *B. cinerea* [32-34], but when berries do not exhibit disease symptoms, that is, in the first stage of the pathogen's internal development, resveratrol content lowers drastically. This phenomenon may be due to the fact that before the fungal presence and before resveratrol synthesis is stimulated, the resveratrol already present in the skin is used by the grape as part of its defense mechanism, i.e., resveratrol would become a stilbene oligomer such as viniferins [35], which are more toxic to the pathogen; thus, the free and glycosylated forms (piceids) of resveratrol decrease. In the second stage of pathogen development, an accumulation of resveratrol takes place until certain levels are reached and maintained throughout its external development. These results are in agreement with those reported by Romero-Pérez *et al.* [20], who indicated that resveratrol and piceid isomers considerably increase in the grape berry skins infected by powdery mildew and that the degree of infection was positively related to the stilbenes content. In principle, it is expected that resveratrol levels diminish laccase performance, although these results seem to indicate that at the skin level, the degree of resveratrol synthesis is greater than the degree of degradation by the enzyme. Consequently, *B. cinerea*'s laccase activity appears to be more important in the pulp than in the skin [23].

Postharvesting Practices

Berry maceration. Increased phenolic concentration in grape juice depends on skin cell wall degradation. Then, a maceration step, either with or without macerating enzymes, may improve the yield and stilbene content of juices. González-Barrio *et al.* [36] smashed and macerated grapes (white table grapes cv. Superior) under different conditions: 25 °C or 45 °C for 0, 1, 2 and 3 h. The best results for the extraction of phenolic compounds were obtained for 2 h of maceration at 45 °C. These authors also observed a synergic positive effect between maceration and the addition of $Na_2S_2O_5$. Under such conditions, the concentration of most phenolic compounds increases from 2 to 3-fold, but differences are more pronounced for stilbenes since the total concentration is 35-fold higher in the macerated-derived juice compared to the juice obtained without maceration.

Different enzymatic preparations (cellulytic and pectolytic enzymes) have been reported for juice production during the maceration process of different berries, such as grape [36, 37], blackcurrant and blueberry [38]. In all cases, a better juice yield is observed which increases from 10% to 30% higher than in the control macerations without enzymes. The higher or lesser effectiveness of the enzymatic treatment seems to be due to the variable composition and the cell wall thickness in the different types of berries extracted.

Clarification of juices and wines. Clarification with some fining agents (used in wine clarification and filtration operations) can lower resveratrol and piceid levels [39-42]. Some of these clarifying agents are also employed in commercial grape juice making. The levels of the four compounds (*trans*- and *cis*-resveratrol and piceids) in red samples are on average 10-fold higher than in white juices and show greater variability. The total resveratrol content in red samples varies from 0.69 to 14.47 mg/L, whereas the range in white samples goes from non detection to 1.44 mg/L.

The levels of total resveratrol found in red and white grape juices are similar to those described for Spanish red and white wines (5.65 and 0.48 mg/L, respectively) by Lamuela-Raventos *et al.* [39] and Romero-Pérez *et al.* [20]. It is interesting to note that the fresh juices extracted from winemaking grape varieties present a total average resveratrol content of 0.72 mg/L, which is more than two-fold the average content measured in commercial juices (0.29 mg/L). It is difficult to tell whether this difference is due to the grape variety used, to changes during storage, or to different practices employed for juice production. The different resveratrol contents in white and red wines have been previously described [20], and the lower levels found in white wines are due to the absence of skin contact during the fermentation process. In white and red grape juices, however, differences in resveratrol content have been attributed to the juice processing technology (i.e., pressing and skin color extraction procedures) because *trans*-resveratrol levels in grape skins are similar for red and white berries [41]. On the other hand, the high occurrence of free resveratrol in extracts is linked to the presence of endogenous β-D-glucosidases, which are likely to remain active during the extraction process [43].

Alcoholic and malolactic fermentations. Pezet and Cuenat [44] analyzed resveratrol in the skin, seeds and must of Gamay grape berries in the different winemaking process steps as well as in wines after malolactic fermentation. They observed that resveratrol levels remain quite constant in seeds, but increase in musts and decrease in skins during alcoholic fermentation. They also observed that resveratrol extraction from skins correlates well with the increase of ethanol concentration in musts until day 6. After malolactic fermentation, the amount of resveratrol in wine is about twice that measured at the end of alcoholic fermentation, thus indicating a pool of resveratrol, probably as piceids and/or as oligomeric forms (viniferins), from which free resveratrol can be liberated by the enzymatic activity of malolactic bacteria.

Fruit processing. In order to increase the resveratrol content of grape berries, Cantos *et al.* [45] developed an interesting system based in the response of grape berries to ultraviolet-C light. Berry cells face UV light stress by inducing their phytoalexins, mainly the stilbene resveratrol. The aim of this work was to identify and quantify the main inducible stilbenes, and to study their induction kinetics in four red (Red Globe, Flame, Crimson, and Napoleon) and three white (Superior, Dominga, and Moscatel Italica) table grape varieties after postharvest UV-C irradiation. They all induced a number of stilbene derivatives upon irradiation with UV-C, although there were both qualitative and quantitative differences in the grape varieties assayed. Regarding the induction of *trans*-resveratrol, the content of red varieties Crimson and Red Globe increased by more than 100- and 2000-fold, respectively, if compared to untreated grapes. The huge resveratrol induction in Red Globe variety was due to the lack of resveratrol in the control grapes. However, the other two red varieties (Flame and Napoleon) induced 4-fold more resveratrol than their respective untreated grapes. The white varieties increased their *trans*-resveratrol content by about 10- to 50-fold if compared to untreated grapes. The authors concluded that after UV-C treatment, the red grape varieties Flame and Red Globe could supply ca. 5 mg of resveratrol/serving (200 g), which is the same amount supplied by seven glasses of red wine (7 x 200 mL) with a high resveratrol content.

Resveratrol Preservation at Home

As mentioned above, an increasing demand for juices from berries has been observed globally, with the corresponding development of the juice industry. In line with this, the use of high technology for fruit processing and packaging is particularly interested in the stability of resveratrol in the juices obtained. Shanmuganathan *et al.* [46] found that *trans*-resveratrol disappears from blueberry juices after one week of storage in the refrigerator. In fact, the resveratrol content degrades by half after 3 days of storage. The authors observed that resveratrol in refrigerated samples degrades less rapidly in comparison with juice samples stored at room temperature, in which resveratrol shows an approximate half-life of only 15 h. If we assume that these results reported for blueberry juices can be extended to other resveratrol-containing juices, then it is recommended to store juice in the refrigerator once opened and to finish consuming it within 3 days to gain the maximum benefits from resveratrol.

A different nutritional question concerning resveratrol is whether this natural product is altered, or not, in baked or heat-processed fruits. With this mind, Lyons *et al.* [47] described for the first time how resveratrol content varies in heated fruits. These authors observed that during heating, berries lose a 14-34% of their mass due to evaporation. Moreover, heating berries for 18 min at 190 °C results in the destruction of 17% and 46% of the initial resveratrol in Polish bilberries and highbush Michigan blueberries, respectively. The variability observed in the stability of resveratrol in the two species evaluated is attributed to a probable berry matrix effect [47].

Bioavailability of Resveratrol

Nowadays, nutraceuticals is the major market for *trans*-resveratrol which is produced mainly from field cultures of *Polygonum cuspidatum* in China. The demand of resveratrol has rapidly increased and new sources of this natural product such as berries, and particularly grapes, have become a genuine reality. *Trans*-resveratrol was first detected in grapevines in 1976 by Langcake and Pryce [2], and their finding overlapped the epidemiological studies that led to the well-known "French Paradox" concerning phenolic compounds, mainly resveratrol, as antioxidants with benefits for human health. Consequently, a large number of studies have been carried out which clarify resveratrol health benefits are related to the bioavailability of this compound.

Several studies have simulated different conditions for resveratrol administration in human volunteers, and it seems that the matrix or fed/fasting conditions may result in discrepancy between data. Vaz-da-Silva *et al.* [48] administered a single dose of resveratrol to human volunteers following a standard high fat content meal or 8 h of fasting. They observed that the absorption rate of *trans*-resveratrol is significantly delayed by the presence of food, although the extent of absorption is not affected in a clinically relevant way. Furthermore, Hollman *et al.* [49] and Paganga and Rice-Evans [50] noted that the absorption of some phenols deriving from diet is enhanced by conjugation with glucose. If glucoside facilitates absorption, then piceids may be more efficiently absorbed than aglycons. In fact, Burkon and Somoza [51] suggested that piceid might prove an alternative soluble form for resveratrol administration instead of a pure compound. On the other hand, Ortuño *et al.* [52] reported a better absorption of resveratrol from a moderate dose of wine or from grape juice than from a grape extract tablets. Another question focuses on its metabolism. Likes most dietary polyphenols, resveratrol absorption is good, but its bioavailability is very poor given its rapid and extensive metabolism [52], where sulfates and glucuronides are the most frequently reported metabolites in the data [53].

References

[1] Takaoka, M.J. Of the phenolic substances of white hellebore (*Veratrum grandiflorum* Loes. Fil.). Hokkaido Imperial University. *Hokkaido Imperial University*, 1940, *3*, 1-16.

[2] Langcake, P.; Pryce, R.J. The production of resveratrol by *Vitis vinifera* and other members of the *Vitaceae* as a response to infection or injury. *Physiological Plant Pathology*, 1976, *9*, 77-86.

[3] Fan, E., Zhang, L., Jiang, S.; Bai, Y. Beneficial effects of resveratrol on atherosclerosis. *Journal of Medicinal Food*, 2008, *11*, 610-614.

[4] Jang, M.; Cai, L.; Udeani, G.O.; Slowing, K.V.; Thomas, C.F.; Beecher, C.W.W.; Fong, H.H.S.; Farnsworth, N.R.; Kinghorn, A.D.; Mehta, R.G.; Moon, R.C.; Pezzuto, J.M. Cancer chemopreventive activity of resveratrol, a natural product derived from grapes. *Science*, 1997, *275*, 218-220.

[5] Thomasset, S.C.; Berry, D.P.; Garcea, G.; Marczylo, T.; Steward, W.P.; Gescher, A.J. Dietary polyphenolic phytochemicals - promising cancer chemopreventive agents in humans? A review of their clinical properties. *International Journal of Cancer*, 2007, *120*, 451-458.

[6] Goldberg, D.M.; Tsang, E.; Karumanchiri, A.; Diamandis, E.P.; Soleas, G.; Ng, E. Method to assay the concentrations of phenolic constituents of biological interest in wines. *Analytical Chemistry*, 1996, *68*, 1688-1694.

[7] Romero-Pérez, A.I.; Lamuela-Raventós, R.M.; Andrés-Lacueva, C.; de la Torre-Boronat, M.C. Method for the quantitative extraction of resveratrol and piceid isomers in grape berry skins. Effect of powdery mildew on the stilbene content. *Journal of Agricultural and Food Chemistry*, 2001, *49*, 210-215.

[8] Meng, X.M.; Maliakal, P.; Lu, H.; Lee, M.J.; Yang, C.S. Urinary and plasma levels of resveratrol and quercetin in humans, mice, and rats after ingestion of pure compounds and grape juice. *Journal of Agricultural and Food Chemistry*, 2004, *52*, 935-942.

[9] Rodríguez-Delgado, M.A.; Malovaná, S.; Pérez, J.P.; Borges, T.; García Montelongo, F.J. Separation of phenolic compounds by high-performance liquid chromatography with absorbance and fluorimetric detection. *Journal of Chromatography A*, 2001, *912*, 249-257.

[10] Tokuşoglu, O.; Unal, M.K.; Yemiş, F. Determination of the phytoalexin resveratrol (3,5,4'-trihydroxystilbene) in peanuts and pistachios by high-performance liquid chromatographic diode array (HPLC-DAD) and gas chromatography-mass spectrometry (GC-MS). *Journal of Agricultural and Food Chemistry*, 2005, *53*, 5003-5009.

[11] Careri, M; Corradini, C.; Elviri, L.; Nicoletti, I. Direct HPLC Analysis of quercetin and *trans*-resveratrol in red wine, grape, and winemaking byproducts. *Journal of Agricultural and Food Chemistry*, 2003, *51*, 5226-5231.

[12] Schröder, G.; Brown, J.W.; Schröder, J. Molecular analysis of resveratrol synthase. cDNA, genomic clones and relationship with chalcone synthase. *European Journal of Biochemistry*, 1988, *172*, 161-169.

[13] Donnez, D., Jeandet, P., Clément, C., Courot, E. Bioproduction of resveratrol and stilbene derivatives by plant cells and microorganisms. *Trends in Biotechnology*, 2009, *27*, 706-713.

[14] Pastrana-Bonilla, E.; Akoh, C.C.; Sellappan, S.; Krewer, G. Phenolic content and antioxidant capacity of muscadine grapes. *Journal of Agricultural and Food Chemistry*, 2003, *51*, 5497-5503.

[15] Navarro, S.; León, M.; Roca-Pérez, L.; Boluda, R.; García-Ferriz, L.; Pérez-Bermúdez, P.; Gavidia, I. Characterisation of Bobal and Crujidera grape cultivars in comparison with Tempranillo and Cabernet Sauvignon: Evolution of leaf macronutrients and berry composition during grape ripening. *Food Chemistry*, 2008, *108*, 182-190.

[16] Creasy, L.L.; Coffee, M. Phytoalexin production potential of grape berries. *Journal of the American Society for Horticultural Science*, 1988, *113*, 230-234.

[17] Stervbo, U.; Vang, O.; Bonnesen, C. A review of the content of putative chemopreventive phytoalexin resveratrol in red wine. *Food Chemistry*, 2007, *101*, 449-457.

[18] Jeandet, P.; Bessis, R.; Sbaghi, M.; Meunier, P.; Trollat, P. Resveratrol content of wines of different ages: Relationship with fungal disease pressure in the vineyard. *American Journal of Enology and Viticulture*, 1995, *46*, 1-4.

[19] Romero-Pérez, A.I.; Ibern-Gómez, M.; Lamuela-Raventós, R.M.; de la Torre-Boronat, M.C. Piceid, the major resveratrol derivative in grape juices. *Journal of Agricultural and Food Chemistry*, 1999, *47*, 1533-1536.

[20] Romero-Pérez, A.I.; Lamuela-Raventós, R.M.; Waterhouse, A.L.; de la Torre-Boronat, M.C. Levels on *cis*- and *trans*-resveratrol and their glucosides in white and rosé *Vitis vinifera* wines from Spain. *Journal of Agricultural and Food Chemistry*, 1996, *44*, 2124-2128.

[21] Jeandet, P.; Bessis, R.; Gautheron, B. The production of resveratrol (3,5,4'-trihydroxystilbene) by grape berries in different developmental stages. *American Journal of Enology and Viticulture*, 1991, *42*, 41-46.

[22] Threlfall, R.T.; Morris, J.R.; Mauromoustakos, A. Effect of variety, ultraviolet light exposure, and enological methods on the *trans*-resveratrol level of wine. *American Journal of Enology and Viticulture*, 1999, *50*, 57-64.

[23] Roldán, A.; Palacios, V.; Caro, I.; Pérez, L. Resveratrol content of Palomino fino grapes: Influence of vintage and fungal infection. *Journal of Agricultural and Food Chemistry,* 2003, *51*, 1464-1468.

[24] Mattivi, F. Solid phase extraction of *trans*-resveratrol from wines for HPLC analysis. *Zeitschrift für Lebensmitteluntersuchung und Forschung A*, 1993, *196*, 522-525.

[25] Rimando, A.M.; Kalt, W.; Magee, J.B.; Dewey, J.; Ballington, J.R. Resveratrol, pterostilbene, and piceatannol in vaccinium berries. *Journal of Agricultural and Food Chemistry*, 2004, *52*, 4713-4719.

[26] Wang, S.Y.; Chen, C.; Wang, C.Y.; Chen, P. Resveratrol content in strawberry fruit is affected by preharvest conditions. *Journal of Agricultural and Food Chemistry*, 2007, *55*, 8269-8274.

[27] Song, W.; Wang, H.J.; Bucheli, P.; Zhang, P.F.; Wei, D.Z.; Lu, Y.H. Phytochemical profiles of different mulberry (*Morus sp.*) species from China. *Journal of Agricultural and Food Chemistry*, 2009, *57*, 9133-9140.

[28] Bavaresco, L.; Vezzulli, S.; Civardi, S.; Gatti, M.; Battilani, P.; Pietri, A.; Ferrari, F. Effect of lime-induced leaf chlorosis on ochratoxin A, trans-resveratrol, and ε-viniferin production in grapevine (*Vitis vinifera* L.) berries infected by *Aspergillus carbonarius. Journal of Agricultural and Food Chemistry*, 2008, *56,* 2085-2089.

[29] Chung, Y.H.A.; Hoitink, J.; Lipps, P.E. Interactions between organic matter decomposition level and soilborne disease severity. *Agriculture, Ecosystems & Environment*, 1988, *24*, 183-193.

[30] Rynk, R. (Ed.) *Northeast regional agricultural engineering service. On-Farm composting handbook, NRAES-54*. Ithaca, NY: Riley Robb Hall, Coop. Ext.; 1992.

[31] Palacios, V.M.; Nebot, E.; Pérez, L. Uses of factor analysis for the characterization and modelling of maturation of Palomino fino grapes in the Jerez region. *American Journal of Enology and Viticulture*, 1997, *48*, 317-322.

[32] Goldberg, D.M.; Ng, E.; Karumanchiri, A.; Yan, J.; Diamandis, E.P.; Soleas, G.J. Assay of resveratrol glucosides and isomers in wine by direct-injection high-performance liquid chromatography. *Journal of Chromatography A*, 1995, *708*, 89-98.

[33] Hoos, G.; Blaich, R. Metabolism of stilbene phytoalexins in grapevines: Oxidation of resveratrol in sail-cell cultures. *Vitis*, 1988, *27*, 1-12.

[34] Sotheeswaran, S.; Pasupathy, V. Distribution of resveratrol oligomers in plants. *Phytochemistry*, 1993, *32*, 1083-1092.

[35] Bavaresco, L.; Petegolli, D.; Cantú, E.; Fregoni, M.; Chiusa, G.; Trevisan, M. Elicitation and accumulation of stilbene phytoalexins in grapevine berries infected by *Botrytis cinerea*. *Vitis*, 1997, *36*, 77-83.

[36] González-Barrio, R.; Vidal-Guevara, M.L.; Tomás-Barberán, F.A.; Espín, J.C. Preparation of a resveratrol-enriched grape juice based on ultraviolet C-treated berries. *Innovative Food Science and Emerging Technologies*, 2009, *10*, 374-382.

[37] Haight, K.G.; Gump, B.H. The use of macerating enzymes in grape juice processing. *American Journal of Enology and Viticulture*, 1994, *45*, 113-116.

[38] Buchert, J., Koponen, J.M.; Suutarien, M., Mustranta, A.; Lille, M.; Törrönen, R.; Poutanen, K. Effect of enzyme-aided pressing on anthocyanin yield and profiles in bilberry and blackcurrant juices. *Journal of the Science of Food and Agriculture*, 2005, *85,* 2548-2556.

[39] Lamuela-Raventós, R.M.; Romero-Pérez, A.I.; Waterhouse, A.L.; de la Torre-Boronat, M.C. Direct HPLC analysis of *cis*- and *trans*-resveratrol and piceid isomers in spanish red *Vitis vinifera* wines. *Journal of Agricultural and Food Chemistry*, 1995, *43*, 281-283.

[40] Soleas, G.J.; Goldberg, D.M.; Diamandis, E.P.; Karumanchiri, A; Yan, J.; Ng, E. A derivatized gas chromatographic-mass spectrometric method for the analysis of both isomers of resveratrol in juice and wine. *American Journal of Enology and Viticulture*, 1995, 46, 346-352.

[41] Tobella, N.N.; Waterhouse, A.L. Fining effects on resveratrol and piceid isomer concentrations in red wine. *American Journal of Enology and Viticulture*, 1996, *47*, 352.

[42] Vrhovsek, U.; Wendelin, S.; Eder, R. Effects of various vinification techniques on the concentration of *cis*- and *trans*-resveratrol and resveratrol glucoside isomers in wine. *American Journal of Enology and Viticulture*, 1997, *48*, 214-219.

[43] Ayran, A.; Wilson, B.; Strauss, C.; Williams, P. The properties of glycosidases of *Vitis vinifera* and a comparison of their ß-glucosidase activity with that of exogenous enzymes. An assessment of possible applications in ecology. *American Journal of Enology and Viticulture*, 1987, *38*, 182-188.

[44] Pezet, R.; Cuenat, P. Resveratrol in wine: Extraction from skin during fermentation and post-fermentation standing of must from Gamay grapes. *American Journal of Enology and Viticulture,* 1996, 47, 287-290.

[45] Cantos, E.; Espín, J.C.; Tomás-Barberán, F.A. Postharvest stilbene-enrichment of red and white table grape varieties using UV-C irradiation pulses. *Journal of Agricultural and Food Chemistry*, 2002, *50*, 6322-6329.

[46] Shanmuganathan, M.; Li, P.C.H. Resveratrol analysis and degradation study in blueberry samples by HPLC with fluorescence detection. *Journal of Liquid Chromatography & Related Technologies*, 2009, *32*, 3038–3048.

[47] Lyons, M.; Yu, C.; Toma, R.B.; Chi, S.Y.; Reiboldt, W.; Lee, J.; Van Breemen, R.B. Resveratrol in raw and baked blueberries and bilberries. *Journal of Agricultural and Food Chemistry*, 2003, *51*, 5867-5870.

[48] Vaz-da-Silva, M.; Loureiro, A.I.; Falcao, A.; Tunes, T.; Rocha, J.F.; Fernandes-Lopes, C.; Soares, E.; Wright, L.; Almeida, L.; Soares-da-Silva, P. Effect of food on the pharmacokinetic profile of *trans*-resveratrol. *International Journal of Clinical Pharmacology and Therapeutics*, 2008, *46*, 564-570.

[49] Hollman, P.C.; de Vries, J.H.; van Leeuwen, S.D.; Mengelers, M.J.; Katan, M.B. Absorption of dietary quercetin glycosides and quercetin in healthy ileostomy volunteers. *The American Journal of Clinical Nutrition*, 1995, *62*, 1276-1282.

[50] Pagangaa, G.; Rice-Evans, C.A. The identification of flavonoids as glycosides in human plasma. *Federation of European Biochemical Societies Letters*, 1997, *401*, 78-82.

[51] Burkon, A.; Somoza, V. Quantification of free and protein-bound *trans*-resveratrol metabolites and identification of *trans*-resveratrol-C/O-conjugated diglucuronides. Two novel resveratrol metabolites in human plasma. *Molecular Nutrition & Food Research*, 2008, *52*, 549-557.

[52] Ortuño, J.; Covas, M.I.; Farre, M.; Pujadas, M.; Fito, M.; Khymenets, O.; Andres-Lacueva, C.; Roset, P.; Joglar, J.; Lamuela-Raventós, R.M.; de la Torre,R. Matrix effects on the bioavailability of resveratrol in humans. *Food Chemistry*, 2010, *120*, 1123-1130.

[53] Cottart, C.H.; Nivet-Antoine, V.; Laguillier-Morizot, C.; Beaudeux, J.L. Resveratrol bioavailability and toxicity in humans. *Molecular Nutrition & Food Research*, 2010, *54*, 7-16.

[54] Burns, J.; Yokota, T.; Hiroshi, A.; Lean, M.E.J.; Crozier, A. Plant foods and herbal sources of resveratrol. *Journal of Agricultural and Food Chemistry*, 2002, *50*, 3337-3340.

[55] Wang, Y.; Catana, F.; Yang, Y.; Roderick, R.; van Breemen, R.B. Analysis of resveratrol in grape products, cranberry juice and wine using liquid chromatography–mass spectrometry. *Journal of Agricultural and Food Chemistry*, 2002, *50*, 431-435.

[56] Fornara, V.; Onelli, E.; Sparvoli, F.; Rossoni, M.; Aina, R.; Marin, G.; Citterio, S. Localization of stilbene synthase in *Vitis vinifera* L. during berry development. *Protoplasma*, 2008, *233*, 83-93.

[57] Shrikhande, A.J. Wine by-products with health benefits. *Food Research International*, 2000, *33*, 469-474.

[58] Palomino, O.; Gómez-Serranillos, M.P.; Slowing, K.; Carretero, E.; Villar, A. Study of polyphenols in grape berries by reversed-phase high-performance liquid chromatography. *Journal of Chromatography A*, 2000, *870*, 449-451.

[59] Chafer, A.; Pascual-Mart, M.C.; Salvador, A.; Berna, A. Supercritical fluid extraction and HPLC determination of relevant polyphenolic compounds in grape skin. *Journal of Separation Science*, 2005, *28*, 2050-2056.

[60] Keskin, N.; Noyan, T.; Kunter, B. Health from grape by resveratrol: review. *Turkiye Klinikleri Journal of Medical Sciences*, 2009, *29*, 1273-1279.

In: Berries: Properties, Consumption and Nutrition
Editor: Carlo Tuberoso

ISBN 978-1-61470-257-3

Chapter III

Conjugated Polysaccharides as Potential Health Promoting Compounds in Berries and Cherries

Kelly Ross [*] ***and Giuseppe Mazza*** [‡]
Pacific Agri-Food Research Centre, Agriculture and Agri-Food Canada, Summerland, British Columbia, Canada

Abstract

In recent years, polysaccharides and their conjugates, which are present in plant materials, have emerged as an important class of compounds that possess biological activities. Polysaccharide conjugates isolated from a variety of plant sources have been identified as bioactive components. Polysaccharides-protein conjugates (i.e. glycoproteins) from wolfberry (*Lycium barbarum* L.), commercially called goji berry, have been reported to possess important bioactive functions, including hypoglycemic and hypolipidemic activities, immuno-modulating action, and antioxidant activity. Conjugated polysaccharides isolated from sweet cherries (*Prunus avium* L.) and cranberries (*Vaccinium macrocarpon* Aiton) have been shown to possess antioxidant activity. Polysaccharide-lipid conjugates (i.e. glycolipids) represent another class of conjugated polysaccharides that exhibit bioactive properties. Galactolipids, a specific type of glycolipid, have been shown to possess in vitro and in vivo anti-tumour promoting activity. Galactolipids have been reported to be present in edible plants such as common beans (*Phaseolus vulgaris*), bell peppers (*Capsicum annuum*), kiwi (*Actinidia deliciosa*), grapes (*Vitis vinifera*) and strawberries (*Fragaria x ananassa*). The bioactivity of polysaccharide conjugates depends on their chemical and structural characteristics. This chapter focuses on: the state of knowledge of different types of conjugated polysaccharides, the bioactivity of naturally occurring conjugated polysaccharides, different types of isolation and purification techniques, the relationships

[*] E-mail: Kelly.Ross@AGR.GC.CA.
[‡] E-mail: Giuseppe.Mazza@AGR.GC.CA.

between their bioactive functions, chemical composition, and the structure of conjugated polysaccharides along with the distribution of conjugated polysaccharide in berries and cherries in comparison to other plant sources.

Introduction

Increasing knowledge regarding the impact of diet on human health at the genetic and molecular levels is changing current nutritional approaches [1]. Diet not only provides adequate nutrients to meet metabolic needs, but can also enhance human health. Epidemiological evidence exists indicating that a diet high in fruits and vegetables reduces risk for the development of cancer, cardiovascular diseases, diabetes and other degenerative diseases [2]. The documented relationship between diet and health has lead consumers to demand more information about foods, such as fruits and vegetables, with health benefits [3]. Phenolic compounds are the major group of phytochemicals in berries and cherries, including: flavonoids (anthocyanins, flavonols, flavones, flavanols, flavanones,), tannins, and phenolic acids. Antioxidant, anti-allergic, anti-carcinogenic, anti-microbial, anti-mutagenic, and anti-inflammatory properties are some of the biological activities phenolics exhibit [4,5]. The effects of these bioactivities are manifested through various health benefits such as a reduced the risk of chronic and degenerative diseases [6,7].

It is well established that fruits such as berries and cherries may be important components of health promoting diets as they contain a wide variety of phenolic compounds [8-10]. However, in recent years, conjugated polysaccharides, which are present in plants materials, have emerged as an important class of compounds that possess biological activities [11-14]. To a limited extent, work characterizing the conjugated polysaccharides present in fruits, such as berries and cherries, has been performed [14-16]. However, the majority of information regarding the bioactivity of conjugated polysaccharides has been documented for non-fruit plant materials such as tea [17]. Regarding identification of the compounds responsible for bioactivity, a similar situation may exist for conjugated polysaccharides in berries and cherries as has been documented for conjugated polysaccharides present in tea. Research performed on tea during the past two decades has revealed that tea possesses beneficial effects, including reduction of cholesterol, depression of hypertension, anti-oxidation, anti-microbial, protection against cardiovascular disease, and anti-cancer [17,18]. These beneficial effects have been mainly attributed to polyphenols (catechins and flavonoids) [19, 20]. However, more recent studies have shown that water-soluble tea polysaccharide protein conjugates (i.e. glycoproteins) may be responsible for the demonstrated bioactivities, such as, anti-oxidant, immunological, anti-blood coagulation, anti-cancer, anti-HIV, anti-atherogenic and hypoglycaemic activities [12,17,21]. Based on these facts, polysaccharide protein conjugates may also contribute to the health effects of fruits such as berries and cherries. Furthermore, polysaccharide lipid conjugates (i.e. glycolipids) have been identified as another class of compounds in plant tissues that may contribute significantly to the health effects associated with consumption of foods of plant origin [2].

The relationships between the bioactivities, chemical composition, and structure of conjugated polysaccharides present in plant materials are not well established and it is an area of research that requires further study. The overall goal of this chapter is to: 1) introduce conjugated polysaccharides as health promoting compounds in plant materials; 2) present evidence supporting the concept that conjugated polysaccharides may act as potential health promoting compounds in berries and cherries; and 3) serve as an impetus for further work in this area. With this aim, the chapter focuses on: the state of knowledge of polysaccharide protein conjugates and polysaccharide lipid conjugates, the bioactivity of naturally occurring conjugated polysaccharides, methodologies for the extraction and characterization of these compounds, the relationships between bioactive functions and the structure of conjugated polysaccharides along with the distribution of conjugated polysaccharides in berries and cherries in comparison to other plant sources.

State of Knowledge of Conjugated Polysaccharides

Analysis of conjugated polysaccharides in various types of biological samples has attracted major interest in recent years [22]. Polysaccharide protein conjugates (i.e. glycoproteins) consist of a protein chain to which one or more carbohydrate chains are covalently attached. The carbohydrates are usually connected through N- or O-linkages, but also other types occur like C-glycosyl linkages [23,24,25]. In N-glycosylation, the addition of sugar chains can happen at the amide nitrogen on the side chain of the amino acid asparagine. In O-glycosylation, the addition of sugar chains can happen on the hydroxyl oxygen on the side chain of hydroxylysine, hydroxyproline, serine, or threonine. Examples of these linkages are provided in Figure 1. Key monosaccharides found in common glycoproteins include: β-D-glucose (Glc); β-D-galactose (Gal); β-D-mannose (Man); α-L-fucose (Fuc) a deoxyhexose type sugar, N-acetylgalactosamine (GalNAc) an aminohexose type sugar, N-acetylglucosamine (GlcNAc) an aminohexose type sugar; and xylose (Xyl) a pentose type sugar [25]. Polysaccharide protein conjugates have a wide variety of biological functions. These functions may be dependent on either the protein part or the carbohydrate part or on both [24,26].

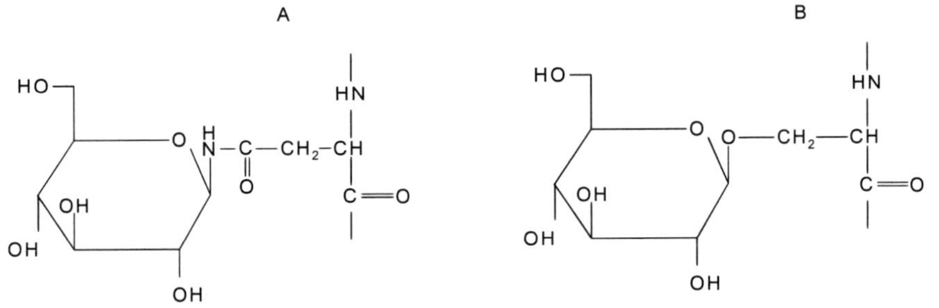

Figure 1. Glucose linked to asparagine:N-linkage (A); Glucose linked to serine: O-linkage (B). Adapted from Berg *et al.* [25].

Polysaccharide lipid conjugates (i.e. glycolipids) are a diverse class of heterogeneous conjugates composed of sugars and lipids that are found in many species ranging from bacteria to human beings [27]. They are amphipathic molecules, existing mainly in the plasma membrane, which contains one or more monosaccharide residues bound by a glycosidic lingkage to a hydrophobic moiety such as an acylglycerol, sphingoid, ceramide or prenyl phosphate group. Polysacchride lipid conjugates in higher plants mainly consist of steryl glucosides, sphingoglycolipids, and glyceroglycolipids. These glycolipids are widely distributed in edible plants such as cereals, legumes, vegetables, and fruits [28]. The content of the glycolipids varies among different plant cell types.

Sterol glucosides consist of a glucose unit linked to the hydroxyl group of one sterol molecule. Sterols in foods exist as free sterols, glycosides, fatty acid esters and acylated steryl glycosides [29]. Spingolipids are a class of complex membrane lipids found in all eukaryotic and some prokaryotic cells [30]. Sphingolipids comprise a range of lipids in which fatty acids are linked via amide bonds to a long-chain base or "sphingoid base" backbone. The long-chain sphingnoid bases are the defining structural unit of the sphingolipids. Sphingosine (D-erythro-1,3-dihydroxy, 2-aminooctadec-4-ene), is the simplest functional sphingolipid, but ceramides, which are composed of sphingosine and a fatty acid linked by an amide bond, are important molecules. Ceramides that possess a carbohydrate headgroup are glycolipids. Figure 2 depicts the basic structure of a ceramide hexose sphingolipid (i.e. a cerebroside). Galactose is the carbohydrate headgroup; galactosylceramide is shown [31].

Galactolipds, which represent a type of glyceroglycolipids, occur in plants mainly as monogalactosyldiacylglycerols (MGDGs) and digalactosyldiacylglycerols (DGDGs). These glycolipids contain one or two saturated and/or unsaturated fatty acids, with chain lengths typically varying from C16 to C20, linked to a glycerol moiety [2,32,33].

Figure 3 shows the chemical structures of MGDGs (A) and DGDGs (B) occurring in plants. Table 1 provides a summary of the common fatty acids present in MGDGs and DGDGs.

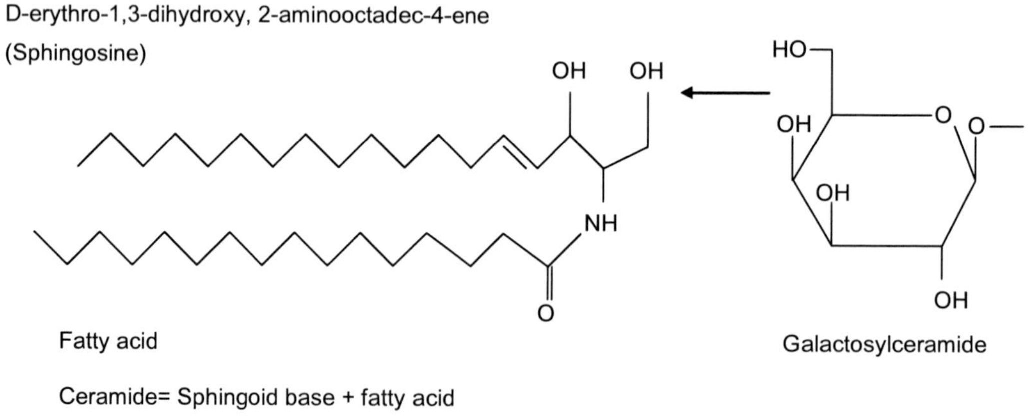

Figure 2. Ceramide is composed of a long-chain sphingoid base (the most common is sphingosine) and an amide-linked, long chain fatty acid. Ceramides that possess a carbohydrate headgroup are glycolipids. A ceramide hexose sphingolipid (i.e. a cerebroside) is shown. Galactose is the carbohydrate headgroup, thus galactosylceramide is shown. Adapted from Merrill *et al.* [31].

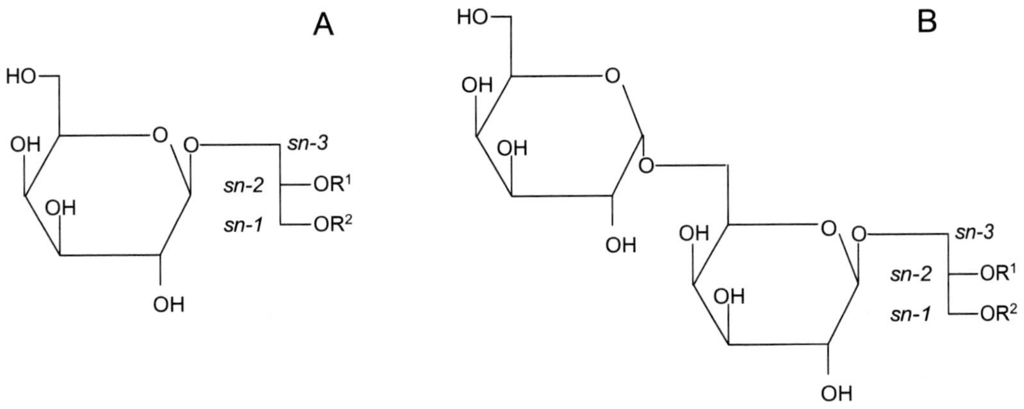

Figure 3. Chemical structures of common MGDGs (A) and DGDGs (B) occurring in plants (R1 and R2 denote specific fatty acids MGDG-monogalactosyldiacylglycerol and DGDG-digalactosyldiacylglycerol, respectively; Carbon 1, 2, and 3 on the glycerol moiety are represented by *sn-1*, *sn-2*, and *sn-3*, respectively). Adapted from Christensen [2].

Table 1. Summary of Common Fatty Acid Present in Monogalactosyldiacylglycerol (MGDG) and Digalactosyldiacylglycerol (DGDG) Glycoplipds.

Galactolipid Type	R^1	R^2
MGDG	α-Linolenoyl (C18:3)	α-Linolenoyl (C18:3)
MGDG	Linoleoyl (C18:2)	α-Linolenoyl (C18:3)
MGDG	Oleoyl (C18:1)	α-Linolenoyl (C18:3)
MGDG	Stearoyl (C18:0)	α-Linolenoyl (C18:3)
MGDG	(7Z, 10Z, 13Z)-Hexadecatrienoyl (C16:3)	α-Linolenoyl (C18:3)
MGDG	Palmitoyl (C16:0)	α-Linolenoyl (C18:3)
MGDG	Palmitoyl (C16:0)	Linoleoyl (C18:2)
DGDG	α-Linolenoyl (C18:3)	α-Linolenoyl (C18:3)
DGDG	Linoleoyl (C18:2)	α-Linolenoyl (C18:3)
DGDG	Oleoyl (C18:1)	α-Linolenoyl (C18:3)
DGDG	Stearoyl (C18:0)	α-Linolenoyl (C18:3)
DGDG	Palmitoyl (C16:0)	α-Linolenoyl (C18:3)
DGDG	Stearoyl (C18:0)	Linoleoyl (C18:2)
DGDG	Palmitoyl (C16:0)	Linoleoyl (C18:2)

Note: R^1 and R^2 refer to the fatty acid present in the glycerol backbone of galactolipd
Adapted from Christensen [2].

Biological Activities of Polysaccharide Protein Conjugates

Research on the biological activity of polysaccharide protein conjugates present in green tea (*Camellia sinesis*) accounts for a large portion of the work that has been performed in this area [12,17,21]. Polysaccharide protein conjugates isolated from green tea have been reported to possess antioxidant activities as determined by a variety of in vitro assays including: deoxyribose, photoreduction of nitro blue tetrazolium (NBT), lipid peroxidation inhibition, superoxide radical scavenging, β-carotene-linoleate, and 1,1-diphenyl-2 picrylhydrazyl (DPPH$^{\bullet}$) free radical scavenging [12,34]. Polysaccharide protein conjugates present in hot water extracts of green tea have been shown to possess hypolipidemic and antiatherogenic effects [17]. Studies performed using rats showed that oral doses of tea polysaccharide protein conjugates at levels of 25-100 mg/kg: reduce plasma total cholesterol and triglyceride levels; lower low-density lipoprotein and neutral fat levels; and increase high-density lipoprotein levels. Also, intra-peritoneal injection of tea polysaccharide protein conjugates at the dose of 50 mg/kg, increased high-density lipoprotein cholesterol levels, yet no significant effect was found on the serum cholesterol and serum triglyceride. Administration of tea polysaccharide protein conjugates at a treatment level of 160 mg/mL was shown to increase the activity of lipoprotein lipase by 7%, which may be useful for the prevention of atherosclerosis [17]. Polysaccharide protein conjugates from water and alkaline extracts of green tea have been shown to demonstrate hypoglycaemic effects [35]. Research by Chen *et al.* [35] confirmed that oral administration of polysaccharide protein conjugates from water and alkaline extracts of green tea suppressed diabetes mellitus in non-obese diabetic mice from the development of autoimmune diabetes.

Tea polysaccharide protein conjugates have been shown to significantly increase blood clotting time as assessed by in vivo and in vitro methods [17]. Also, the anti-cancer activity of the polysaccharide protein conjugates from hot water extracts of green tea at different concentrations has been established by determining the degree of inhibition of cell proliferation (MTT assay) using two kinds of colon cancer cell lines (HCT-15, Caco-2). Polysaccharide protein conjugates from hot water extracts of green tea displayed good dose dependent anti-proliferation activity to HCT-15 while polysaccharide conjugates exhibited very weak anti-proliferation activity to Caco-2. [17,34]. An acidic polysaccharide from green tea was shown to exhibit selective anti-adhesive effects against pathogenic bacteria, namely *Helicobacter pylori*, *Propionibacterium acnes*, and *Staphylococcus aureus*, while exerting no effects against beneficial bacteria [36]. Polysaccharide protein conjugates present in the alkaline extracts from Rooibos (*Aspalathus linearis*) tea leaves have been shown to demonstrate anti-HIV activity as exposure to polysaccharide conjugates inhibited binding of HIV-1 to MT-4 cells [17].

Polysaccharide protein conjugates isolated from plant materials other than tea have been shown to demonstrate biological activity. Nearly 35 years ago researchers showed that polysaccharides extracted from edible mushrooms exhibited anti-tumour activity [37]. Polysaccharide protein conjugates isolated from lemon peels and were shown to exhibit hypotensive properties [38]. Other work has shown the antioxidant activity of polysaccharide-protein conjugates isolated from the fungus *Ganoderma atrum* [13]. The bioactivity of conjugated polysaccharides present in *Glinus oppositifolius* (L.), an annual herb used in folk medicine to treat various types of illnesses related to the immune response, like joint pains, inflammations, fever, malaria and wounds has been reported [11]. Two acidic polysaccharide protein conjugates isolated from this herb were proven to exhibit immuno-modulating properties, such as potent dose-dependent complement fixating activities, and chemotaxis of macrophages, T cells and NK cells [11]. Water-soluble polysaccharide fractions from the hot-water-extract of rice bran (proteoglycans) and rice endosperm showed potent in vitro immuno-modulating properties [39]. Polysaccharides present in the hot water extracts of ginseng roots were reported to exhibit antioxidant activity, as determined with a variety of in vivo methods such as: hydroxyl radical scavenging assay, superoxide radical scavenging assay, and scavenging activity of self-oxidation of 1, 2, 3-phentriol assay [40].

With regards to fruits and berries, polysaccharide protein conjugates from wolfberry (*Lycium barbarum*), commercially called goji berry have been shown to demonstrate bioactive properties [15,16,41,42]. Administration of wolfberry polysaccharide protein conjugates to alloxan-induced diabetic or hyperlipidemic rabbits, reduced blood glucose levels, serum total cholesterol, and triglyceride concentrations while concurrently increasing high density lipoprotein cholesterol levels [15]. Also polysaccharide protein conjugates from wolfberry have been shown to exhibit in vitro antioxidant activity as determined with a variety of assays measuring: Trolox equivalent antioxidant capacity (TEAC), oxygen radical absorbance capacity (ORAC), superoxide radical scavenging activity, reducing power, β-carotene-linoleate model, inhibition of mice erythrocyte hemolysis mediated by peroxyl free radicals, DPPH$^{\bullet}$ radical scavenging, and metal chelating activity [15,16]. Recent work by Fan *et al.* [14] has demonstrated the in vitro antioxidant activity of polysaccharides from cherry, cranberry and kiwi fruits using ORAC and 2,2'-azino-bis(3-ethylbenzthiazoline-6-sulphonic acid (ABTS) assays. This is very promising in terms of linking some of the health benefits associated with fruit consumption with the bioactivity of conjugated polysaccharides.

Biological Activities of Polysaccharide Lipid Conjugates

Phytosterols, including steryl glucosides and acylated steryl glucosides have been the subject of much interest with respect to their hypocholesterolemic effect [43-45]. Also, phytosterols have been shown to demonstrate anti-carcinogenic and immune-modulating properties [46]. Acylated steryl glucosides isolated from pre-germinated brown rice bran have been shown to possess anti-diabetic properties [47] and acylated steryl glucosides isolated form the plant *Blutaparon portulacoides* have been shown to possess antiparasitic and antibacterial properties [48]. With respect to human nutrition, there is no known nutritional requirement for sphingolipids, yet they are hydrolyzed throughout the gastrointestinal tract to metabolites (ceramides and sphingoid bases) that are used by cells to regulate growth, differentiation, apoptosis and other cellular functions [31]. Studies with experimental animals have shown that feeding sphingolipids inhibits colon carcinogenesis, reduces serum low density lipoprotein cholesterol and elevates high density lipoprotein, suggesting that sphingolipids represent a functional constituent of food [30,31,49,50]. Several galactolipids such as, MGDG galactolipid 1,2-di-O-α-linolenoyl-3-O-β-D-galactopyranosyl-*sn*-glycerol, have been shown to possess in vitro and/or in vivo anti-tumor activity and anti-inflammatory activity [33, 51]. Additionally, MGDG galactolipid (2S)-1,2-di-O-[(9Z,12Z,15Z)-octadeca-9,12,15-trienoyl]-3-O-β-D-galactopyranosyl glycerol isolated from dried and milled fruits of rose hips (*Rosa canina*) has shown anti-inflammatory activity with inhibitory effects on chemotaxis of human peripheral blood neutrophils in vitro [52]. Further, it has been demonstrated that MGDG galactolipid 1,2-di-O-α-linolenoyl-3-O-β-D-galactopyranosyl-*sn*-glycerol may be responsible for the anti-tumor-promoting activity of *Citrus hystrix*, a traditional herb in Thailand [53] and may also contribute to the inhibitory effects of spinach (*Spinacia oleracea*) on human cancer cell proliferation [54- 56].

Analysis of Conjugated Polysaccharides

Extraction of Polysaccharide Protein Conjugates

Conjugated polysaccharides exist as a structural constituent of the cell wall of plant materials thus the analysis of conjugated polysaccharides, usually consists of three procedures: extraction, purification and characterization. Literature indicates that plant materials, [11-13,15,41,42,57] require drying and particle size reduction as a pre-extraction step. Also, prior to extraction, removal of the lipids and polyphenolic molecules is performed. A variety of solvents including dichloromethane, chloroform, methanol, and ethanol (80-100%) are used [11-13,15,16,39,40]. For the extraction procedure, water, dilute basic solutions and organic solvents at different temperatures have been used [11-14,16,17,26,35,57-61] however, conjugated polysaccharides have mainly been isolated and purified from hot (50-100 °C) water extracts [11-16,26,35,37,39,40,57-59]. The crude conjugated polysaccharides are liberated from the extraction medium by precipitation with ethanol or filtration [11-16,40]. Extraction of polysaccharide protein conjugates from fresh cherries, cranberries, and kiwis without a drying step has been reported. These materials were pitted (where required), macerated into a wet slurry and subjected to subsequent hot water extraction and purification procedures [14]. An alternative method for preparation of conjugated polysaccharide from green tea was described by Fang *et al.* [58]. The green tea powder was subjected to hot (100 °C) water extraction. The aqueous extract was then subjected to extraction with ethyl acetate to remove polyphenols. Ethanol was added to the aqueous layer to precipitate the conjugated polysaccharides while the water layer was subjected to dialysis to obtain free proteins.

Purification of Polysaccharide Protein Conjugates

After extraction, the crude polysaccharide protein conjugates are typically subjected to purification and fractionation. Removal of free proteins from the crude conjugated polysaccharides has been performed via the Sevag procedure, which involves extracting with 5:1 chloroform:*n*-butanol [13,26,62].

In some cases [59] the crude conjugated polysaccharides are applied to a polyamide absorption resin column with water as the elution solvent to further remove any residual polyphenolics and polar impurities. Typically conjugated polysaccharides are purified and fractionated using anion-exchange chromatography with a diethylaminoethyl (DEAE) Sepharose fast flow column, DEAE cellulose column or a Hiload 26/60 Superdex-200 column using aqueous NaCl in increasing concentration (0 to 2M) as eluent [11-14,16,35,57-61].

Characterization of Polysaccharide Protein Conjugates

Characterization of the composition and physicochemical properties of the conjugated polysaccharides is essential for defining the relationship between structure and function. A key step in this process is determination of carbohydrate content and monosaccharide composition. Colorimetry with different chromogenic systems, such as carbazole–sulfuric acid, anthracenone–sulfuric acid, phenol–sulfuric acid are commonly applied to determine the total sugar content (including uronic acid content) of polysaccharides [59,63]. Gas chromatography (GC) is commonly used to identify the constituent sugars/monosaccharides present in the polysaccharides. However, prior to constituent monosaccharide identification of oligosaccharides and polysaccharides by GC, the samples are hydrolyzed in a sealed container under the protection of N_2 with acidic reagents such as sulfuric acid, hydrochloric acid or trifluoroacetic acid [63]. Derivatization of monosaccharides to enhance volatility is an important procedure for GC analysis of sugars. There are two main species of derivatives of sugars in GC analysis, one species are trimethylsilyl ether derivatives, which are formed by reacting sugars with hexamethyldisilane (HMDS), trimethylchlorosilane (TMCS), trimethylsilyl (TMS) in nonaqueous organic solvents such as pyridine or dimethyl sulfoxide. The other species are acetate derivatives, which include: trifluoroacetate alditol derivatives, trifluoroacetic acid alditol derivatives, acetic acid oxime derivatives and acetic acid nitrile derivatives. These derivatives are usually formed in pyridine, butylene oxide or methyl imidazole solvents. In GC analysis of sugars, both flame ionization detection (FID) and the GC–MS combination detection are used to identify and quantify monosaccharides. Typically capillary columns, such as OV-1, OV-1701, OV-225, SP-2100, SE-30, etc. are used to separate and identify constituent monosaccharide during GC analysis [12,63]. The protein contents of the polysaccharide conjugate fractions are typically measured according to Bradford's method [12,64].

Further contribution to the understanding of the relationship between structure and function necessitates determination of the molecular weight and homogeneity of the crude polysaccharide conjugates and polysaccharide fractions. Typically high performance size exclusion chromatography (HPSEC) is employed as this method is rapid, highly selective and highly repeatable. In brief, the polysaccharides conjugates in aqueous solution are typically injected into a column and species elute through the column in the order of molecular weights, which are determined via a calibration curve from a series of standard samples such as dextran samples. In size exclusion chromatography, the general packing materials are typically rigid or half-rigid water soluble gels, such as Sephadex, TSK, Macrosphere, Bio-Gel, Bondagel, etc. and the eluents are typically distilled water, sodium chloride, and phosphate [14,63].

Isolation and Characterization of Polysaccharide Lipid Conjugates

Isolation of polysaccharide lipid conjugates from plant materials has been described in the literature [28,65,66]. The initial step is homogenization of the plant material followed by freeze drying to remove water [66]. Following drying, the material is subjected to extraction with chloroform/methanol (2:1, v/v) to remove all of the lipids. After extraction, the total lipids are dissolved in chloroform and subjected to silica gel column chromatography with sequential elution with chloroform, acetone, and methanol to separate out the neutral lipids, glycolipids, and phospholipids, respectively. The glycolipids are fractionated, into steryl glucosides, spingholipids, and glyceroglycol lipids, with silica gel column chromatography by sequential elution with increasing the methanol concentration in mixtures of chloroform/methanol [66,67]. Using this procedure, the glycolipids present in the fruit pastes of red bell pepper [66] were separated into 6 fractions, acylated steryl glucoside, steryl glucoside, monogalactosyldiacylglycerol, digalactosyldiacylglycerol, and glucocerebroside (a ceramide monohexoside).

Fatty acid composition of the glycolipids is typically determined by gas chromatography (GC) after transmethylation with 5% HCl in methanol. The sugar composition of the glycolipids is determined by GC as alditol acetates after hydrolysis. The sterol composition is determined by GC as trimethylsilyl derivatives and derivatization has been performed using a mixture of pyridine, HMDS (hexamethyldisilazane) TMCS (trimethylchlorosilane) (5:2:1 v/v/v) [68,69]. HPLC-MS is typically used as a fractionation and identification method [28,66].

Conjugated Polysaccharides: Composition, Distribution and Structure-Function Relationships

Protein Polysaccharide Conjugates in Plant Non-Fruit Material

The bioactivities of polysaccharides and their conjugates are affected by many factors including chemical components, conformation, molecular weight, and, even the extraction and isolation methods [12]. Numerous researchers have reported on the chemical composition of the tea polysaccharide conjugates [12,17,26,35,60,61,70] and knowledge gained from this work is undoubtedly valuable for future studies defining the polysaccharide protein conjugates present in fruits such as berries and cherries. The work of Chen *et al.* [12] isolated three polysaccharide protein conjugate fractions, TPC-1, TPC-2, and TPC-3, from the hot water extract of green tea with the following yields, 0.1, 0.2 and 0.2%, respectively. The neutral sugars contents of the fractions were reported to be 46.9, 45.3, and 39.8 %, respectively. These fractions differed in sugar composition and molar (%) ratio. Fraction TPC-1 was composed of 6 sugars, arabinose, ribose, xylose, glucose, galactose and mannose with molar ratios of 3.3:2.0:2.7:4.1:1.0:2.5. Fraction TPC-2 only contained four monosaccharides: arabinose, ribose, glucose and mannose with molar ratios of 1.9:1.6:2.7:2.7:1 while fraction TPC-3 contained 5 monosaccharides arabinose, ribose, xylose, glucose, and galactose with molar ratios 4.5:2.0:2.8:1.8:1. Chen *et al.* [35] used sequential hot water and alkaline extraction to obtain water and alkali soluble polysaccharide protein conjugates, TPC-W and TPC-A, respectively from green tea. Both the water and alkali soluble polysaccharide protein conjugates, contained seven monosaccharides, namely rhamnose, fucose, arabinose, xylose, mannose, glucose and galactose with molar (%) ratios of 8.74:4.69:29.04:0.42:7.11:14.10:35.89 and 13.81:1.43:36.07:5.24:4.89:6.28:32.27, respectively. The difference in monosaccharide composition of the water and alkali soluble polysaccharide protein conjugates indicates the effect of isolation procedure. Arabinose and galactose were dominant monosaccharide components present in the water and alkali soluble polysaccharide protein conjugates.

The protein content of the polysaccharide protein conjugate fractions obtained from green tea by Chen *et al.* [12] was 2.8, 3.8, and 4.0%. Their work showed that as protein content increased, the antioxidant activities of the three polysaccharide-protein conjugates increased. The uronic acid content of the three fractions was also measured and ranged from 30.0 to 51.8%; a direct relationship between the uronic acid contents and antioxidant activity of tea polysaccharide conjugates was observed [12,59].

The molecular weights of the polysaccharide protein conjugate fractions from green tea have been characterized and the molecular weights of the three fractions were determined to be: 268, 118, and 42 kDa, respectively [12]. These researchers reported that the fraction with the lowest molecular weight exhibited the highest antioxidant activity which was in agreement with the work of Zhang *et al.* [71] which also reported that molecular weight affected the anti-tumour bioactivity of mushroom polysaccharides. Based on these results, Chen *et al.* [12] speculated that tea polysaccharide conjugates with low molecular weight and high protein contents may bind free radicals more easily. Chen *et al.* [35] examined the distribution proportion and molecular weight of homogeneous components in the water and alkali soluble polysaccharide protein conjugates from green tea. The water soluble conjugated polysaccharide protein conjugates were found to have a total of three homogeneous components with the molecular weights of 4550, 48.5, and 6.62 kDa in mass proportion of 37.38, 6.54 and 56.07% respectively. The alkali soluble conjugated polysaccharide protein conjugates consisted of four homogeneous components with the molecular weights and mass proportions of 4940 (68.57%), 67.7 (2.86%), 11.2 (11.43%) and 4.13 (17.14%) kDa, respectively. Chen *et al.* [35] confirmed that oral administration of water and alkali soluble polysaccharide protein conjugates prevented non-obese diabetic mice from the developing of autoimmune diabetes yet only water soluble polysaccharide protein conjugates had a dose-dependent effect on blood glucose thereby showing better potential for delaying diabetes onset. There was little difference in molecular weight between water and alkali soluble polysaccharide protein conjugates. Differences in fine chemical structure due to compositional variation may have elicited these different responses [72] as the bioactivity of polysaccharide protein conjugated may be affected by a specific conformational feature [73,74].

Work has been performed on characterizing the polysaccharide protein conjugates present in non-fruit plant material other than tea. Information on the structural identification of polysaccharides isolated from ginseng root was presented by Luo *et al.* [40]. A crude polysaccharide was isolated from the hot water extract of ginseng with a yield of 28.05%. The crude polysaccharide was fractionated and two fractions, namely GPII and GPIII were obtained in the yields of 3.7 and 7.78 %, respectively. The average molecular weight of the two fractions, GPII and GPII, were about 300 and 400 kDa, respectively. The polysaccharide contents of GPII and GPIII were 99.8 and 96.5%, and protein contents were 0 and 3.4%. Notably, both GPII and GPIII consisted mainly of glucose and were identified as neutral polysaccharides. GPII was composed of 60.06% (1→)- or (1→6)-glycosidic linkages and 39.94% (1→3)-glycosidic linkages, and GPIII 16.23% (1→)- or (1 → 6)-glycosidic linkages, 25.98% (1 →2)-glycosidic linkages, and 57.79% (1 →3)-glycosidic linkages. Although both GPII and GPIII fractions exhibited strong antioxidant activities further work examining how composition and structure affected bioactivities is required as there is no clear information on how a polysaccharide is structurally designed to have optimal bioactivity.

Polysaccharide protein conjugates were isolated from *Glinus oppositifolius* (L.), an annual herb, via extraction and fractionation [11]. Three fractions were obtained, a neutral fraction (GON) and two acidic fractions (GOA1 and GOA2). The total carbohydrate content of the GON, GOA1 and GOA2 fractions were reported as 65.7, 52.6, and 45%, respectively. No protein was detected in GON while the protein content of the GOA1 and GOA2 were 10, and 1.5%, respectively. All three polysaccharide conjugate fractions contained neutral sugars in varying amounts arabinose (5.5-26.4 mol%), rhamnose (trace-10.3 mol%), xylose (0.5-3.9 mol%), mannose (0.6-4.6%), galactose (9.7-42.9 mol%), glucose (3.3-23.7 mol%). The neutral polysaccharide conjugate fraction did not contain any galacturonic acid while both acidic fractions contained appreciable amounts of galacturonic acid (12.1-68.3 mol%) and also contained some 4-O-methyl-glucuronic acid (0.4-2.9 mol%). Regarding amino acid profile, GOA1 had a high content of hydroxyproline, alanine and serine while GOA2 was shown to contain small amounts of hydroxyproline compared to GOA1. This work mainly focussed on characterizing the acid polysaccharide protein conjugate fractions. The acidic fractions exhibited a potent dose dependent effect on immunomodulating activity.

A water-soluble protein-bound polysaccharide was extracted from the fruiting bodies of the fungus *Ganoderma atrum*. This glycoprotein, coded PSG-1, was obtained in a yield of 2.1% [13]. The polysaccharide portion was mainly composed of mannose, galactose and glucose in a molar ratio of 1:1.28:4.91 while the protein content was 10.1%. The glycoprotein contained 17 general amino acids and was rich in glutamic acid, asparagic acid, alanine, glycine, threonine methionine, and serine. The high concentration of threonine and serine indicated the possibility of the existence of the O-glycosidic linkages. The glycoprotein exhibited an average molecular weight of about 1013 kDa. The antioxidant activity of the purified polysaccharides was evaluated in vitro by the DPPH$^{\bullet}$ free radical scavenging and scavenging activity of self-oxidation of 1, 2, 3-phentriol assays. A dose dependent response on antioxidant activity was found. Again although this conjugated polysaccharide displayed antioxidant activity more work is required to examine the effects of composition and structure.

A variety of polysaccharide protein conjugates have been obtained from hot water extracts of rice (bran and endosperm) [39,75]. Endosperm polysaccharide conjugates contained 85% carbohydrates and 5.2% protein. The carbohydrate composition was galactose (24.1 mol %), mannose (18.3 mol %), arabinose (15.1 mol %), glucose (11.2 mol %) and xylose (8.1 mol%), fucose (3.8 mol%), rhamnose (4.5mol %), and galacturonic acid (14.9 mol%). The carbohydrate composition of the bran polysaccharide conjugates (proteoglycans) presented by Yamagishi *et al.* [75] varied according to fraction: galactose (10-45 mol %), glucose, (5-60 mol %), arabinose (7-44 mol %), xylose (4-33 mol %) and rhamnose (8-22 mol%). The protein content ranged from 11.8-27.4% depending on the fraction. The endosperm polysaccharide conjugates and the bran proteoglycans displayed anti-complementary/immunomodulating activity. The different fractions of bran proteoglycans and endosperm polysaccharides exhibited dissimilarity in their sugar compositions which may affect anti-complementary activity. The bran proteoglycan fraction with a high content of galactose and arabinose monomer possessed a greater anti-complementary activity than the bran proteoglycan fraction with a high content of xylose and galactose monomer. The endosperm polysaccharide contained mannose, fructose, and uronic acid in addition to sugars present in bran proteoglycans; this fraction displayed anti-complementary activity values comparable to the bran proteoglycan faction that possessed high galactose and arabinose contents. Again, differences in fine chemical structure due to compositional variation may have elicited these different responses [72].

Polysaccharide Protein Conjugates in Plant Fruit Material

Compared to the work performed characterizing non-fruit polysaccharide protein conjugates much less has been performed on fruit protein conjugates. Nevertheless, some information is present in current literature. Table 2 provides a summary of the characteristics of the polysaccharide protein conjugates identified in plant non-fruit and fruit material. The glycoconjugates present in gogi berry/wolfberry (*Lycium barbarum*) fruit has been examined [15,16,70]. Luo *et al.* [15] showed that polysaccharide protein conjugates are major bioactive constituents in *Lycium barbarum* fruits. A purified fraction, LBP-X, was identified as the major fraction of *Lycium barbarum* polysaccharides by Luo *et al.* [15]. It was determined that LBP-X contains six monosaccharides, including rhamnose, galactose, glucose, arabinose, mannose, and xylose in a molar ratio of 4.22:2.43:1.38:1.00:0.95:0.38.

Amino acid analysis revealed that LBP-X contains 17 amino acids and the total protein content was 8.46%. The monosaccharides and amino acids were both implicated as bioactive constituents contributing to antioxidant activity along with the observed hypoglycaemic and hypolipidemic effects [15]. Li *et al.* [16] demonstrated that polysaccharide protein conjugates isolated from *Lycium barbarum* possess antioxidant activity. The carbohydrate content of the conjugate was 97.5% and exhibited a molecular weight of 157.3 kDa. The monosaccharide profile was reported to be composed of D-rhamnose, D-xylose, D-arabinose, D-fucose, D-glucose, D-galactose with a molar ratio of 1:1.07:2.14:2.29:3.59:10.06; the monosaccharides were linked together by β-glycosidic linkages.

Fan *et al.* [14] extracted, purified, and characterized water-soluble polysaccharides obtained from wolfberry (*Lycium barbarum* L.), three sweet cherry (*Prunus avium* L.) cultivars, Sweetheart, Lapins, and Skeena, kiwi (*Actinidia chinensis* L.) and cranberry fruits (*Vaccinium macrocarpon* Aiton). The yields of the crude polysaccharides conjugates obtained from the hot water extract of wolfberries, kiwi, cranberries, Sweetheart cherries, Lapins cherries, and Skeena cherries were 8.4, 9.8, 10.6, 4.7, 5.4, and 11.0 %, respectively. The crude polysaccharide yield for Lapins cherries was affected by harvest time (i.e. maturity level) as the yield of crude polysaccharides decreased with ripening, indicating that polysaccharides were converted to low molecular sugars during ripening. The crude polysaccharide conjugates from hot water extracts were also purified and fractionated with ion exchange column chromatography into fractions (F2, F3, and F4).

The results of Fan *et al.* [14] indicate that the crude polysaccharides and fractions obtained from the four fruits are heterogeneous. Rhamnose, arabinose, xylose, galactose and glucose were reported as the predominant component sugars present in the polysaccharides from wolfberry, cherry and kiwi while fucose and mannose were reported as minor sugar constituents.

Table 2. Summary of Characteristics of Polysaccharide Protein Conjugates Identified in a Variety of Plant Foods

Plant Food Source for Polysaccharide Protein Conjugates*	Ref.	Yield (%)	Carbohydrate (%)	Protein (%)	Molecular Weight Average (kDa)	Sugar Composition (Monomer Ratio, mol %)	Uronic Acid Content (%)	Reported Bioactivity	Extraction & Purification Methods**
Green tea (*Camellia sinensis*)	[12]							Antioxidant activity	Pre-extraction with ethanol followed by extraction with 70 °C water; precipitation with ethanol; purification with a DEAE-cellulose column with 0.1 to 1.0M NaCl eluent
Fraction TPC-1		0.1	46.9[a]	2.8	268	Ara:Rib:Xyl:Glc:Gal:Man (3.3:2.0:2.7:4.1:1.0:2.5)	30.0		
Fraction TPC-2		0.2	45.3[a]	3.8	118	Ara:Rib:Glc:Man (1.9:1.6:2.7:2.7:1)	47.6		
Fraction TPC-3		0.2	39.8[a]	4.0	42	Ara:Rib:Xyl:Glc:Gal (4.5:2.0:2.8:1.8:1)	51.8		
Green tea (*Camellia sinensis*)	[35]							Suppression of diabetes in mice via oral dosing	Sequential extraction with 90° C water followed by 50 °C, 1.0% NaOH
Fraction TPC-W		-	23.3[a]	2.1	6.6-4550	Rha:Fuc:Ara:Xyl:Man:Glc:Gal (8.7:4.7:29.0:0.42:7.1:14.1:35.9)	8.8		
Fraction TPC-A		-	8.5[a]	10.5	4.1-4940	Rha:Fuc:Ara:Xyl:Man:Glc:Gal (13.8:1.4:36.1:5.2:4.9:6.3:32.3)	13.5		
Ginseng root (*Panax quinquefolium*)	[40]							Antioxidant activity	Pre-extraction with ethanol; extraction with 80 °C water; precipitation with ethanol; purification with a DEAE-Sepharose CL-6B column with 0 to 1.0M NaCl eluent
Crude fraction		28.1	-	-	-	-	-		
Fraction GPII		3.7	99.8[b]	0	300	-	-		
Fraction GPIII		7.8	96.5[b]	3.4	400	-	-		
Herb (*Glinus oppositifolius*)	[11]							Immuno-activity	Pre-extraction with dichloromethane, methanol, and ethanol; extraction with 50 °C water; filtration; purification with a DEAE-Sepharose fast flow column with 0 to 2.0M NaCl eluent
Fraction GON: Neutral		-	65.7[b]	-	-	Ara:Rha:Fuc:Xyl:Man:Gal:Glc (36.1:t:0.5:2.6:4.6:32.5:23.7)	-		
Fraction GOA1: Acidic		-	52.6[b]	10	70	Ara:Rha:Xyl:Man:Gal:Glc:MGlcA:GalA (26.4:4.2:3.9:4.3:42:9:3.5:2.9:12.1)	-		
Fraction GOA2: Acidic		-	45[b]	1.5	30-39	Ara:Rha:Fuc:Xyl:Man:Gal:Glc:MGlcA:GalA (5.5:10.3:1.3:0.5:0.6:9.7:3.3:0.4:68.3)	-		

Plant Food Source for Polysaccharide Protein Conjugates*	Ref.	Yield (%)	Carbohydrate (%)	Protein (%)	Molecular Weight Average (kDa)	Sugar Composition (Monomer Ratio, mol %)	Uronic Acid Content (%)	Reported Bioactivity	Extraction & Purification Methods**
Fungus(*Ganoderma atrum*) Fraction PGS-1	[13]	2.1	-	10.1	1013	Man:Gal:Glc (1:1.28:4.91)	15.6	Antioxidant activity	Pre-extraction with ethanol; extraction with 100 °C water; precipitation with ethanol; purification with a Hiload 26/60 Superdex-200 column with water eluent
Rice (milled) (*Oryza sativa*) Fractions from bran	[39, 75]	-	-	11.8-27.4	-	Gal:Glc:Ara:Xyl:Rha (10-45:5-60:7-44:4-33:8-22)	-	Immuno-activity	Pre-extraction with ethanol:ether (1:1) to remove lipids; glucoamylase treatment in 90 °C aqueous solution to remove water soluble endosperm fraction; extraction with 70° C water to obtain crude bran fraction; precipitation with ammonium sulphate to yield bran fractions; purification with a DEAE-Sepharose column with 0.2 NaCl and 0.5M $(NH_4)_2CO_3$ eluents
Fraction from endosperm		-	85[b]	5.2	-	Gal:Man:Ara:Glc:Xyl:Fuc:Rha:GalA (24.1:18.3:15.1:11.2:8.1:3.8:4.5:14.9)	-		
Wolberry/gogi berry (*Lycium barbarum* L) Fraction LBP-X	[15]	-	-	8.46	-	Rha:Gal:Glc:Ara:Man:Xyl (4.22:2.43:1.38:1.0:0.95:0.38)	-	Hypo-glycemic, hypo-lipidemic and antioxidant activity	Pre-extraction with chloroform, methanol, and ethanol to remove lipids; extraction with 50 °C water; precipitation with ethanol and acetone; purification with a DEAE-cellulose column with 0.05 to 0.5M NaCl eluent
Wolberry/gogi berry (*Lycium barbarum* L) Fraction from berry	[16]	-	97.5[b]	-	157	Rha:Xyl:Ara:Fuc:Glc:Gal (1:1.07:2.14:2.29:3.59:10.06)	-	Antioxidant activity	Pre-extraction with 100 ° C water to obtain crude fraction, removal of lipids with chloroform, methanol, and ethanol, extraction with 90 °C water; precipitation with ethanol and acetone to obtain purified fraction

Table 2. (continued)

Plant Food Source for Polysaccharide Protein Conjugates*	Ref.	Yield (%)	Carbohydrate (%)	Protein (%)	Molecular Weight Average (kDa)	Sugar Composition (Monomer Ratio, mol %)	Uronic Acid Content (%)	Reported Bioactivity	Extraction & Purification Methods**
Wolberry/gogi berry (*Lycium barbarum* L)	[14]					Rha:Fuc:Ara:Xyl:Man:Gal:Glc		Antioxidant activity	Extraction with 100 °C water to obtain a raw extract; precipitation with ethanol; washing with ethanol and acetone; further extraction with 80 °C water; purification with a DEAE Sepharose Fast Flow column with 0, 0.05, 0.1, 0.25M NaCl eluent to yield, crude fraction, F2, F3, and F4, respectively
Crude raw fraction		8.4	-	-	58-604	(0.47:0.1:8.8:0.57:0.22:1.65:1)	26.9		
Fraction F2		-	-	-	57	(0.32:0.45:6.46:0.83:0.25:1.57:1)	-		
Fraction F3		-	-	-	76	(0.82:0.52:11.8:0.83:0.27:3.29:1)	-		
Fraction F4		-	-	-	95-537	(1.98:0.77:17.2:0.98:0.15:2.74:1)	36.6		
Cherry (*Prunus avium* L)	[14]							Antioxidant activity	Extraction with 100 °C water to obtain a raw extract; precipitation with ethanol; washing with ethanol and acetone; further extraction with 80 °C water; purification with a DEAE Sepharose Fast Flow column with 0, 0.05, 0.1, 0.25M NaCl eluent to yield, crude fraction, F2, F3, and F4, respectively
Lapins-variety						Rha:Fuc:Ara:Xyl:Man:Gal:Glc			
Crude raw fraction		5.4	-	-	19.4-1422	(0.75:0.16:18.5:0.61:0.41:2.48:1)	43.0		
Fraction F2		-	-	-	18.1-106	(0.79:0.17:6.12:0.59:0.94:3.69:1)	43.9		
Fraction F3		-	-	-	190	(2.58:0.97:19.9:1.24:0.81:4.13:1)	43.6		
Fraction F4		-	-	-	160-1111	(4.78:0.67:38.9:1.1:0.59:6.78:1)	57.4		
Skeena-variety									
Crude raw fraction		11.0	-	-	18.5-1282	(1.12:0.24:10.9:0.49:0.59:2.89:1)	49.8		
Fraction F2		-	-	-	14.5	(0.54:0.12:1.5:0.29:0.76:1.3:1)	-		
Fraction F3		-	-	-	112	(0.67:0.11:3.45:0.37:0.76:2.01:1)	54.1		
Fraction F4		-	-	-	159-880	(1.69:0.29:28.7:0.87:0.81:6.47:1)	55.5		
Sweetheart-variety									
Crude raw fraction		4.7	-	-	117-999	(1.02:0.09:6.65:0.33:0.46:2.2:1)	35.2		
Fraction F2		-	-	-	17.7-94	(0.42:0.08:2.16:0.45:0.88:2.19:1)	-		
Fraction F3		-	-	-	118	(1.18:0:7.9:0.68:0.85:5.35:1)	57.7		
Fraction F4		-	-	-	142-801	(3.62:0.24:32.11:0.87:0.4:7.28:1)	58.8		

Plant Food Source for Polysaccharide Protein Conjugates*	Ref.	Yield (%)	Carbohydrate (%)	Protein (%)	Molecular Weight Average (kDa)	Sugar Composition (Monomer Ratio, mol %)	Uronic Acid Content (%)	Reported Bioactivity	Extraction & Purification Methods**
Cranberry (*Vaccinium macrocarpon* Aiton)	[14]					Rha:Fuc:Ara:Xyl:Man:Gal:Glc		Antioxidant activity	Extraction with 100 °C water to obtain a raw extract; precipitation with ethanol; washing with ethanol and acetone; further extraction with 80 °C water; purification with a DEAE Sepharose Fast Flow column with 0, 0.05, 0.1, 0.25M NaCl eluent to yield, crude fraction, F2, F3, and F4, respectively
Crude raw fraction		10.6	-	-	310	(0.16:t:4.38:1.5:t:2.01:1)	45.4		
Fraction F2		-	-	-	320	(0.37:t:3.17:0.71:0.08:1.26:1)	41.3		
Fraction F3		-	-	-	350	(0.57:0:4.78:1.06:0:2.77:1)	60.4		
Fraction F4		-	-	-	104-581	(2.991.4:25.6:1.31:0.2:18.9:1)	43.9		
Kiwi (*Actinidia deliciousa*)	[14]					Rha:Fuc:Ara:Xyl:Man:Gal:Glc		Antioxidant activity	Extraction with 100 °C water to obtain a raw extract; precipitation with ethanol; washing with ethanol and acetone; further extraction with 80 °C water; purification with a DEAE Sepharose Fast Flow column with 0, 0.05, 0.1, 0.25M NaCl eluent to yield, crude fraction, F2, F3, and F4, respectively
Crude raw fraction		9.8	-	-	137	(0.40:0.26:7.14:0.71:0.30:2.64:1)	52.1		
Fraction F2		-	-	-	-	(-)	-		
Fraction F3		-	-	-	125	(0.93:0:12.8:0.85:0.33:2.81:1)	52.2		
Fraction F4		-	-	-	250	(3.16:1.17:19.88:2.03:0.49:8.48:1)	51.6		

*Nomenclature for polysaccharide protein conjugates presented is consistent with the notation used in the referenced work.

** Referenced work should be consulted for detailed extraction and purification procedures.

[a] Values presented on neutral sugars basis

[b] Values presented on total carbohydrate basis

Arabinionse (Ara); Ribose (Rib); Xylose (Xyl); Glucose (Glc); Galactose (Gal); Mannose (Man); Rhamnose (Rha); Fucose (Fuc); 4-O-methyl-glucuronic acid (MGlcA); Galacturonic Acid (GalA).

- = data not available/data not explicitly presented in referenced work.

t = trace.

Diethylaminoethyl= DEAE.

For the cranberry polysaccharides, arabinose, xylose, and galactose were the major sugar constituents. The monosaccharide profile for the crude extracts from wolfberry was given as: rhamnose, fucose, arabinose, xylose, mannose, galactose, glucose, with molar (%) ratios of 0.47:0.10:8.84:0.57:0.22:1.65:1, respectively.

These monosaccharides were present in all of the wolfberry fractions as well. The monosaccharide profile for the crude extracts from kiwi was given as: rhamnose, fucose, arabinose, xylose, mannose, galactose, and glucose with molar (%) ratios of 0.40:0.26:7.14:0.71:0.30:2.64:1, respectively. No fucose was detected in F3 of the kiwi polysaccharides. The monosaccharide profile for the crude extracts from cranberry was given as: rhamnose, arabinose, xylose, galactose, glucose with molar (%) ratios of 0.16:4.38:1.5:2.01:1, respectively. Neither fucose nor mannose was detected in F3 of cranberry polysaccharides. The monosaccharides rhamnose, fucose, arabinose, xylose, mannose, galactose, and glucose were present in the crude cherry extracts of all varieties tested; arabinose was the main sugar in each extract.

The uronic acid content was determined for the crude polysaccharides and each fraction. For wolfberry fruit the uronic acid content of the crude polysaccharide and F4 is 26.9 and 36.6%, respectively. No uronic acid was detected in F2 and F3. For kiwi fruit the uronic acid content of the crude polysaccharide, F3 and F4 was 52.1, 52.2, and 51.6%, respectively. No uronic acid was detected in F2. For the cranberry fruit the uronic acid content of the crude polysaccharide, F2, F3, and F4 was 45.4, 41.3, 60.4, and 43.9%, respectively. For the cherry fruits, the uronic acid content ranged from 35-43% in the crude polysaccharide, 43.6-57.7 in F3, and 55.5-58.8% for F4 depending on variety. The Lapin cherries were the only variety to contain uronic acid (43.9%) in F2. Antioxidant activity of raw polysaccharides extracts and their fractions from the four different fruits was evaluated by ORAC and ABTS assays. All raw polysaccharide extracts and their fractions (F2, F3 and F4) had antioxidant activity. Unlike the work of Chen *et al.* [12,59] there was no observed relationship between uronic acid content and antioxidant activity. Fan *et al.* [14] did not determine the protein content nor assess the amino acid profile of the hot water polysaccharide extracts thus it was difficult to determine whether different monosaccharide and amino acid profiles and contents may have elicited these different bioactivities as was suggested in the work of Chen *et al.* [35]. However for each fraction type there appears to be a positive relationship between arabinose content and antioxidant activity. Differences in fine chemical structure due to compositional variation may have elicited these different responses [72] and therefore more study is needed in this area.

With respect to molecular weight two size fractions of polysaccharides were present in the crude extracts from wolfberry; molecular weights are 604.5 and 57.6 kDa, respectively [14]. The crude extracts from Lapins cherries contained three different size fractions of polysaccharides; molecular weights are 1422.7, 174.1 and 19.4 kDa, respectively. Crude extracts from Skeena cherries and Sweetheart cherries displayed molecular weight distribution patterns similar to Lapins cherries except that raw extracts of Sweetheart cherries did not show the low molecular population, which possibly reflected cultivar differences and/or differences in maturity. The crude extracts from kiwi and cranberries displayed a narrower molecular weight distribution range. The molecular weights of the cranberry and kiwi fruit polysaccharides were reported as 313 and 136.6 kDa, respectively. The authors suggested that the molecular weights of the polysaccharides may play an important role on their antioxidant activity. A relatively higher molecular weight of the cherry and cranberry polysaccharides may have resulted in an increase in the antioxidant activity which was in contrast to the findings of Chen *et al.* [12,59] and Zhang *et al.* [71]. However these works also indicated the concomitant effect of high protein content and low molecular weight which may help to explain the different results. The antioxidant activity results obtained in the study of Fan *et al.* [14] clearly established the antioxidant potency of the polysaccharides extracted from wolfberry, cherry, kiwi and cranberry fruits, however, the relationship between the structure polysaccharide protein conjugates and antioxidative mechanisms requires further studies [76].

Polysaccharide Lipid Conjugates in Edible Plant Material

Quantitative analysis of glycolipids in edible parts of plants has been performed by high-performance liquid chromatography (HPLC) using ultraviolet (UV) and evaporative light-scattering detection (ELSD) [28]. Sterols in foods exist as free sterols, steryl glycosides, fatty acid esters and acylated steryl glycosides [29]. The following are values for the amount acylated steryl glucosides (ASG) and steryl glucosides (SG) in a variety of plant tissues: wheat (flour) contains 256 and 54 mg/kg (dry matter, DM), acylated steryl glucosides and steryl glucoside, respectively. Soybean contains 380 and 116 mg/kg (DM), acylated steryl glucosides and steryl glucoside, respectively; rice (milled) contains 236 and 19 mg/kg, (DM), acylated steryl glucosides and steryl glucoside, respectively; spinach contains 235 and 123 mg/kg, (FW, fresh weight), acylated steryl glucosides and steryl glucoside, respectively; tomato contains 86 and 12 mg/kg, (FW), acylated steryl glucosides and steryl glucoside, respectively; grape contains 32 and 31 mg/kg, (FW), acylated steryl glucosides and steryl glucoside, respectively; kiwi contains 79 and 38 mg/kg, (FW), acylated steryl glucosides and steryl glucoside, respectively; and strawberry contains 53 and 19 mg/kg, (FW), acylated steryl glucosides and steryl glucoside, respectively [28]. Bishop and Wade [77] reported extracting 123 mg lipid per 100g fresh cherries and indicated that acylated sterol glycoside was present at a level of 2.6 mg sugar per 100mg total lipid.

Sphingolipids present in legumes, vegetables, and fruits are mainly cerebrosides containing glucose, galactose, mannose, and inositol headgroups. Values of ceramide monohexosides (i.e. cerebrosides) for some plant tissues were provided by Sugawara and Miyazawa [28]. Wheat (flour) has a ceramide monohexoside content of 210 mg/kg (dry matter, DM). Rice (milled) has a ceramide monohexoside content of 25 mg/kg (DM). Soybean has a ceramide monohexoside content of 80 mg/kg (DM). Spinach has a ceramide monohexoside content of 139 mg/kg (fresh weight, FW). The ceramide monohoxide content of tomato, grape, kiwi, and strawberry have been reported as: 34, 79, 62, and 34 mg/kg (FW), respectively.

The content of galactolipids (monogalactosyldiacylglycerols, MGDG and digalactosyldiacylglycerols, DGDG) in legumes, vegetables, and some fruits has been reported [2, 33]. The fresh weight (FW) concentration of MGDGs and DGDGs in spinach was high ranging from 546-850 mg/kg and 563 mg/kg, respectively. The fresh weight concentration of MGDGs in bell pepper ranged from 377-243 mg/kg. No DGDGs were reported in bell peppers. The fresh weight concentration of these galactolipids in most fruits is relatively lower ranging from 0 to 100 mg/kg. Kiwi fruit was reported to contain between 45-65 mg MGDG/kg FW and 79 mg DGDG/kg FW. Grapes were reported to contain 10 mg MGDG/kg and 9 mg DGDG/kg FW, strawberries were reported to contain 11 mg MGDG/kg and 10 mg DGDG/kg FW. No MGDG or DGDG was detected in sweet cherries [2,28]. However, Bishop and Wade [77] reported that monoglycosyldiacylglycerol and diglycosyldiacylglycerol were present in sweet cherries at levels of 0.4 and 1.62 mg sugar per 100 mg total lipid. Also, it was reported that the glycolipids present in sweet cherries contained a high content of fatty acid 18:3 (α-linolenic acid) which is a fatty acid characteristic of plant galactosyldiacylglycerols (i.e. galactolipids). Galactolipids have been isolated from gogiberries/wolfberries [78].

An investigation of MGDG in bell peppers revealed that both the green and red varieties had a relatively high content of this galactolipid while the content in the more mature yellow variety was considerably lower, indicating that the concentration of galactolipids may decrease with maturity [2,33]. The composition and concentration of plant metabolites are significantly influenced by the stage of maturity, cultivars, cultural practices, geographic origin, growing season, climatic conditions, postharvest storage conditions, and food-processing procedures [5] therefore these variables may affect and must be accounted for in the determination of polysaccharide lipid conjugates present in plant materials such as berries and cherries.

Conclusion

The compounds responsible for the health promoting properties of plant materials including berries and cherries are still in need of further study as several groups of natural products have been identified as important potential contributors to the health effects of plant based foods. With respect to fruits such as berries and cherries, polysaccharide protein conjugates (i.e. glycoproteins) and polysaccharide lipid conjugates (i.e. glycolipids) have not received much attention in relation to potential health effects and represents an area that requires further study. However, a body of research demonstrating that these compounds may be responsible for some of the health benefits associated with the consumption of plant foods exists. The majority of research studying the potential health benefits of polysaccharide protein conjugates in plant materials has been performed on non-fruit sources such as tea, herbs, and fungi. Protein polysaccharide conjugates have been identified and characterized in wolfberry/gogi berries and some exploratory work examining the presence of polysaccharide protein conjugates in kiwi fruit and cherries has been performed. Glycoproteins present in tea have been reported to: lower blood pressure, slow heartbeat, prevent blood coagulation, possess anti-tumor activity, possess anti-HIV, and enhance immunity. Fruits such as cherry, cranberry, kiwi, and wolfberry have been shown to possess polysaccharide protein conjugates with antioxidant activity and these compounds may contribute to the health benefits obtained from eating a diet high in fruits. In order to fully understand their biological activities, it is essential to elucidate the chemical structures and chain conformations of polysaccharide protein conjugates present in berries and cherries. Glycolipids including acylated and steryl glucosides, ceramide hexosides, and galactolipids have received limited attention in relation to the health effects of fruit and vegetable foods. The presence of glycolipids has been documented in some fruits including grapes, strawberries and wolf/gogi berries, however a comprehensive survey on their presence and levels in a wide variety of fruits and berries is required. Also, an examination on of the effects of genotype, environment, maturity, storage, and processing conditions is necessary. The biological activities of glycolipids, as demonstrated in animal studies and in vitro studies suggests that polysaccharide lipid conjugates may be used in the treatment and prevention of inflammatory conditions and cancer and that they may be considered as an important group of nutraceuticals. In all, a good opportunity exists for scientists to elucidate the biological roles of polysaccharide protein conjugates and protein lipid conjugates in fruits such as berries and cherries.

References

[1] Biesalski, H.K.; Dragsted, L.O.; Elmadfa, I.; Grossklaus, R.; Muller, M.; Schrenk, D.; Walter, P.; Weber, P. Bioactive compounds: Definition and assessment of activity. *Nutrition*, 2009, *25*, 1202–1205.

[2] Christensen, L.P. Galactolipids as potential health promoting compounds in vegetable foods. *Recent Patents on Food, Nutrition & Agriculture*. 2009, *1*, 50-58.

[3] Paredes-Lopez, O.; Cervantes-Ceja, M.L.; Vigna-Perez, M.; Hernandez-Perez, T. Berries: Improving human health and health and healthy aging, and promoting quality life-A review. *Plant Foods for Human Nutrition*, 2010, *65*, 299-308.

[4] Wang, J.; Mazza G. Inhibitory effects of anthocyanins and other phenolic compound on nitric oxide production in LPS/IFN-γ-Activated RAW 264.7 macrophages. *Journal of Agricultural and Food Chemistry*, 2002, *50*, 850-857.

[5] Kim, D.O.; Heo, H.J.; Young, J.K.; Yang, S.H.; Lee, C.Y. Sweet and sour cherry phenolics and their protective effects on neuronal cells. *Journal of Agricultural and Food Chemistry*, 2005, *53*, 9921-9927.

[6] Kaur, C.; Kapoor, H.C. Antioxidants in fruits and vegetables: The millennium's health. *International Journal of Food Science and Technology*, 2001, *36*, 703-725.

[7] Commenges, D.; Scotet, V.; Renaud, S.; Jacqmin-Gadda, H.; Barberger-Gateau, P; Dartigues, J.F. Intake of flavonoids and risk of dementia. *European Journal of Epidemiology*, 2000, *16*, 357-363.

[8] Kahhonen, M.P.; Hopia, A.I.; Heinonen, M. Berry phenolics and their antioxidant activity. *Journal of Agricultural and Food Chemistry*, 2001, *49*, 4076-4082.

[9] Serrano, M.; Diaz-Mula, H.M.; Zapata, P.J.; Castillo, S.; Guillen, F.; Martinez-Romero, D.; Valverde, J.M.; Valero, D. Maturity stage at harvest determines the fruit quality and antioxidant potential after storage of sweet cherry cultivars. *Journal of Agricultural and Food Chemistry*, 2009, *57*, 3240-3246.

[10] Fazzari, M.; Fukumoto, L.; Mazza, G.; Livrea, M.; Tesoriere, L.; Marco, L.D. In vitro bioavailability of phenolic compound from five cultivars cultivars of frozen sweet

cherries (*Prunus avium* L.). *Journal of Agricultural and Food Chemistry*, 2008, *56*, 3561-3568.

[11] Inngjerdingen, K.T.; Debes, S.C.; Inngjerdingen, M.; Hokputsa, S.; Harding, S.E.; Rolstad, B.; Michaelsen, T.E.; Diallo, D.; Paulsen, B.S. Bioactive pectic polysaccharides from *Glinus oppositifolius* (L.) Aug. DC., a Malian medicinal plant, isolation and partial characterization, *Journal of Ethnopharmacology*, 2005, *101*, 204-214.

[12] Chen, H.; Zhang, M.; Zhishuang, Q.; Bijun, X. Antioxidant activities of different fractions of polysaccharide conjugates from green tea (*Camellia sinensis*). *Food Chemistry*, 2008, *106*, 559-563.

[13] Chen, Y.; Xie, M.Y.; Nie, S.P.; Li, C.; Wang, Y.X. Purification, composition analysis and antioxidant activity from the fruiting bodies of *Ganoderma atrum*. *Food Chemistry*, 2008, *107*, 231-241.

[14] Fan, H.; Mazza, G.; Liao, X. Purification, composition and antioxidant activity of polysaccharides from wolfberry, cherry, kiwi, and cranberry fruits. *Croatian Journal of Food Science and Technology*, 2010, *2*, 9-17.

[15] Luo, Q.; Cai, Y.; Yan, J.; Sun, M.; Corke, H. Hypoglycemic and hypolipidemic effects and antioxidant activity of fruit extracts from *Lycium barbarum*. *Life Sciences*, 2004, *76*, 137-149.

[16] Li, X.M.; Li, X.L.; Zhou, A.G. Evaluation of antioxidant activity of the polysaccharides extracted from *Lycium barbarum* fruits in vitro. *European Polymer Journal,* 2007, *43*, 488-497.

[17] Nie, S.P.; Xie, M.Y. A review on the isolation and structure of tea polysaccharides and their bioactivities. *Food Hydrocolloids*, 2011, *25*, 144-149.

[18] Béliveau, R.; Gingras, D. Green tea: prevention and treatment of cancer by nutraceuticals. *The Lancet*, 2004, *364*, 1021-1022.

[19] Bravo, L. Polyphenols: chemistry, dietary sources, metabolism, and nutrition significance. *Nutrition Reviews*, 1998, *56*, 317-333.

[20] Dell'Aica, I.; Dona, M.; Tonello, F.; Piris, A.; Mock, M.; Montecucco, C. Potent inhibitors of anthrax lethal factor from green tea. *EMBO Reports*, 2004, *5*, 418-422.

[21] Xie, M.Y.; Nie, S.P. A review of the research progress on tea polysaccharide. *Journal of Food Science and Biotechnology*, 2006, *25*, 107-114.

[22] Demarco, M.L.; Woods, R.J. Structural glycobiology: A game of snakes and ladders. *Glycobiology*, 2008, *18*, 426–440.

[23] Ajit, V.; Richard, C.; Jeffrey, E.; Hudson, F.; Gerald, H.; Jamey, M. *Essentials of glycobiology*. New York, USA: Cold Spring Harbour Laboratory Press. 1997.

[24] Vliegenthart, J.F.G. Studies on the structure of glycoproteins. *Carbohydrate Polymer*, 1998, *34*, 427.

[25] Berg, JM; Tymoczko, JL; Stryer, L. *Biochemistry* 5th ed., W.H. Freeman; 2002.

[26] Nie, S.P.; Xie, M.Y.; Fu, Z.H.; Wan, Y.Q.; Yan, A.P. Study on the purification and chemical compositions of tea glycoprotein. *Carbohydrate Polymers,* 2008, *71*, 626-633.

[27] Malhotra, R.; Singh, B. Glycolipids of *Saccharomyces cerevisiae* cells. *Journal of Biological Sciences*, 2005, *5*, 253-256.

[28] Sugawara, T.; Miyazawa, T. Separation and determination of glycolipids from edible plant sources by high-performance liquid chromatography and evaporative light-scattering detection. *Lipids,* 1999, *34*, 1231-1237.

[29] Grunwald, C.; Huang, L.S.; 1989. Analysis of steryl glycosides. In: W.D. Nes and E.J. Parish, eds. *Analysis of Sterols and Other Biologically Significant Steroids*. New York; Academic Press; 1989; 49–60.

[30] Vesper, H.; Schmelz, E.M.; Nikolova-Karakashian, M.N.; Dillehay, D.L.; Lynch, D.V.; Merrill, A.H. Sphingolipids in food and the emerging importance of sphingolipids to nutrition. *Journal of Nutrition*, 1999, *129*, 1239–1250.

[31] Merrill, A.H.; Schmelz, E.M.; Wang, E.; Dillehay, D.L.; Rice, L.G.; Filmore, M.; Riley, R.T. Importance of sphingolipids and inhibitors of sphingolipid metabolism as components of animal diets. *Journal of Nutrition,* 1997, *127*, 830S–833S.

[32] Dörmann, P.; Benning, C. Galactolipids rule in seed plants. *Trends Plant Science*, 2002, *7*, 112–118.

[33] Larsen, E.; Christensen, L.P. Common vegetables and fruits as a source of 1,2-Di-O-α-Linolenoyl-3-O-β-D-Galactopyranosyl-sn-Glycerol, a potential anti-inflammatory and antitumor agent. *Journal of Food Lipids*, 2007, *14*, 272-279.

[34] Nie, S.P.; Xie, M.Y.; Zhou, P.; Cao, S.W. In vitro antioxidative and anticancer activities of tea glycoprotein in green tea. *European Food Research and Technology,* 2007, *224*, 437-442.

[35] Chen, X.; Lin, Z.; Ye, Y.; Zhang, R.; Yin, J.; Jiang, Y.; Wan, H. Suppression of diabetes in non-obese diabetic (NOD) mice by oral administration of water-soluble and alkali-soluble polysaccharide conjugates prepared from green tea. *Carbohydrate Polymers,* 2010, *82*, 28–33.

[36] Lee, J.H.; Shim, J.S.; Lee, J.S.; Kim, J.K.; Yang, I.S.; Chung, M.S. Inhibition of pathogenic bacterial adhesion by acidic polysaccharide from green tea (*Camellia sinensis*). *Journal of Agricultural and Food Chemistry*, 2006, *54*, 8717-8723.

[37] Chihara, G.; Hamuro, J.; Maeda, Y.Y.; Arai, Y.; Fukuoka, F. Fractionation and purification of the polysaccharides with marked antitumor activity, especially Lentinan, from *Lentinsu edodes* (Berk.) Sing. (an edible mushroom). *Cancer Research*, 1975, *30*, 2276-2781.

[38] Matsubara, Y.; Sawabe, A.; Iizuka, Y. Structures of new limonoid glycoside in lemon (*Citrus limon* BURM. *f.*) peelings. *Agricultural and Biological Chemistry,* 1990, *54*, 1143-1148.

[39] Yamagishi, T.; Tsuboi, T.; Kikuchi, K. Potent natural immunomodulator, rice water-soluble polysaccharide fractions with anticomplementary activity. *Cereal Chemistry,* 2003, *80*, 5-8.

[40] Luo, D.; Fang, B. Structural identification of ginseng polysaccharides and testing of their antixoxidant activities. *Carbohydrate Polymers*, 2008, *72*, 376-381.

[41] Gan, L.; Zhang, S.H.; Liu, Q.; Xu, H.B. A polysaccharide-protein complex from *Lycium barbarum* upregulates cytokine expression in human peripheral blood mononuclear cells. *European Journal of Pharmacology,* 2003, *471*, 217-222.

[42] Gan, L.; Zhang, S.H.; Yang, X.L.; Xu, H.B. Immunomodulation and antitumor activity by a polysaccharide-protein complex from *Lycium barbarum*. *International Immunopharmacology*, 2004, *4*, 563-569.

[43] Jones, P.J.; Raeini-Sarjaz, M.; Ntanios, F.Y.; Vanstone, C.A.; Feng, J.Y.; Parsons, W.E. Modulation of plasma lipid levels and cholesterol kinetics by phytosterol versus phytostanol esters. *Journal of Lipid Research*, 2000, *41*, 697-705.

[44] Katan, M.B.; Grundy, S.M.; Jones, P.; Law, M.; Miettinen, T.; Paoletti, R. Efficacy and safety of plant stanols and sterols in the management of blood cholesterol levels. *Mayo Clinic Proceedings*, *78*, 965-978.

[45] Gyles, C.L.; Carlberg, J.G.; Gustafson, J.; Davlut, D.A.; Jones, P.J.H. Economic valuation of the potential health benefits from foods enriched with plant sterols in Canada. *Food and Nutrition Research*, *54*, 5113-5119.

[46] Phillips, K.M.; Ruggio, D.M.; Ashraf-Khorassani, M. Analysis of steryl glucosides in foods and dietary supplements by solid-phase extraction and gas chromatography. *Journal of Food Lipids*, 2005, *12*, 124–140.

[47] Usuki, S.; Ariga, T.; Dasgupta, S.; Kasama, T.; Morikawa, K.; Nonaka, S.; Okuhara, Y.; Kise, M.; Yu, R.K. Structural analysis of novel bioactive acylated steryl glucosides (ASGs) in pre-germinated brown rice bran. *Journal of Lipid Research*, 2008, *49*, 2188-2196.

[48] Salvador, M.J.; Ferreira, E.O.; Pral, E.M.F.; Alfieri, S.C.; Albuquerque, S.; Ito, I.Y.; Dias, D.A. Bioactivity of crude extracts and some constituents of *Blutaparon portulacoides* (*Amaranthaceae*). *Phytomedicine,* 2002, *9*, 566–571.

[49] Berra, B.; Colombo, I.; Sottocornola, E.; Giacosa, A. Dietary sphingolipids in colorectal cancer prevention. *European Journal of Cancer Prevention*, 2002, *11*, 193-197.

[50] Schmelz, E.M. Sphingolipids in the chemoprevention of colon cancer. *Frontiers in Bioscience*, 2004, *9*, 2632-2639.

[51] Hou, C.C.; Chen, Y.P.; Wu, J.H. A galactolipid possesses novel cancer chemopreventive effects by suppressing inflammatory mediators and mouse B16 melanoma. *Cancer Research*, 2007, *67*, 6907-6915.

[52] Larsen, E.; Kharazmi, A.; Christensen, L.P; Christensen, S.B. An antiinflammatory galactolipid from rose hip (*Rosa canina*) that inhibits chemotaxis of human peripheral blood neutrophils in vitro. *Journal of Natural Products*, 2003, *66*, 994–995.

[53] Murakami, A., Nakamura, Y., Koshimizu, K. and Ohigashi, H. 1995. Glyceroglycolipids from *Citrus hystrix*, a traditional herb in Thailand, potently inhibit the tumor-promoting activity of 12-O-tetradecanoylphorbol 13-acetate in mouse skin. *Journal of Agricultural and. Food Chemistry*, 1995, *43*, 2779–2783.

[54] Wang, R.; Furumoto, T.; Motoyama, K.; Okazaki, K.; Kondo, A.; Fukui, H. Possible anti-tumor promoters in *Spinacia oleracea* (spinach) and comparison of their contents among cultivars. *Bioscience Biotechnology and Biochemistry*, 2002, *66*, 248–254.

[55] Murakami, C.; Kumagai, T.; Hada, T.; Kanekazu, U.; Nakazawa, S.; Kamisuki, S.; Maeda, N.; Xu, X.; Yoshida, H.; Sugawara, F. Effects of glycolipids from spinach on mammalian DNA polymerases. *Biochemical Pharmacology*, 2003, *65*, 259–267.

[56] Kuriyama, I.; Musumi, K.; Yonezawa, Y. Inhibitory effects of glycolipids fraction from spinach on mammalian DNA polymerase activity and human cancer cell proliferation. *Journal of Nutritional Biochemistry*, 2005, *16*, 594-601.

[57] Yuan, J.F.; Zhang, Z.Q.; Fan, Z.C.; Yang, J.X. Antioxidant effects and cytotoxicity of three purified polysaccharides from *Ligusticum chuanxiong* Hort, *Carbohydrate Polymers*, 2008, *74*, 822-827.

[58] Fang, Y.; Sheng, J.; Xu, J.; An, X,; Hu, Q. Antioxidant activities of crude tea polyphenols, polysaccharides and proteins of selenium-enriched tea and regular green tea. *European Food Research and Technology Journal*, 2007, *225*, 843–848.

[59] Chen, H.X.; Zhang, M.; Xie, B.J. Quantification of uronic acids in tea polysaccharide conjugates and its antioxidant properties. *Journal of Agricultural and Food Chemistry*, 2004, *52*: 3333–3336.

[60] Chen, H.X.; Zhang, M.; Qu, Z.S.; Xie, B.J. Compositional analysis and preliminary toxicological evaluation of a tea polysaccharide conjugate. *Journal of Agricultural and Food Chemistry*, 2007, *55*, 2256-2260.

[61] Chen, H.X.; Wang, Z.S.; Lu, X.M.; Xie, B.J. Isolation and chemical characterisation of a polysaccharide from green tea (*Camellia sinensis* L.). *Journal of the Science of Food and Agriculture*, 2008, *88*, 2523-2528.

[62] Staub, A.M. Removal of protein – Sevag method. *Methods in Carbohydrate Chemistry*, 1965, *5*, 5–6.

[63] Wang, Q.; Fang, Y. Analysis of sugars in traditional Chinese drugs. *Journal of Chromatography B*, 2004, *812*, 309–324.

[64] Bradford, M.M. A rapid and sensitive method for the quantitation of microgram quantities of protein utilizing the principle of protein binding. *Analytical Biochemistry*, 1977, *72*, 248–254.

[65] Folch, J.; Lees, M.; Sloane-Stanley, G.H. A simple method for the isolation and purification of total lipids from animal tissues. *Journal of Biological Chemistry*, 1957, *226*, 497-509.

[66] Yamauchi, R.; Aizawa, K.; Inakuma, T.; Kato, K. Analysis of molecular species of glycolipids in fruit pastes of red bell pepper (*Capsicum annuum* L.) by high performance liquid chromatography-mass spectrometry. *Journal of Agricultural and Food Chemistry*, 2001, *49*, 622-627.

[67] Wang, L.; Wang, T.; Fehr, W.R. HPLC quantification of sphingolipids in soybeans with modified palmitate content. *Journal of Agricultural and Food Chemistry*, 2006, *54*, 7422-7428.

[68] Sweeley, C.C.; Bentley, R.; Makita, M.; Wells, W.W. Gas liquid chromatography of trimethylsilyl derivatives of sugar and related substances. *Journal of the American Chemical Society*, 1963, *85*, 2497.

[69] Bortolomeazzi, R.; De Zan, M.; Pizzale, L.; Conte, L.S. Mass spectrometry characterization of the 5α-, 7α-, and 7β-hydroxy derivatives of β-Sitosterol, Campesterol, Stigmasterol, and Brassicasterol. *Journal of Agricultural and Food Chemistry*, 1999, *47*, 3069-3074.

[70] Peng, X.; Tian, G. Structural characterization of the glycan part of glycoconjugate LbGp2 from *Lycium barbarum* L., *Carbohydrate Research*, *331*, 95-99.

[71] Zhang, M.; Cheung, P.C.K; Zhang, L. Evaluation of mushroom dietary fiber (nonstarch polysaccharides) from sclerotia of *Pleurotus tuber-regium* (Fries) Singer as a potential antitumor agent. *Journal of Agricultural and Food Chemistry*, 2001, *49*, 5059–5062.

[72] Yamada, H. Pectic polysaccharides from Chinese herbs: structure and biological activity. *Carbohydrate Polymers*, 1994, *25*, 269-276.

[73] Wagner, H.; Kraus, S.; Jurcic, K. Search for potent immunostimulating agents from plants and other natural sources. In: Wagner, H. (Ed.), *Immunomodulatory Agents from Plants*. Basel: Birkhauser Verlag; 1999, 1–39.

[74] Alban, S.; Classen, B.; Brunner, G.; Blaschek, W. Differentiation between the complement modulating effects of an arabinogalactanprotein from *Echinacea purpurea* and heparin. *Planta Medica,* 2002, *68*, 1118–1124.

[75] Yamagishi, T.; Matsuda, K.; Watanabe, T. Isolation and partial characterization of proteoglycans from rice bran. *Carbohydrate Research*, 1975, *43*, 321-333.

[76] Ajisaka, K.; Agawa, S.; Nagumo, S.; Kurato, K.; Yokoyama, T.; Arai, K.; Miyazaki, T. Evaluation and comparison of the antioxidative potency of various carbohydrate using different methods. *Journal of Agricultural and Food Chemistry*, 2009, *57*, 3102-3107.

[77] Bishop, D.G.; Wade, N.L. Lipid composition of sweet cherries. *Phytochemistry*, 1977, *16*, 67-68.

[78] Gao, Z.; Ali, Z.; Khan, I.A. Glycerogalactolipids from the fruit of *Lycium barbarum*. *Phytochemistry*, 2008, *69*, 2856–2861.

In: Berries: Properties, Consumption and Nutrition
Editor: Carlo Tuberoso
ISBN 978-1-61470-257-3

Chapter IV

Blueberries: Major Phytochemicals and Potential Health Effects in Cardiovascular Diseases

Xianli Wu** *and Jie Kang
USDA Arkansas Children's Nutrition Center,
Department of Physiology and Biophysics
University of Arkansas for Medical Sciences,
Little Rock, AR, USA

Abstract

Consumption of blueberries has increased rapidly over the past decade, as have the numbers of studies suggesting health benefits. Now the blueberry is a commonly consumed berry in the United States. They are used in jellies, jams, and pies, baked into muffins, and are an ingredient of many other snacks and delicacies or baby foods. The major phytochemicals in blueberries are polyphenols, including anthocyanins, proanthocyanidins, other flavonoids, phenolic acids and stilbene derivatives. A diet rich in fruits and vegetables has long been recognized to reduce the risk of cardiovascular diseases. In recent years, evidence has emerged suggesting that some phytochemicals in plant foods, polyphenols in particular, may be largely responsible for their protective activities against cardiovascular diseases, mainly through antioxidant and anti-inflammatory activities. Blueberries are rich in polyphenols and exhibit extremely high antioxidant capacity. They have been implicated in preventing cardiovascular diseases for many years. Recent studies, including animal and human studies, have found the beneficial effects of blueberries in cardiovascular diseases from different aspects: preventing development of atherosclerotic lesions, protecting the myocardium from induced ischemic damage, having positive effects on the course of chronic heart failure,

* USDA Arkansas Children's Nutrition Center, Department of Physiology and Biophysics University of Arkansas for Medical Sciences, 15 Children's Way, Little Rock, AR 72202 USA, E-mail: wuxianli@uams.edu.

lowering blood pressure and improving selected features of metabolic syndrome and related cardiovascular risk factors. The possible underlying mechanisms included but not limited to reducing oxidation of lipoproteins, improving serum antioxidant status and lipid levels, improving endothelial dysfunction and inhibiting inflammation on the vascular system.

1. Introduction

It has long been recognized that a diet rich in fruits and vegetables has protective effects on chronic diseases such as cancer and heart diseases from epidemiological studies [1-4]. Fruits and vegetables are rich in nutrients and non-nutrient phytochemicals. In recent years, different lines of evidences have been accumulated and pointed out that phytochemicals, polyphenolic compounds in particularly, may be largely responsible for their cardio-protective effects mainly through antioxidant and anti-inflammatory activities [5]. Among all the fruits and vegetables, berries, especially dark color berries such as blueberries, were found to contain extremely high level of polyphenols and show strong antioxidant capacities and potential anti-inflammatory effects [6,7].

The blueberry of the genus *Vaccinium* is a native American species. In fact the blueberry is one of the few fruits native to North America. *Vaccinium* is the family of all blueberries and includes more than 450 plants. This plant grows wild around the world and there are many names given to different blueberries. Blueberries may be cultivated, or they may be picked from semi-wild or wild bushes. In North America, the most common cultivated species is *V. corymbosum*, which is also called Northern highbush blueberry. Hybrids of this with other *Vaccinium* species adapted to southern U.S. climates are known collectively as Southern highbush blueberries, of which *V. ashei*. (Southern Rabbiteye) is the most common variety. So-called "wild" (lowbush) blueberries are found from the Atlantic provinces westward to Quebec and southward to Michigan and West Virginia. They are smaller than cultivated highbush blueberries and are prized for their intense color.

Consumption of blueberry increased rapidly with more and more studies revealed its health effects. Now blueberry is among the most commonly consumed berries in the US. Blueberries are used in jellies, jams, and pies, baked into muffins, and are an ingredient of many other snacks and delicacies. In the last few years, blueberry juice has entered the market and is considered a growing category of juice in consumer stores. According to a recent comparison of commonly consumed polyphenol-rich beverages in the US, blueberry juice was ranked the top 4 after pomegranate juice, red wine and concord grape juice [8]. Blueberries have been implicated in preventing cardiovascular diseases for many years. Several recent reports, including animal and human studies, have largely contributed to our understanding of the health effects of blueberries in preventing cardiovascular diseases and the underlying mechanism. Since the majority of the studies about cardio-protective effects of blueberries have been focused on three major varieties in North America, Northern highbush blueberry (*V. corymbosum*), "rabbiteye" blueberries (*V. ashei*) and "wild" (lowbush) (*V. angustifolium*) blueberries, we therefore restrict our discussions on the data from these three species in this chapter.

2. Major Phytochemicals in Blueberries

Blueberries contain high levels of polyphenols as their major phytochemicals, including anthocyanins, proanthocyanidins, phenolic acids, other flavonoids and other phenolic compounds.

2.1. Anthocyanins

Anthocyanins are water soluble plant secondary metabolites responsible for the blue, purple, and red color of many plant tissues. They occur primarily as glycosides of their respective aglycone anthocyanidin-chromophores (Figure 1), with the sugar moiety mainly attached at the 3-hydroxyl group on the C-ring or the 5- or 7-hydroxyl group on the A-ring.

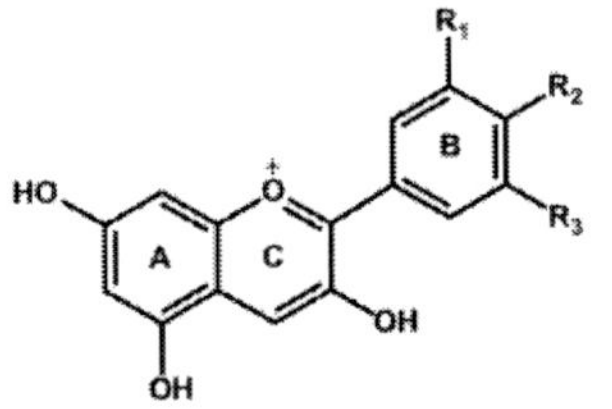

anthocyanidin	R_1	R_2	R_3	MW
pelargonidin	H	OH	H	271
cyanidin	OH	OH	H	287
delphinidin	OH	OH	OH	303
peonidin	OMe	OH	H	301
petunidin	OMe	OH	OH	317
malvidin	OMe	OH	OMe	331

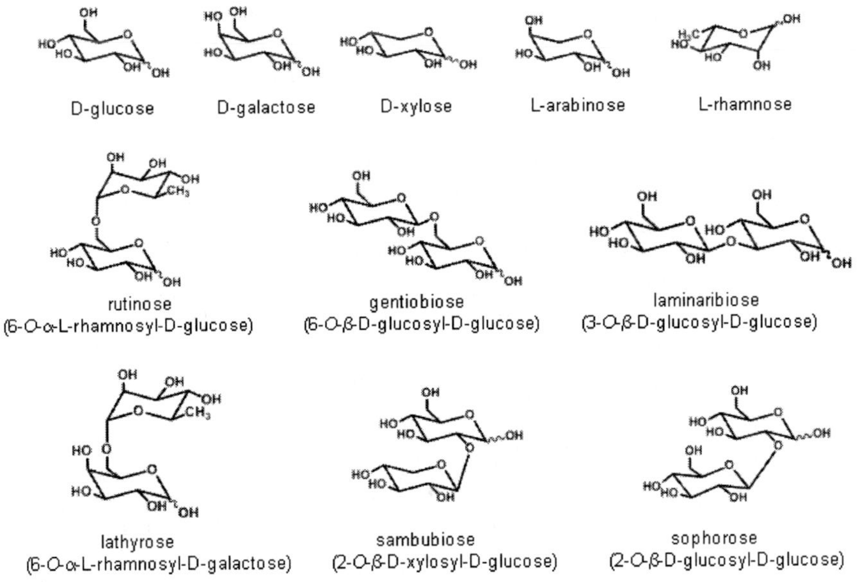

Figure 1. Structures of six common anthocyanidins and the sugar moieties.

Glycosylation at 3', 4' or 5'-hydroxyl group of the B-ring, although very rare, has also been observed. Glucose, galactose, arabinose, rhamnose and xylose are the most common sugars that are bonded to anthocyanidins as mono-, di- or trisaccharide forms. Aglycones are rarely found in fresh plant materials. There are about seventeen anthocyanidins found in nature, whereas only six of them, cyanidin, delphinidin, petunidin, peonidin, pelargonidin, and malvidin are ubiquitously distributed (Figure 1). The differences in chemical structure of these six common anthocyanidins occur at the 3' and 5' positions of the B-ring (Figure 1). The sugar moieties may also be acylated by a range of aromatic or aliphatic acids. Most studies on anthocyanins focus on fruits and vegetables, especially edible dark color berries.

Different blueberry cultivars were found to contain twenty to twenty-seven anthocyanins, which included five common aglycones. The lowbush blueberry was found to contain twenty-seven anthocyanins, and the highbush blueberry contained twenty-five, whereas only twelve anthocyanins were detected in the rabbiteye blueberry [9-11](Table 1).

Table 1. Identification of anthocyanins from three varieties of blueberry.

No.	$[M]^+$ (*m/z*)	MS/MS (*m/z*)	Anthocyanin	Blueberry species
1	465	303	delphinidin-3-*O*-galactoside	highbush, lowbush and rabbiteye
2	465	303	delphinidin-3-*O*-glucoside	highbush, lowbush and rabbiteye
4	435	303	delphinidin-3-*O*-arabinoside	highbush, lowbush and rabbiteye
3	449	287	cyanidin-3-*O*-galactoside	highbush, lowbush and rabbiteye
5	449	287	cyanidin-3-*O*-glucoside	highbush, lowbush and rabbiteye
6	419	287	cyanidin-3-*O*-arabinoside	highbush, lowbush and rabbiteye
7	479	317	petunidin-3-*O*-galactoside	highbush and lowbush
8	479	317	petunidin-3-*O*-glucoside	highbush, lowbush and rabbiteye
9	449	317	petunidin-3-*O*-arabinoside	highbush, lowbush and rabbiteye
10	463	301	peonidin-3-*O*-glucoside	highbush, lowbush and rabbiteye
11	463	301	peonidin-3-*O*-galactoside	highbush and lowbush
12	433	301	peonidin-3-*O*-arabinoside	highbush
13	493	331	malvidin-3-*O*-galactoside	highbush, lowbush and rabbiteye
14	493	331	malvidin-3-*O*-glucoside	highbush, lowbush and rabbiteye
15	463	331	malvidin-3-*O*-arabinoside	highbush, lowbush and rabbiteye
16	535	287	cyanidin-3-*O*-(malonyl)glucoside	lowbush
17	491	287	cyanidin-3-*O*-(6"-*O*-acetyl)glucoside	highbush and lowbush
18	491	287	cyanidin-3-*O*-(6"-*O*-acetyl)galactoside	highbush and lowbush
19	491	287	cyanidin-3-*O*-(6"-*O*-acetyl)glucoside	highbush
20	551	303	delphinidin-3-*O*-(malonyl)glucoside	lowbush
21	507	303	delphinidin-3-*O*-(6"-*O*-acetyl)glucoside	highbush and lowbush
22	521	317	petunidin-3-*O*-(6"-*O*-acetyl)glucoside	highbush and lowbush
23	521	317	petunidin-3-*O*-(6"-*O*-acetyl)galactoside	highbush
24	449	317	petunidin + pentose	lowbush
25	505	301	peonidin-3-*O*-(6"-*O*-acetyl)galactoside	highbush and lowbush
26	505	301	peonidin-3-*O*-(6"-*O*-acetyl)glucoside	highbush and lowbush
27	535	331	malvidin-3-*O*-(6"-*O*-acetyl)glucoside	highbush and lowbush
28	535	331	malvidin-3-*O*-(6"-*O*-acetyl)galactoside	highbush and lowbush
29	579	331	malvidin-3-*O*-(malonyl)glucoside	lowbush
30	535	331	malvidin + acetyl + hexose	lowbush

2.2. Proanthocyanidins

Proantocyanidins present in a lot of common foods including cereals, fruits, vegetables and wines [12]. Proanthocyanidins represent a group of condensed flavan-3-ols. (+)-Catechin and (-)-epicatechin are the basic monomeric units of this group for blueberry (Figure 2).

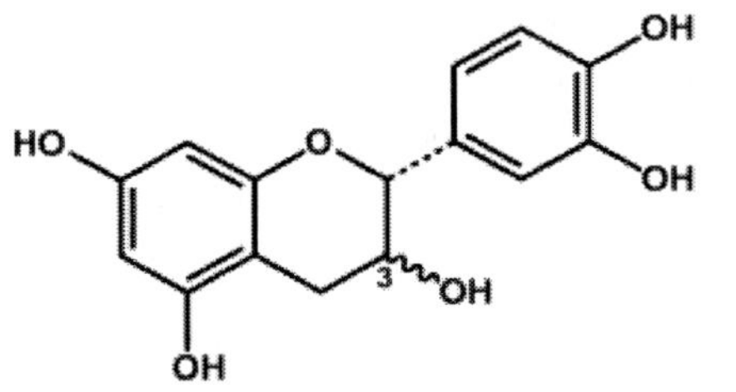

monomer:

(+)-catechin (3S)
(-)-epicatechin (3R)

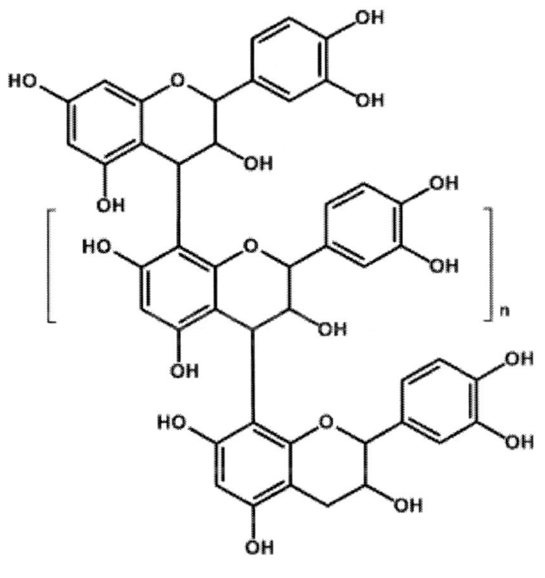

oligomer (n = 0-3) (DP = 2 -5)
polymer (n > 3) (DP > 5)

Figure 2. Structures of proantocyanidins in blueberries.

The molecular weight of proantocyanidins expressed as degree of polymerization (DP) is one of the most important properties: 1 unit for monomer (DP = 1), 2-5 units for oligomers (DP = 2-5), over 5 units for polymers (DP > 5) [13] (Figure 2). Compared with the lower molecular proanthocyanidins with DP < 10, there are few reports of polymeric proanthocyanidins (DP > 10), partially due to lack of powerful analytical methods to get the pure higher polymers [14]. Proanthocyanidins are usually divided into A and B types. For B-type, the monomeric units are mainly linked through C4 → C8 or sometimes C4 → C6 bonds. If an additional ether linkage between C2 and O7 is formed, they are called A-type proanthocyanidins [14,15].

Only B type proanthocyainidin were found in blueberries [16]. The relative contents are monomers 0.18 mg/g, oligomers (DP = 2-5) 1.81 mg/g, polymers (DP = 6-10) 2.71 mg/g, and polymers (DP > 10) 15.28 mg/g [14].

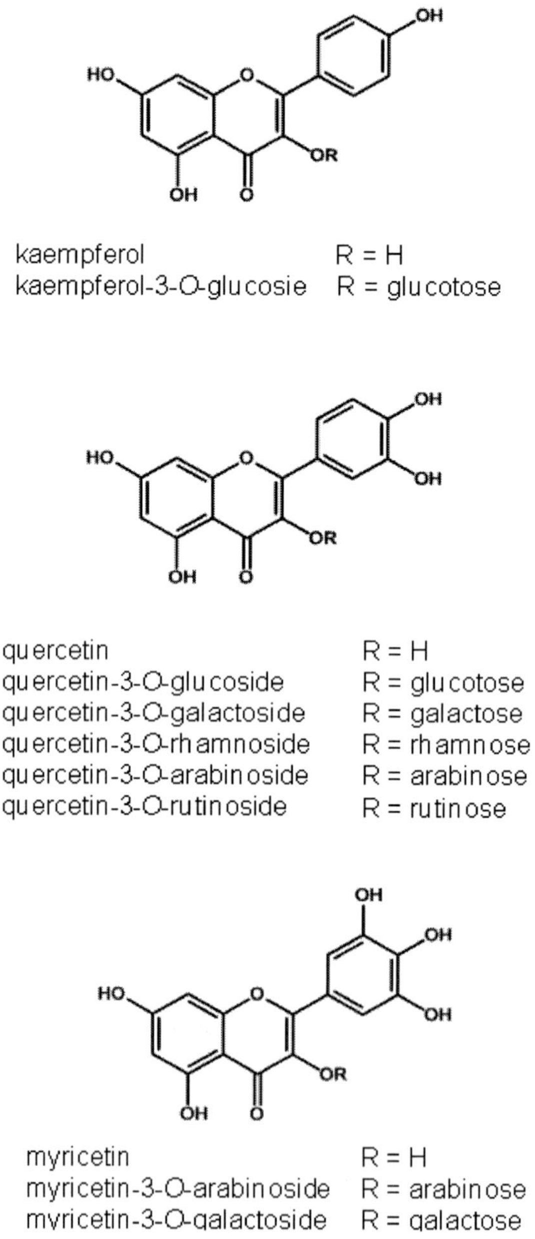

Figure 3. Structures of flavonols in blueberries.

2.3. Other Flavonoids

Except for anthocyanins and flavan-3-ols, flavonols and their glycosides were also found in blueberries. Three types of aglycones were reported: kaempferol, quercetin and myricetin [17] (Figure 3). The differences of these compounds are the numbers of hydroxyl groups on the ring B. The sugar chains of flavonol glycosides include glucose, galactose, rhamnose, arabinose and rutinose [17-19].

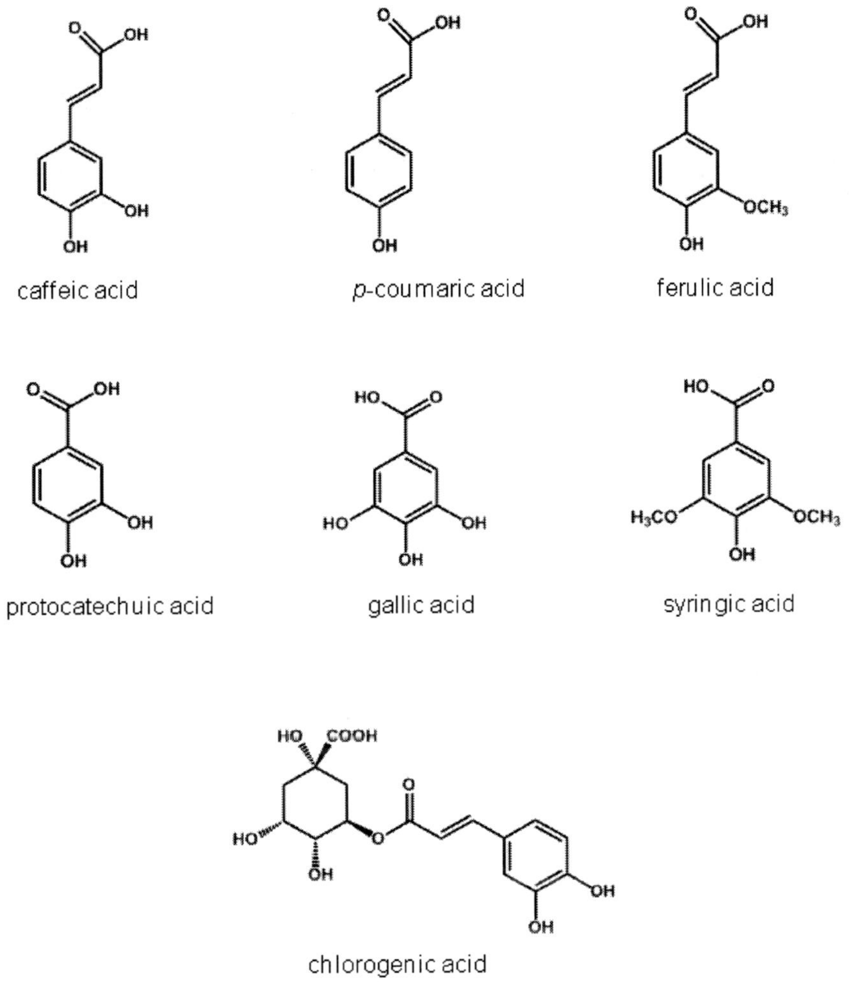

Figure 4. Structures of phenolic acids in blueberries.

2.4. Phenolic Acids

Phenolic acids are another group of important phenolic compounds in blueberries. They share a phenolic ring and an organic carboxylic acid group (Figure 4). The chlorogenic acid is the principle phenolic acid in all the most common cultivated *Vaccinium* species, and indeed it is the most abundant single phytochemical in blueberries [11,20,21].

2.5. Stilbenes

Resveratrol, pterosilbene, and piceatannol are naturally occurring compounds considered as derivatives of stilbenes, which have an ethane double bond substituted with a phenyl group on both carbon atoms of the bond.

The name stilbene is derived from Greek, which means “shining” partly because of the red to brown bright color of these conjugated compounds. The stilbene has two configurational isomers, *trans*- and *cis*- stilbenes. Due to phenyl groups are big substituting groups, *trans*- isomers are much more stable than *cis*- stilbenes. The three compounds mentioned above are all *trans*- stilbenes.

Resveratrol, which was found in considerable quantities in grapes, was detected in all three blueberry varieties (highbush, lowbush and rabbiteye blueberries). The other two stilbenes, pterostilbene and piceatannol were found in rabbiteye and highbush blueberries, respectively [22] (Figure 5).

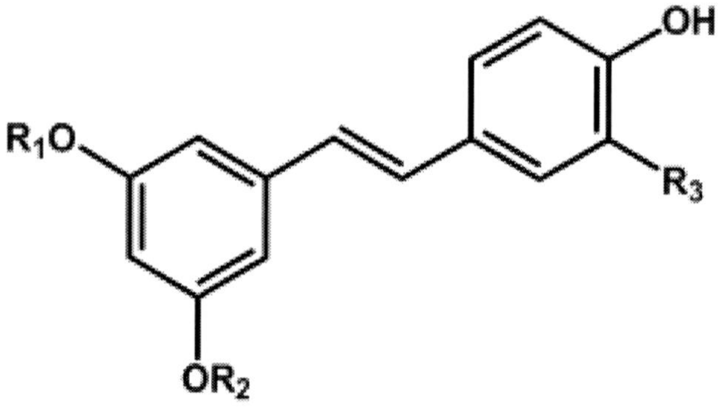

resveratrol	$R_1 = R_2 = R_3 = H$
pterostilbene	$R_1 = R_2 = CH_3, R_3 = H$
piceatannol	$R_1 = R_2 = H, R_3 = OH$

Figure 5. Structures of stilbenes in blueberries.

2.6. Other Compounds

Two triterpenoids, ursolic acid and 3β,19α-dihydroxy-urs-12-en-28-oic acid, and one common sterol glycoside, sitosterol-3-*O*-glucoside, were isolated from the dried fruit of highbush blueberries [23] (Figure 6).

Four fatty acids, quinic, shikimic, malic and citric acids, were only reported from the lowbush blueberries [20], whereas succinic acid was found in both highbush and rabbiteye blueberries, but were not found in lowbush blueberries [20] (Figure 7).

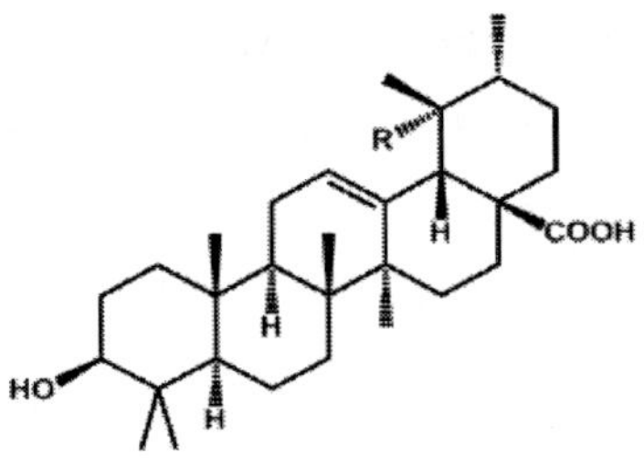

ursolic acid R = H
3β,19α-dihydroxy-urs-12en-28-oic acid R = OH

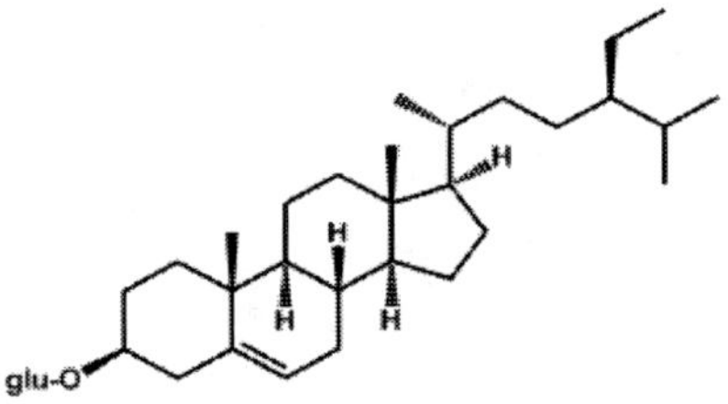

sitosterol-3-O-glucoside

Figure 6. Structures of triterpenoids in blueberries.

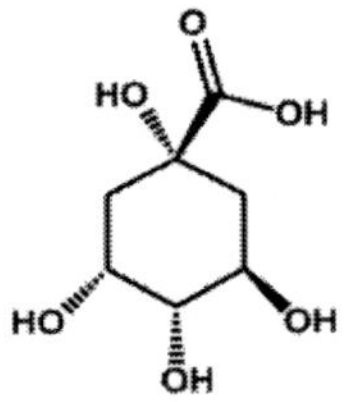

quinic acid

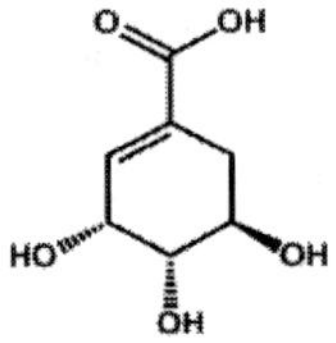

shikimic acid

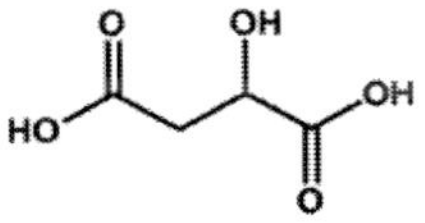

malic acid

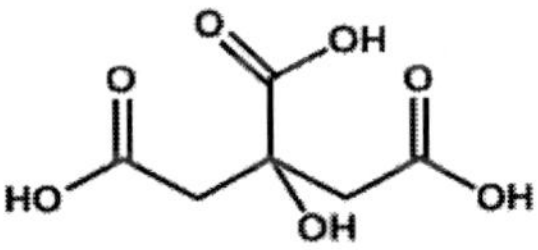

citric acid

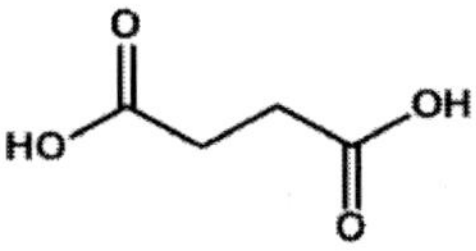

succinic acid

Figure 7. Structures of organic acids in blueberries.

3. Health Effects in Preventing Cardiovascular Diseases

Cardiovascular disease (CVD) continues to be the leading cause of death in the US [24]. Atherosclerosis (thickening of arterial intima) is one of the most common causes of CVD. Thickening of arteries, also known as atherosclerosis, result in CVD [25]. Atherosclerosis is a disease that usually does not become clinically apparent until later in life, but can begin in childhood. Hypercholesterolemia has been implicated a risk factor for the initiation of atherosclerosis. Interventions that promote lowering of low-density lipoprotein (LDL) cholesterol or inhibiting accumulation of lipids in artery wall, such as diet, exercise and medications, have the long-term potential of decreasing the frequency and extent of CVD in adulthood [26-28].

Epidemiological studies have suggested that dietary factors play a pivotal role in prevention of CVD [29]. It was estimated that five of the ten leading causes of death are related to diet. Our understanding of mechanisms of atherosclerosis has been changed dramatically over last decades. It has been widely accepted that atherosclerosis is an inflammatory disease and is initiated as response-and-injury pattern [30,31]. Oxidized LDL (oxLDL) is one of the major driven agents leading to inflammatory process. Thus, hypercholesterolimia and inflammation were regarded as "partners in crime" [32]. The dietary factors that can regulate LDL metabolism, LDL oxidation and modulate the immune system are of great clinical significance in the prevention of atherosclerosis [1,33-35].

Blueberries were found containing extremely high level of polyphenols and exhibit strong antioxidant capacities [5,6]. Prevention of cardiovascular diseases by blueberries has been implicated for many years. Nevertheless, it was until recent years that the evidence from animal and human studies started to rapidly accumulate showing the cardio-protective effects and revealing the underlying mechanisms. Here we will summarize the cardio-protective effects of blueberries and the underlying mechanism from the publications during last few years in this chapter.

3.1. Evidence from Animal Studies

From the animal studies, especially those published most recently, we've learned that blueberries showed the promising cardio-protective effects from several aspects.

3.1.1. Affecting Plasma Lipid Status

Polyphenols have been suggested as strong antioxidant and thus may act to inhibit LDL oxidation. There were evidence showing that polyphenols may affect reverse cholesterol transport to decrease total and LDL-cholesterol. In a study using pig model [36], lowbush blueberry supplementation in the basal diets, either containing a high or low level of plant-based components, resulted in a decrease in total, LDL- and HDL-cholesterol. However, Blueberry supplementation had no effect on the susceptibility of leukocyte DNA to oxidation and no effect on the susceptibility of LDL to oxidation. These suggested that blueberries can beneficially affect plasma lipid status. But the effects were in relation to the basal diet compositions.

3.1.2. Managing Hypertension

Hypertension, defined as blood pressure (BP) 140/90 mm Hg or higher, is associated with an increased risk of cardiovascular disease [37]. Strategies to manage hypertension are considered the key in controlling mortalities from CVD. The exact cause of the development of essential hypertension remains unknown, although it has become evident that oxidative stress plays a role in human and experimental hypertension. Given the presence of oxidative stress, antioxidants may be useful in the treatment of hypertension by slowing the onset or retarding the progression of elevated BP. In one recent study [38], eight-week-old normotensive rats and spontaneously hypertensive stroke-prone (SHRSP) rats were fed either a control diet or a diet enriched with 3% freeze-dried lowbush blueberries for 8 weeks. Systolic blood pressure (SBP) was measured and urine was collected for biomarker analysis. In SHRSP consuming diet containing blueberries, SBP was 19% lower at week 4 and 30% lower at week 6, relative to SHRSP on control diet. Maximum SBP was 216 ± 11 mm Hg in SHRSP rats consuming control diet vs 178 ± 15 mm Hg in the blueberry-fed group ($P = 0.036$). SHRSP rats had elevated levels of urine F_2-isoprostanes/creatinine relative to normotensive rats, indicating systemic oxidative stress in this strain. Blueberry feeding had no effect on urinary excretion of F_2-isoprostanes; therefore, it is unlikely that a systemic antioxidant effect of blueberries is responsible for the antihypertensive effects. Blueberry-fed rats had reduced markers of renal oxidative stress, such as proteinuria and kidney nitrites. Thus, blueberry diet may be capable of protecting the kidneys from oxidative damage in SHRSP rats, thereby reducing the magnitude of hypertension.

3.1.3. Improving Vascular Reactivity and Vascular Tone

CVD occurs as a result of chronic injury to the dynamic vascular endothelium that constitutes the inner layer of blood vessels [39-41]. A functional endothelium depends on the balance between secretion of vasodilator and vasoconstriction mediator. Endothelial dysfunction has been described as an imbalance between vasodilator and vasoconstrictor mediators that results in altered vascular tone, organ blood flow, and peripheral vascular resistance. It is one of the earliest events that occurs in the development of CVD even before the onset of atherosclerosis and has been related to aging and hypertension. In the last five years, a series of studies about consumption of lowbush blueberries and endothelial functions, vascular reactivity and vascular tone in rat models have been conducted by Klimis-Zacas *et al.* [42-47].

In their first report [47], they indicated for the first time that wild blueberries incorporated into the diet affect the vascular smooth muscle contractile machinery by suppressing the $\alpha 1$-adrenergic receptor agonist L-phenylephrine (Phe) mediated contraction while having no effects on membrane sensitivity of the endothelial or vascular smooth muscle cell layer. The mechanism of action seems to be accomplished through an endothelium-dependent pathway. The follow-up study [44] was designed to evaluate vascular function and responsiveness in aortas of weanling male Sprague-Dawley rats fed a control or a blueberry diet for seven weeks. A significantly diminished vasoconstrictor response to Phe was observed in aortic rings from rats fed the blueberry diet. Inhibition of nitric oxide (NO) synthase but not cyclooxygenase (COX) caused a significant increase in the constrictor response in both dietary groups, with the blueberry group having the greater response. Similarly, the participation of the NO pathway in endothelium-dependent vasorelaxation induced by acetylcholine (ACh) was greater in the rats fed a blueberry diet, while COX inhibition showed no effect on maximum ACh induced vasorelaxation in any diet group. The vessel sensitivity of aortic rings from blueberry fed rats to the vasoconstrictor and vasodilator was significantly reduced when compared to controls. Another study from this group was performed to evaluate the effects of the dietary enrichment with wild blueberries on aortic function and reactivity in the developmental phase of essential hypertension in spontaneously hypertensive rats (SHR) [45]. Spontaneously hypertensive rats (SHR) are extensively used as an animal model of endothelial dysfunction in various experimental designs, including pharmacological and dietary studies. In the SHR, endothelial dysfunction is attributed to the concomitant reduction in the availability of endothelium-derived vasodilator factors and increased production of vasoconstrictors. The major findings in this study were that in Phe-induced vasoconstriction, SHR-blueberry aortas relaxed to a greater degree in comparison to controls when mefenamic acid (MFA) was present and that the incubation with this COX inhibitor failed to restore - and in fact decreased - the maximum vasodilator response to ACh, in comparison to controls. The vessel reactivity index (pD2) observations indicate that blueberries appear to modulate cell membrane agonist interactions primarily in response to ACh in the young SHR model, but not to the α1-adrenoreceptor agonist. Similar study was also conducted in adult (20 weeks old) SHR, with established endothelial dysfunctions [46]. Twenty-week-old SHR were fed a control or an 8% lowbush blueberry diet after 8 weeks. The vasoconstriction elicited by Phe was reduced in the blueberry group, attributed to the NO pathway, favoring a lower vascular tone under basal conditions. Acetylcholine-induced vasorelaxation in the blueberry group was possibly mediated through the COX, but not the NO pathway. These findings document the potential of wild blueberries to modify major pathways of vasomotor control and improve the vascular tone in the adult SHR with endothelial dysfunction. Most recently, a study of the duration of dietary intervention necessary to induce the positive changes on vasomotor tone was reported by the same group [42]. In this study, forty male Sprague-Dawley rats were randomly assigned to a control or a lowbush blueberry diet for four or seven weeks. Vascular ring studies were conducted in 3-mm isolated rat aortic rings to investigate vasoconstriction induced by six doses of the α1-adrenergic agonist Phe alone or in the presence of the NOS inhibitor, L-NMMA. The maximum force of contraction (F_{max}) and vessel sensitivity (pD2) were determined. There were no significant differences on F_{max} after four weeks of the blueberry diet but only a significant increase in pD2 in the absence of L-NMMA. Seven week blueberry consumption significantly attenuated contraction in response to Phe and resulted in lower pD2. Inhibition of NOS induced a significant increase in the constrictor response in both diet groups at both time periods, with the blueberry group fed for seven weeks having the greater response. Thus wild blueberries incorporated into the diet at 8% w/w positively affect vascular smooth muscle contractility and sensitivity but these effects are evident only after 7 weeks of blueberry consumption.

According to Klimis-Zacas *et al.* [43], compounds in lowbush blueberries can alter the composition of glycosaminoglycans (GAGs), a structurally diverse group of macromolecules produced by vascular endothelial and smooth muscle cells. GAGs participate in organization of the extracellular matrix and by their interaction with other molecules, regulate functions as diverse as cell proliferation, migration and adhesion, cell signaling, blood coagulation, and lipoprotein metabolism [48,49]. An abundance of oversulfated GAGs has been linked to chronic inflammation and the progression of atherosclerosis [50]. The feeding study employing Sprague-Dawley rats investigated the effect of wild blueberry consumption over 13 weeks on the composition and abundance of GAGs in the aorta [43]. The study found the concentration of GAGs in the aortas of blueberry-fed rats significantly higher than that from rats fed control diet with an overall decrease in the sulfation level of GAG disaccharides, which may be expected to affect the structure of the extracellular matrix, lipoprotein lipase activity, and signal transduction in vascular endothelial and smooth muscle cells.

3.1.4. Positive Effects on the Course of Chronic Heart Failure

Reactive oxygen species (ROS) play a major role in ischemia-related myocardial injury. In a recent study [51] designed to evaluate the effects of lowbush blueberries to block the detrimental effects of ROS in ischemia-related myocardial injury, young male Fischer-344 rats were fed diet supplemented with blueberry or a regular control diet for three months. The threshold for mitochondrial permeability transition was measured in isolated cardiomyocytes. The increased myocardial tolerance to ischemic damage was observed. At a cellular level, the blueberry diet increased cardiomyocyte survival by elevating the mitochondrial permeability transition ROS threshold. *In vivo* experiments, this diet reduced the size of myocardial infarction induced by a permanent coronary ligation by attenuating necro-apoptosis and inflammation in the area at risk. The beneficial effects of the blueberry diet were extended after coronary ligation by continuing the attenuation of the post-myocardial infarction (MI) remodeling and MI expansion.

Another study from the same group was conducted to test the hypothesis that lowbush blueberry diet attenuated the course of chronic heart failure (CHF), including mortality and cardiac remodeling during the first year after induction of MI in rats [52]. Two weeks after coronary artery ligation, rats were divided into two groups of similar average MI size, measured by echocardiography, and then twelvemonths dietary regimens were initiated as follows: *ad libitum* regular control diet and isocaloric food with 2% blueberry supplement also available *ad libitum*. These dietary groups were compared to each other and to sham groups. Mortality over the twelve-months was reduced by 22% in blueberry diet compared with control diet ($p < 0.01$). In the course of developing CHF, blueberry diet had no effect on the body weight, heart rate or blood pressure. Bimonthly Echo revealed significant attenuation of the left ventricular chamber remodeling, left ventricular posterior wall thinning, and MI expansion in blueberry diet compared with control diet. In fact, blueberry diet arrested the MI expansion. This is the first experimental evidence that a blueberry-enriched diet has positive effects on the course of CHF.

3.1.5. Preventing Development of Atherosclerotic Lesions

Previous *studies* have suggested that blueberries may help to prevent cardiovascular disease, but there was no direct evidence that eating blueberries could cause plaque in arteries to regress until a most recent paper published by Wu, *et al.* [53]. In this paper, 30 apolipoprotein-E deficient mice (apo$E^{-/-}$ mice) were divided into two groups. The apo$E^{-/-}$ mouse model has been widely used in cardiovascular research [54, 55]. ApoE deficiency in mice leads to the development of atherosclerotic lesions resembling those in humans [56]. The mice were fed either AIN-93G diet as control diet or AIN-93G diet supplemented with 1% freeze-dried lowbush blueberries for 20 weeks. At the end of the study, the plaques measured at two sites on the aorta (arteries leading from the heart) were 39 and 58 percent smaller in the mice who ate the blueberry powder compared to the plaque lesions in the animals whose diet did not contain blueberry powders. Comparing to control diet, adding blueberries did not change the lipid profile, nor did they change the overall antioxidant activity in the serum measured by ORAC. But blueberry diet lowered the concentration of a biomarker of lipid peroxidation, F_2-isoprostane, as well as boosted the activity of antioxidant enzymes superoxide dismutase (SOD) 1, SOD2, glutathione reductase (GSR), thioredoxin reductase 1 and paraoxonase 1. The potential mechanisms may involve reduction in oxidative stress by both inhibition of lipid peroxidation and enhancement of antioxidant defense.

3.2. Evidence from Human Studies

Evidence from human studies showing cardio-protective effects of blueberries are still very rare until now. There is only one study directly related to cardio-protective benefits. In this recent published study [57], 48 participants with metabolic syndrome consumed freeze-dried highbush blueberry beverage (50 g freeze-dried blueberries, ~350 g fresh blueberries) or equivalent amounts of fluids (controls, 960 mL water) daily for eight weeks in a randomized controlled trial. Anthropometric and blood pressure measurements, assessment of dietary intakes, and fasting blood draws were performed at screening and at week 4 and 8 of the study. The decreases in systolic and diastolic blood pressures were greater in the blueberry-supplemented group (26% and 24%, respectively) than in controls (21.5% and 21.2%) ($P < 0.05$), whereas the serum glucose concentration and lipid profiles remained unchanged. The decreases in plasma oxidized LDL and serum malondialdehyde and hydroxynonenal concentrations were greater in the blueberry group (228% and 217%, respectively) than that in the control group (29% and 29%) ($P < 0.01$). This study showed that blueberries may improve selected features of metabolic syndrome and related cardiovascular risk factors at dietary achievable doses.

3.3. Mechanisms of Cardio-Protective Effects of Blueberries

Blueberries contain high levels of polyphenols and appear to have extremely high antioxidant capacities [6,58].

A number of studies that conducted in cell line, animals as well as human subjects suggested that blueberries affected events related to occurrence in the progression of cardiovascular diseases, included reducing oxidation of lipoproteins, improving serum antioxidant status and lipid levels, improving endothelial dysfunction and inhibiting inflammation on the vascular system.

3.3.1. Reducing Lipid Peroxidation

LDL oxidation is a key step in early stage of atherosclerosis development. OxLDL initiates a series of inflammatory events leading to the recruiting leukocytes including monocyte and T-lymphocyte into intima and differentiation of monocyte into macrophages [59,60]. Unlike native LDL, oxLDL is not taken by macrophage through LDL receptor, but scavenger receptor without down regulation. The rapid uptake of oxLDL particles by macrophage leads to foam-cell formation, which is characterized as early event of atherosclerosis. In addition to being taken up rapidly by macrophage to form foam cells, oxLDL was shown to be atherogenic through other mechanisms. For example, oxLDL is itself a chemotactic agent for monocyte and for T cells. OxLDL was also shown the cytoxicity for endothelial cells, resulting in loss of endothelial integrity.

Blueberry has been shown to inhibit human LDL and liposome oxidation in cell culture and significantly reduce lipid hydroperoxides in human subjects as well [61-63]. These studies indicated that reducing oxidative stress might be one important mechanism of the anti-atherogenic effects of blueberries.

3.3.2. Improving Serum Antioxidant Status

Increasing the serum antioxidant status has been implicated as a possible preventative means to reduce the development of cardiovascular disease. A single blinded crossover study was performed in a group of eight middle-aged male subjects (38–54 years) [64]. Subjects consumed a high-fat meal and a control supplement followed one week later by the same high-fat meal supplemented with 100 g freeze-dried lowbush blueberry powder. Serum antioxidant status was determined using the oxygen radical absorbance capacity (ORAC) assay and the total antioxidant status (TAS) assay. The wild-blueberry treatment was associated with a significant treatment effect as determined by the ORAC assay (water-soluble fraction $ORAC_{perchloric\ acid\ (PCA)}$, $P = 0.04$). Significant increases in serum antioxidant status above the controls were observed at 1 h ($ORAC_{PCA}$ (8.5% greater), $P = 0.02$; TAS (4.5% greater), $P = 0.05$), and 4 h ($ORAC_{total}$ (15.0% greater), $P = 0.009$; $ORAC_{acetone}$ (16.0% greater), $P = 0.007$) post-consumption of the high-fat meal. It was concluded that the consumption of wild blueberries, a food source with high in vitro antioxidant properties, was associated with a diet-induced increase *in vivo* serum antioxidant status. A few years later, a similar study was conducted [65]. Changes in plasma antioxidant capacity (AOC) following consumption of a single meal of different berries or fruits including lowbush blueberry were studied in five clinical trials with six to ten subjects per experiment. Consumption of blueberries in two studies increased the value of hydrophilic AOC. This study also demonstrated consumption of blueberries was associated with increased plasma AOC in the postprandial state and consumption of an energy source of macronutrients containing no antioxidants was associated with a decline in plasma AOC.

3.3.3. Improving Endothelial Dysfunction

Endothelial dysfunction, including impaired vasomotor disturbance, abnormal coagulation and increased vascular proliferation, is closely associated with the development of atherosclerosis and precedes the clinical manifestations of atherosclerosis [39,41,66,67]. Many functions of the endothelium are influenced by nitric oxide (NO), which is synthesized by endothelial NO synthase (eNOS). Endothelial dysfunction in hypercholeserolemic patients is in large part due to a reduced bioavailability of NO. However, NO is produced by one of the three distinct isoforms of the enzyme nitric oxide synthase. These three isoforms have different locations and show different effects in atherosclerosis. For examples, studies demonstrated that eNOS driven NO synthesis causes development of major cardiovascular risk factors (insulin resistances, arterial hypertension and dyslipidaemia). Whereas stimulation of inducible NOS (iNOS) and NO overproduction causes metabolic insulin resistance and characterizes atherosclerosis, heart failure and cardiogenic shock in humans, suggesting a "Yin-Yang" effect of NO in the cardiovascular homeostasis. The unique role of NO in maintaining endothelial function and associated with other risk factors made it become an important target for nutritional intervention on prevention of atherosclerosis [68].

Blueberry polyphenol extracts were shown to afford protection to endothelial cells against stressor induced up-regulation of oxidative and inflammatory insults [69], and to reduce lipopolysaccharide (LPS)-induced pro-inflammatory mediators such as NO and iNOS [70]. These beneficial effects of blueberries might involve direct modulation of oxidative stress and/or inflammatory signaling cascades.

3.3.4. Mediating Inflammatory Factors

Inflammation is central to cardiovascular disease. It often begins with inflammatory changes in the endothelium, which can express the adhesion molecules such as VACM-1 and ICAM-1. Adhesion molecules attract monocytes, which then migrate through the endothelial layer under the influence of various pro-inflammatory chemoattractants. Once within the arterial intima, the monocytes continue to undergo inflammatory changes, transform into macrophages, engulf lipids, and become foam cells. T lymphocytes also migrate into the intima, where they release pro-inflammatory cytokines that amplify the inflammatory activity. Through these inflammatory processes, the initial lesion of atherosclerosis, the fatty streak, is formed [71,72].

Blueberry polyphenols have been shown to reduce tumor necrosis factor-alpha (TNF-α), induced up-regulation of various inflammatory mediators (IL-8, MCP-1 and ICAM-1) involved in the recruitment of leukocytes to sites of damage or inflammatory along the endothelium [69]. Treatment of BV2 microglial cells with blueberry extracts has been shown to be effective in reducing LPS-induced pro-inflammatory mediators such as NO, TNF-α interleukin-1 beta (IL-1β), iNOS, and cyclooxygenase 2 (COX2) [73]. A column-purified fraction of polyphenol-enriched blueberry extract was used to treat LPS-activated BV2 cells. The results thus far showed that blueberry polyphenols significantly suppressed iNOS and COX 2 promoter activities. In addition, blueberry polyphenols inhibited NF-κB nuclear translocation in LPS-activated BV2 cells. These findings suggested that the beneficial effects of blueberries may involve direct modulation of oxidative stress and/or inflammatory signaling cascades [70].

3.3.5. Other Mechanisms

An *in vitro* study showed that blueberries displayed strong the bile acid binding activities [74]. Binding of bile acids and increasing their fecal excretion has been hypothesized as a possible mechanism by which dietary fiber lowers cholesterol. By binding bile acids, food fractions prevent their reabsorption and stimulate plasma and liver cholesterol conversion to additional bile acids.

Conclusion

Blueberries contain high levels of polyphenols. The major polyphenols in blueberries have been well characterized as anthocyanins, proanthocyanidins, other flavonoids, phenolic acids and stilbene derivatives. Blueberries exhibit extremely high antioxidant capacity and potential anti-inflammatory effects. The experimental evidence supporting cardio-protective effects of blueberries have been rapidly accumulated in last few years. Studies from various *in vitro* models and from animals or human subjects have shown that blueberries have a potential role in the prevention of cardiovascular diseases. Blueberries may act mainly through the mechanisms such as reducing oxidative stress, decreasing inflammation, improving endothelial dysfunction and lowering blood pressure. However, the human studies are still very rare until now. Further research to determine the actual bioactive components in blueberries and their mechanisms are necessary.

References

[1] Bazzano, L.A.; Serdula, M.K.; Liu, S. Dietary intake of fruits and vegetables and risk of cardiovascular disease. *Current Atherosclerosis Reports*, 2003, *5*, 492-499.

[2] Galassetti, P.; Pontello, A. Dietary effects on oxidation of low-density lipoprotein and atherogenesis. *Current Atherosclerosis Reports*, 2006, *8*, 523-529.

[3] Ignarro, L.J.; Balestrieri, M.L.; Napoli, C. Nutrition, physical activity, and cardiovascular disease: an update. *Cardiovascular Research*, 2007, *73*, 326-340.

[4] Parikh, P.; McDaniel, M.C.; Ashen, M.D.; Miller, J.I.; Sorrentino, M.: Chan, V.; Blumenthal, R.S.; Sperling, L.S. Diets and cardiovascular disease: an evidence-based assessment. *Journal of the American College of Cardiology*, 2005, *45*, 1379-1387.

[5] Manach, C.; Mazur, A.; Scalbert, A. Polyphenols and prevention of cardiovascular diseases. *Current Opinion in Lipidology*, 2005, *16*, 77-84.

[6] Wu, X.; Beecher, G.R.; Holden, J.M.; Haytowitz, D.B.; Gebhardt, S.E.; Prior, R.L.; Lipophilic and hydrophilic antioxidant capacities of common foods in the United States. *Journal of Agricultural and Food Chemistry*, 2004, *52*, 4026-4037.

[7] Guo, W.; Kong, E.; Meydani, M. Dietary polyphenols, inflammation, and cancer. *Nutrition and Cancer*, 2009, 61, 807-810.

[8] Seeram, N.P.; Aviram, M.; Zhang, Y.; Henning, S.M.; Feng, L.; Dreher, M, Heber, D, Comparison of antioxidant potency of commonly consumed polyphenol-rich beverages

in the United States. *Journal of Agricultural and Food Chemistry*, 2008, *56*, 1415-1422.

[9] Barnes, J.S; Nguyen, H.P.; Shen, S.; Schug, K.A. General method for extraction of blueberry anthocyanins and identification using high performance liquid chromatography-electrospray ionization-ion trap-time of flight-mass spectrometry. *Journal of Chromatography A*, 2009, *1216*, 4728-4735.

[10] Wu, X.; Prior, R.L. Systematic identification and characterization of anthocyanins by HPLC-ESI-MS/MS in common foods in the United States: fruits and berries. *Journal of Agricultural and Food Chemistry*, 2005, *53*, 2589-2599.

[11] You, Q.; Wang, B.; Chen, F.; Huang, Z.; Wang, X.; Luo, P.G. Comparison of anthocyanins and phenolics in organically and conventionally grown blueberries in selected cultivars. *Food Chemistry*, 2011, *125*, 201-208.

[12] Prior, R.L.; Gu, L. Occurrence and biological significance of proanthocyanidins in the American diet. *Phytochemistry*, 2005, *66*, 2264-2280.

[13] Auger, C.; Al-Awwadi, N.; Bornet, A.; Rouanet, J.-M.; Gasc, F.; Cros, G.; Teissedre, P.-L. Catechins and procyanidins in Mediterranean diets. *Food Research International*, 2004, *37*, 233-245.

[14] Gu, L.; Kelm, M.; Hammerstone, J.F.; Beecher, G.; Cunningham, D.; Vannozzi, S.; Prior, R.L. Fractionation of polymeric procyanidins from lowbush blueberry and quantification of procyanidins in selected foods with an optimized normal-phase HPLC-MS fluorescent detection method. *Journal of Agricultural and Food Chemistry*, 2002, *50*, 4852-4860.

[15] Hummer, W.; Schreier, P. Analysis of proanthocyanidins. *Molecular Nutrition & Food Research*, 2008, *52*, 1381-1398.

[16] Prior, R.L, Lazarus, S.A.; Cao, G.; Muccitelli, H.; Hammerstone, J.F. Identification of procyanidins and anthocyanins in blueberries and cranberries (Vaccinium spp.) using high-performance liquid chromatography/mass spectrometry. *Journal of Agricultural and Food Chemistry*, 2001, *49*, 1270-1276.

[17] Kader, F.; Rovel, B.; Girardin, M.; Metche, M. Fractionation and identification of the phenolic compounds of Highbush blueberries (*Vaccinium corymbosum* L.). *Food Chemistry*, 1996, *55*, 35-40.

[18] Borges, G.; Degeneve, A.; Mullen, W.; Crozier, A. Identification of flavonoid and phenolic antioxidants in black currants, blueberries, raspberries, red currants, and cranberries. *Journal of Agricultural and Food Chemistry*, 2010, *58*, 3901-3909.

[19] Neto, C.C. Cranberry and blueberry: evidence for protective effects against cancer and vascular diseases. *Molecular Nutrition & Food Research*, 2007, *51*, 652-664.

[20] Kalt, W.; McDonald, J.E. Chemical composition of lowbush blueberry cultivars. *Journal of the American Society for Horticultural Science*, 1996, *121*, 142-146.

[21] Wang, S.Y.; Chen, C.-T. Effect of allyl isothiocyanate on antioxidant enzyme activities, flavonoids and post-harvest fruit quality of blueberries (*Vaccinium corymbosum* L., cv. Duke). *Food Chemistry*, 2010, *122*, 1153-1158.

[22] Rimando, A.M.; Kalt, W.; Magee, J.B.; Dewey, J.; Ballington, J.R. Resveratrol, pterostilbene, and piceatannol in vaccinium berries. *Journal of Agricultural and Food Chemistry*, 2004, *52*, 4713-4719.

[23] Wang, M, Li, J, Shao, Y, Huang, TC, Huang, MT, Chin, CK, Rosen, RT, Ho, CT, in: Shahidi, F, Ho, CT (Eds.), Phytochemicals and Phytopharmaceuticals, AOCS Press, Champaign, IL 2000, pp. 271–277.

[24] Heidenreich, P.A.; Trogdon, J.G.; Khavjou, O.A.; Butler, J.; Dracup, K.; Ezekowitz, M.D.; Finkelstein, E.A.; Hong, Y.; Johnston, S.C.; Khera, A.; Lloyd-Jones, D.M.; Nelson, S.A.; Nichol, G.; Orenstein, D.; Wilson, P.W.; Woo, Y.J. Forecasting the future of cardiovascular disease in the United States: a policy statement from the American Heart Association. *Circulation*, 2011, *in press*.

[25] Lusis, A.J. Atherosclerosis. *Nature*, 2000, *407*, 233-241.

[26] Heinecke, J.W. Lipoprotein oxidation in cardiovascular disease: chief culprit or innocent bystander? *Journal of Experimental Medicine*, 2006, *203*, 813-816.

[27] Steinberg, D. Oxidative Modification of LDL in the Pathogenesis of Atherosclerosis. *American Journal of Geriatric Cardiology*, 1993, *2*, 38-41.

[28] Stocker, R.; Keaney, J.F.J. Role of Oxidative Modifications in Atherosclerosis *Physiological Reviews*, 2004, *84*, 1381-1478.

[29] Zarraga, I.G.E.; Schwarz, E.R. Impact of dietary patterns and interventions on cardiovascular health. *Circulation*, 2006, *114*, 961-973.

[30] Hansson, G.K. Inflammation, Atherosclerosis, and Coronary Artery Disease. *New England Journal of Medicine*, 2005, *352*, 1685-1695.

[31] Libby, P. Inflammation in atherosclerosis. *Nature*, 2002, *420*, 868-874.

[32] Steinberg, D. Atherogenesis in perspective: Hypercholesterolemia and inflammation as partners in crime. *Nature Medicine*, 2002, *8*, 1211-1217.

[33] Blomhoff, R. Dietary antioxidants and cardiovascular disease. *Current Opinion in Lipidology*, 2005, *16*, 47-54.

[34] Hu, F.B. Plant-based foods and prevention of cardiovascular disease: an overview. *American Journal of Clinical Nutrition*, 2003, *78*, 544S-515S.

[35] Hung, H.-C.; Joshipura, K.J.; Jiang, R.; Hu, F.B.; Hunter, D.; Smith-Warner, S.A.; Colditz, G.A.; Rosner, B.; Spiegelman, D.; Willett, W.C. Fruit and vegetable intake and risk of major chronic disease. *Journal of the National Cancer Institute*, 2004, *96*, 1577-1584.

[36] Kalt, W.; Foote, K.; Fillmore, S.A.; Lyon, M.; Van Lunen, T.A.; McRae, K.B. Effect of blueberry feeding on plasma lipids in pigs. *British Journal of Nutrition*, 2008, *100*, 70-78.

[37] Vasan, R.S.; Larson, M.G.; Leip, E.P.; Evans, J.C.; O'Donnell, C.J.; Kannel, W.B.; Levy, D. Impact of high-normal blood pressure on the risk of cardiovascular disease. *New England Journal of Medicine*, 2001, *345*, 1291-1297.

[38] Shaughnessy, K.S., Boswall, I.A.; Scanlan, A.P., Gottschall-Pass, K.T.; Sweeney, M.I. Diets containing blueberry extract lower blood pressure in spontaneously hypertensive stroke-prone rats. *Nutrition Research*, 2009, *29*, 130-138.

[39] Cai, H.; Harrison, D.G. Endothelial dysfunction in cardiovascular diseases: the role of oxidant stress. *Circulation Research*, 2000, *87*, 840-844.

[40] Landmesser, U.; Hornig, B.; Drexler, H. Endothelial function: a critical determinant in atherosclerosis? *Circulation*, 2004, 109, II27-33.

[41] Okumura, K.; Imamura, A.; Murakami, R.; Numaguchi, Y.; Matsui, H.; Toyoaki, M. Endothelial function and early atherosclerotic changes. *Future Cardiology*, 2005, *1*, 501-508.
[42] Del Bo, C.; Kristo, A.S.; Kalea, A.Z.; Ciappellano, S.; Riso, P.; Porrini, M.; Klimis-Zacas, D. The temporal effect of a wild blueberry (*Vaccinium angustifolium*)-enriched diet on vasomotor tone in the Sprague-Dawley rat. *Nutrition, Metabolism & Cardiovascular Diseases*, 2010, *in press*.
[43] Kalea, A.; Lamari, F.; Theocharis, A.; Cordopatis, P.; Schuschke, D.A.; Karamanos, N.; Klimis-Zacas, D. Wild blueberry (*Vaccinium angustifolium*) consumption affects the composition and structure of glycosaminoglycans in Sprague-Dawley rat aorta. *Journal of Nutritional Biochemistry*, 2006, *17*, 109-116.
[44] Kalea, A.Z.; Clark, K.; Schuschke, D.A.; Klimis-Zacas, D.J. Vascular reactivity is affected by dietary consumption of wild blueberries in the Sprague-Dawley rat. *Journal of Medicinal Food*, 2009, *12*, 21-28.
[45] Kalea, A.Z.; Clark, K.; Schuschke, D.A.; Kristo, A.S.; Klimis-Zacas, D.J. Dietary enrichment with wild blueberries (*Vaccinium angustifolium*) affects the vascular reactivity in the aorta of young spontaneously hypertensive rats. *Journal of Nutritional Biochemistry*, 2010, *21*, 14-22.
[46] Kristo, A.S.; Kalea, A.Z.; Schuschke, D.A.; Klimis-Zacas, D.J. A wild blueberry-enriched diet (*Vaccinium angustifolium*) improves vascular tone in the adult spontaneously hypertensive rat. *Journal of Agricultural and Food Chemistry*, 2010, *58*, 11600-11605.
[47] Norton, C.; Kalea, A.; Harris, P.; Klimis-Zacas, D. Wild blueberry-rich diets affect the contractile machinery of the vascular smooth muscle in the Sprague-Dawley rat. *Journal of Medicinal Food*, 2005, *8*, 8-13.
[48] Karamanos, N.K. Glycosylation of proteins: specificity, biological role, and analysis of glycan moieties. *Journal of Protein Chemistry*, 1998, *17*, 513-514.
[49] Ohtsubo, K.; Marth, J.D. Glycosylation in cellular mechanisms of health and disease. *Cell*, 2006, *126*, 855-867.
[50] Tovar, A.M.; Cesar, D.C.; Leta, G.C.; Mourao, P.A. Age-related changes in populations of aortic glycosaminoglycans: species with low affinity for plasma low-density lipoproteins, and not species with high affinity, are preferentially affected. *Arteriosclerosis, Thrombosis, and Vascular Biology*, 1998, *18*, 604-614.
[51] Ahmet, I.; Spangler, E.; Shukitt-Hale, B.; Juhaszova, M.; Sollott, S.J.; Joseph, J.A.; Ingram, D.K.; Talan, M. Blueberry-enriched diet protects rat heart from ischemic damage. *PLoS One*, 2009, *4*, e5954.
[52] Ahmet, I.; Spangler, E.; Shukitt-Hale, B.; Joseph, J.A.; Ingram, D.K.; Talan, M. Survival and cardioprotective benefits of long-term blueberry enriched diet in dilated cardiomyopathy following myocardial infarction in rats. *PLoS One*, 2009, *4*, e7975.
[53] Wu, X.; Kang, J.; Xie, C.; Burris, R.; Ferguson, M.E.; Badger, T.M.; Nagarajan, S. Dietary blueberries attenuate atherosclerosis in apolipoprotein E-deficient mice by upregulating antioxidant enzyme expression. *Journal of Nutrition*, 2010, *140*, 1628-1632.

[54] Meir, K.S.; Leitersdorf, E. Atherosclerosis in the apolipoprotein-E-deficient mouse: a decade of progress. *Arteriosclerosis, Thrombosis, and Vascular Biology*, 2004, *24*, 1006-1014.

[55] Wouters, K.; Shiri-Sverdlov, R.; van Gorp, P.J.; van Bilsen, M.; Hofker, M.H. Understanding hyperlipidemia and atherosclerosis: lessons from genetically modified apoe and ldlr mice. *Clinical Chemistry and Laboratory Medicine*, 2005, *43*, 470-479.

[56] Letters, J.M.; Witting, P.K.; Christison, J.K.; Eriksson, A.W.; Pettersson, K.; Stocker, R. Time-dependent changes to lipids and antioxidants in plasma and aortas of apolipoprotein E knockout mice. *Journal of Lipid Research*, 1999, *40*, 1104-1112.

[57] Basu, A.; Du, M.; Leyva, M.J.; Sanchez, K.; Betts, N.M.; Wu, M.; Aston, C.E.; Lyons, T.J. Blueberries decrease cardiovascular risk factors in obese men and women with metabolic syndrome. *Journal of Nutrition*, 2010, *140*, 1582-1587.

[58] Wu, X.; Beecher, G.R.; Holden, J.M.; Haytowitz, D.B.; Gebhardt, S.E.; Prior, R,L. Concentrations of anthocyanins in common foods in the United States and estimation of normal consumption. *Journal of Agricultural and Food Chemistry*, 2006, *54*, 4069-4075.

[59] Hörkköa, S.; Bindera, C.J.; Shawa, P.X.; Changa, M.-K.; Silvermana, G., Palinskia, W.; Witztum, J.L. Immunological responses to oxidized LDL. *Free Radical Biology & Medicine*, 2000, *28*, 1771-1779.

[60] Kita, T.; Kume, N.; Minami, M.; Hayashida, K.; Murayama, T.; Sano, H.; Moriwaki, H.; Kataoka, H.; Nishi, E.; Horiuchi, H.; Arai, H.; Yokode, M. Role of Oxidized LDL in Atherosclerosis. *Annals of the New York Academy of Sciences*, 2001, *947*, 199-206.

[61] Heinonen, I.M.; Meyer, A.S.; Frankel, E.N. Antioxidant activity of berry phenolics on human low-density lipoprotein and liposome oxidation. *Journal of Agricultural and Food Chemistry*, 1998, *46*, 4107-4112.

[62] Marniemi, J.; Hakala, P.; Maki, J.; Ahotupa, M. Partial resistance of low density lipoprotein to oxidation in vivo after increased intake of berries. *Nutrition, Metabolism & Cardiovascular Diseases*, 2000, *10*, 331-337.

[63] McAnulty, S.; McAnulty, L.; Morrow, J.; Khardouni, D.; Shooter, L.; Monk, J.; Gross, S.; Brown, V. Effect of daily fruit ingestion on angiotensin converting enzyme activity, blood pressure, and oxidative stress in chronic smokers. *Free Radical Research*, 2005, *39*, 1241-1248.

[64] Kay, C.D.; Holub, B.J. The effect of wild blueberry (Vaccinium angustifolium) consumption on postprandial serum antioxidant status in human subjects. *British Journal of Nutrition*, 2002, *88*, 389-398.

[65] Prior, R.L.; Gu, L.; Wu, X.; Jacob, R.A.; Sotoudeh, G.; Kader, A.A,; Cook, R.A. Plasma antioxidant capacity changes following a meal as a measure of the ability of a food to alter in vivo antioxidant status. *Journal of the American College of Nutrition*, 2007, *26*, 170-181.

[66] Kawashima, S.; Yokoyama, M. Dysfunction of endothelial nitric oxide synthase and atherosclerosis. *Arteriosclerosis, Thrombosis, and Vascular Biology*, 2004, *24*, 998-1005.

[67] Landmesser, U.; Hornig, B.; Drexler, H. Endothelial dysfunction in hypercholesterolemia: mechanisms, pathophysiological importance, and therapeutic interventions. *Seminars in Thrombosis and Hemostasis*, 2000, *26*, 529-537.

[68] Ignarro, L.; Napoli, C. Novel features of nitric oxide, endothelial nitric oxide synthase, and atherosclerosis. *Current Diabetes Reports*, 2005, *5*, 17-23.

[69] Youdim, K.; McDonald, J.; Kalt, W.; Joseph, J. Potential role of dietary flavonoids in reducing microvascular endothelium vulnerability to oxidative and inflammatory insults. *Journal of Nutritional Biochemistry*, 2002, *13*, 282-288.

[70] Lau, F.C.; Joseph, J.A.; McDonald, J.E.; Kalt, W. Attenuation of iNOS and COX2 by blueberry polyphenols is mediated through the suppression of NF-κB activation. *Journal of Functional Foods*, 2009, *1*, 274-283.

[71] Libby, P. Inflammation and cardiovascular disease mechanisms. *American Journal of Clinical Nutrition*, 2006, *83*, 456S-460S.

[72] Libby, P. Inflammatory mechanisms: the molecular basis of inflammation and disease. *Nutrition Reviews*, 2007, *65*, S140-146.

[73] Lau, F.C.; Bielinski D.F.; Joseph, J.A. Inhibitory effects of blueberry extract on the production of inflammatory mediators in lipopolysaccharide-activated BV2 microglia. *Journal of Neuroscience*, 2007, *85*, 1010-1017.

[74] Kahlon, T.S.; Smith, G.E. In vitro binding of bile acids by blueberries (Vaccinium spp.), plums (Prunus spp.), prunes (Prunus spp.), strawberries (Fragaria x ananassa), cherries (Malpighia punicifolia), cranberries (*Vaccinium macrocarpon*) and apples (*Malus sylvestris*). *Food Chemistry*, 2006, *100*, 1182-1187.

In: Berries: Properties, Consumption and Nutrition
Editor: Carlo Tuberoso
ISBN 978-1-61470-257-3

Chapter V

Flavour Properties and Chemistry of Berries

Mari Sandell*[*1,2], Oskar Laaksonen[1] and Saara Lundén[2]
[1]Department of Biochemistry and Food Chemistry
[2]Functional Foods Forum
University of Turku, Turku, Finland

Abstract

Flavour is a combination of odour, taste and chemesthesis. Various volatile and non-volatile chemical compounds are contributing to berry flavour. To understand the role of those compounds in sensory perception of berries, it is necessary to connect chemico-physical analyses to sensory evaluation. Trained sensory panel is sensitive to describe and rate the intensity of different flavours, but not able to identify the compounds causing the properties. Many factors such as berry genus, variety, growing conditions, stage of ripeness and processing affect flavour. Berries are very sensitive material to quality changes. Different headspace techniques are useful tools to extract the volatile berry compounds. Gas chromatography coupled to sniffing system for instance makes it possible to study the odour active compounds. In the case of non-volatile orosensory contributing compounds the modern methods using liquid chromatography coupled with mass spectrometry are very important. Moreover, it is very important to optimise the sample preparation to be similar both in sensory studies and instrumental measurements. Multiregression methods should be applied to investigate the interaction between perceived flavour and chemical composition. This chapter reviews studies concerning berry odour, taste and astringency. It demonstrates the complexity of berry flavour. The berry samples investigated here are strawberry, black currant, bilberry, crowberry and sea buckthorn and they have been growing in North Europe.

[*] E-mail: mari.sandell@utu.fi.

1. Introduction

Berries in general are rich in bioactive compounds and a good choice for a healthy food [1-8]. Wild and cultivated berries such as strawberry, sea buckthorn, black currant, cloudberry and bilberry are regarded as natural high value food products and sources of many essential nutritional components compared to orange (Table 1). These berries are rich in favourable minerals such as potassium, magnesium and calcium and plant phytonutrients that act as antioxidants [9-13]. They contain a lot of water, they are lactose, gluten and cholesterol free and the content of sodium is very low. Berry seed oils contain a plentiful amount of different functional compounds [14-18]. Cuticula of the berry skin contains in addition to cellulose various nutritionally important polymeric compounds such as cutins and cutans [19].

Food products and food ingredients become nutrition for people after swallowing and ingestion. No matter how healthy or important a food product is, it does not reach its goal if people avoid it. For many people, food flavour has a great impact on food choice, acceptability and eating. Flavour is affected by both the non-volatile and the volatile chemical compounds of food. Flavour is a combination of taste, odour and other chemosensory sensation such as astringency in berries. The American Society for Testing and Materials (ASTM) defines astringency as "the complex of sensations due to shrinking, drawing or puckering of the epithelium as a result of exposure to the substances such as alums or tannic acids".

Table 1. Average amounts (g) of selected nutritional components in 100 g of the edible portion of selected berries compared to orange

	Straw berry	Sea buckthorn	Black currant	Cloud-berry	Bil-berry	Cran-berry	Lingon-berry	Orange
Energy (kJ)	195	377	247	225	184	136	162	197
Fat	0.2	5	0.4	0.5	0.6	0.7	0.5	0.3
Organic acids	1.6	2	2.7	0	1.4	1.4	0	0.6
Sugars	8.4	6.3	7.8	7.8	6.4	3.5	6.7	8.9
Sucrose	2.3	0.1	0.3	0.1	0.5	0.1	0.2	3.6
Fructose	3.0	2.5	4.0	3.7	2.9	0	2.9	2.7
Glucose	3.1	3.7	3.5	4.0	3.0	2.2	3.6	2.6
Fibre	1.9	6	5.8	6.3	3.3	3.3	2.6	2.1
Linoleic acid	0.064	0.250	0.045	0.084	0.123	0.125	0.125	0.032
Linolenic acid	0.064	0.090	0.027	0.075	0.117	0.143	0.143	0.028
Vitamin C	0.060	0.165	0.120	0.100	0.015	0.020	0.0075	0.051
Ca	0.021	0.042	0.072	0.016	0.019	0.013	0.022	0.054
K	0.190	0.133	0.340	0.170	0.110	0.025	0.080	0.150
Mg	0.015	0.030	0.024	0.029	0.009	0.008	0.009	0.013
Na	0.0007	0.0035	0.0050	0.0015	0.0003	0.0009	0.0002	0.0016
NaCl	0.0018	0.0089	0.0013	0.0038	0.0008	0.0023	0.0005	0.0041

Source: National Institute for health and welfare (Finland, 2010).

Berries have characteristic flavour due to numerous volatile compounds and non-volatiles, such as acids, sugars and phenolic compounds [7,20-21]. The characteristics of flavour and aroma vary widely among the berries. This is due to the differences in morphology, structure, and especially due to flavour precursor matrix and genomics of different berry genera and species [21-25]. Also the growing conditions may affect chemical composition [9,24-29]. Berries are very sensitive to quality changes in different ways during their growing, harvest and processing [24-25,28]. This may be perceived as off-flavours also. Although the chemical composition of the berry and the sensory properties of different chemical compounds may be known, the interactions of compounds in matrices are unpredictable without proper research into the berry itself. In order to understand the physiological effects behind the sensory quality of various berries, the composition of berries and their fractions have to be investigated in detail.

The focus of this chapter is on flavour and flavour related volatile and non-volatile chemical compounds in berries such as strawberry, sea buckthorn, black currant, crowberry and bilberry. Our special goal is to identify the interactions between the flavour perception and chemical compounds by using different berries as models.

2. Description of Berries

Most of the berries reviewed in this chapter have been cultivated or grown wild in Finland, handpicked fully ripe and studied at University of Turku. They were frozen (-20 °C) immediately after harvest, pooled and stored for analyses.

Strawberry (*Fragaria* x *ananassa* Duch.) is cultivated world widely. It is considered by many to be their favourite berry crop mainly because of its pleasantness. However, it is a very perishable fruit and sensitive to injuries. In Finland it is the main horticultural crop. This chapter will focus on varieties 'Senga Sengana', 'Jonsok', 'Korona', 'Polka', 'Honeoye', and 'Bounty'.

Sea buckthorn (*Hippophaë rhamnoides* L.) berries have increasing commercial importance among Western consumers. Both the berries and leaves have been used for centuries in traditional Chinese medicine and nutrition to diminish the risk of several diseases and to maintain good health. Sea buckthorn berries occur in several subspecies, of which the commercially most important are Chinese ssp. *sinensis*, Russian ssp. *mongolica* and European ssp. *rhamnoides*. This chapter will focus on the varieties 'Avgustinka', 'Oranzhevaya', 'Botanicheskaya', 'Trofimovskaya', 'Prozcharachnaya', 'Prevoshodnaya' and 'Raisa'.

Black currant (*Ribes nigrum*) is cultivated around the world and the plant belongs to the family *Grossulariaceae*. Black currant is the second biggest cultivated berries in Finland. Cutin composition of black currant is known to be significantly different from many other berries growing in Finland [19]. This chapter will focus more on variety 'Mortti'.

Crowberry (*Empetrum nigrum*) is a small shrub with edible berries growing wild in northern hemisphere. It is one of the biggest and the most stabile wild berry crop in the whole Scandinavia but still under-exploited. It has an intense colour based on anthocyanins of which 50 % is bound in the cuticular skin of the berry [11]. The keeping quality of crowberry is exceptionally good. The unique skin is build up of a complex, three dimensional network that protects the berry flesh.

Bilberry (*Vaccinium myrtillus* L.) belongs to the genus *Vaccinium* along with blueberries (*V. corymbosum* L. and other blueberries), and cranberries (*Vaccinium oxycoccos* L.). Bilberries are traditionally used in juices or jams and as colorants due to their high anthocyanin content. In Finland bilberry is very popular wild berry crop and favoured by consumers.

3. Sensory Evaluation and Statistical Procedures

In this chapter the berry samples were evaluated with trained panels. The assessors were pretrained to recognize sensory stimuli samples, to rank the reference solutions and differentiate samples in triangle tests. Generic descriptive analysis with a structured line scale of 0-10 was used. The evaluation was performed at the sensory laboratory in accordance with the ISO 8589-1988 standard. The general guidelines for the selection, training and monitoring for assessors (ISO 8586-1) and DIS 11035 methodology for the identification of descriptors (ISO/DIS 1992) were followed. Samples were evaluated in randomized order during parallel sessions with the help of anchored reference compounds and by using the Compusense-*five* data collection software (version 4.6, Compusense, Guelph, ON, Canada).

The key compounds contributing to essential sensory properties can be identified using multivariate statistical analyses, especially partial least squares (PLS) regression. The variation of the instrumentally analysed chemical composition may be used to explain the variation of the sensory data.

In the studies discussed in this chapter, the PLS2-method was applied for standardized data to detect the relationships between the two data matrices X and Y. X-variables (predictors) were the chemical compounds and Y-variables (responses) were the sensory properties. Cross validation was used to estimate a number of principal components for statistically reliable models. Multivariate analyses were performed using versions of Unscrambler (Camo Process AS, Oslo, Norway). The differences between various variable groups were also analysed using one-way- and two-way-ANOVAs with suitable post-hoc tests.

4. Odour Properties of Strawberry and Sea Buckthorn

Odour may be a complex group of sensations compromising both the nasal (orthonasal) and oral (retronasal) perception. In general, odour compound needs to be volatile. However, all the volatile compounds are not odour active or aroma compounds. The volatile compounds differ in their molecular weight, polarity and volatility.

In berries the volatiles are so called secondary plant metabolites. They exist in the fruit in their free form or glycosidically bound. They are derived from the fatty acid, the amino acid, the phenylpropanoid (Shikimi), and the terpene metabolism. The contributions of the individual compounds to odour or flavour are depending on their odour threshold, concentration and their relation to the other compounds. Volatiles exist at ppm and sub-ppm levels, and the profile of berry volatiles is usually very complex [30-31].

4.1. Odour Chemistry of the Berries

The method for sampling volatile compounds depends on the analytical problem to be solved. Volatile compounds might be isolated with liquid extraction [32], simultaneous distillation-extraction, solid-phase extraction, supercritical fluid extraction or applying different headspace collection methods [33-34].

With headspace method there is no need to use separate clean up procedures and it allows the study of relatively volatile and free compounds. The advantage of the headspace method compared to conventional extraction techniques such as solvent extraction is its nondestructivity and capability to isolate volatiles in their natural form. Another advantage of the headspace method is that it simulates sniffing, where the sample is also taken from headspace.

All steps of analyses including sample preparation, collection techniques of volatiles, and also respective analytical method can cause the losses of certain compounds or the formation of artefacts. The profiles of volatile compounds in headspace of mashed berries could be analysed with gas chromatography mass spectrometry (GC-MS) applying dynamic purge-and-trap sampling [33-34] or solid phase microextraction (SPME) [35].

To find out the key compounds contributing to odour or aroma there is a need to compare instrumental data to data received with human senses. In case of odours, one suitable tool would be GC-sniffing system where the volatiles will be analysed with gas chromatography coupled to the special sniffing port [36]. The sniffing panellist will be evaluating the eluent odour by odour and describing the quality of odorants. A trained panel will create the odour profile or aromagram finally. After the hard data processing the aromagram will be correlated with the volatile profile of berry sample received with GC to find out the correlation between compounds found in headspace sample and their odours based on sniffing results. In addition to sniffing, the odour profile might be created with a trained sensory panel in the sensory laboratory using descriptive analyses. The interaction between sensory profile and chemical composition needs to be studied with a suitable statistical method, such as multivariate regression analysis.

4.2. Strawberry Odour

Many investigators world widely have studied the aroma of both fresh and frozen strawberries. The main compounds contributing to strawberry odour are esters, furanones, aldehydes, terpenes, sulfur compounds and alcohols. The perceived odour descriptions and some of the measured thresholds of different strawberry volatiles are shown in Table 2.

The variety, maturity and storage conditions affect the composition of strawberry aroma [37]. Over 350 volatile compounds have been identified in strawberries [38-39]. The relationship between the aroma impact volatiles and strawberry varieties has been the subject of numerous investigations [40-43]. Esters in general contribute fruity and floral notes to the overall aroma [44]. Butanoates and hexanoates are the dominating esters.

Table 2. Common strawberry aroma compounds with odour perception description analysed with GC-sniffing

Compound	Odour perception	Odour threshold mg/kg[40]	Reference
γ-Decalactone	Sweet/caramel-like, peach, fruity	0.001 - 0.01	[40,46,52,54]
γ-Dodecalactone	Strawberry-like		[52]
β-Ionone	Nuts/sweet		[52]
2-Heptanone	Blue cheese	0.001-0.01	[40,54]
2-Pentanone	Kerosene, solvent	0.01-0.1	[40,54]
2-Methyl propanoic acid	Burnt	0.01-0.1	[40]
2-Methyl butanoic acid	Fruity	0.01-0.1	[40,54]
3-Methylbutanoic acid	Sweaty		[53]
2,5-Dimethyl-4-methoxy-3(2H)-furanone (DMMF, Mesifuran)	Caramel like, bread, fusty	0.1-1.0	[40,52,53,54]
2,5-Dimethyl-4-hydroxy-3(2H)-furanone (DMHF, Furaneol®)	Burnt, sweet caramel	0.001-0.01	[40,53,54]
3-Methyl-2-heptanol	Parsley		[52]
Acetic acid	Vinegar, sour	10-100	[40,53]
Pentyl acetate	Fruity		[52]
Benzaldehyde	Lecherous		[52]
Butyl acetate	Apple, glue	0.01-0.1	[40,54]
Butanoic acid	Sour, sweaty	0.1-1	[40,53,54]
2,3-butanedione	Buttery		[53]
Cinnamyl acetate	Cooked sugar		[52]
Cis-3-hexenol	Green, leaf-like		[53,54]
Cyclohexyl acetate	Fruity		[52]
Ethyl 2-butenoate	Cooked apple		[52]
Ethyl acetate	Chemical	0.1-1.0	[40,52]
Ethyl butanoate	Vanilla-like, fruity, sweet, cheese	$0.1 \times 10^{-5-4}$	[40,46,52,53,54]
Ethyl hexanoate	Fruity, acid, fresh, sweet	$0.1 \times 10^{-4-3}$	[40,46,52,54]
Ethyl cinnamate	Caramel-like		[52]
Ethyl 2-methylpropanoate	Fruity		[52,53]
Ethyl 3-methylbutanoate	Cooked apple, fruity		[52,53]
Ethyl 2-methylbutanoate	Fruity, sweet		[53,5]
Ethyl propanoate	Sweet-caramel		[52]
Hexanoic acid	Fatty, stuffy, sour sweet	1-10	[40,52,54]

3-Methylbutyl acetate	Fruity		[52]
3-Methylbutyl alcohol	Apple jam		[52]
1-Methylethyl hexanoate	Sweet, fresh		[5]
Linalool	Floral, lemon peel, sweet	$0.1x10^{-3-2}$	[40,52,54,5]
Methyl 2-methylbutanoate	Cooked apple, fruity		[52,53]
Methyl butanoate	Fruity, cheese	0.001-0.01	[40,54,5]
Methyl hexanoate	Fruity/pineapple	0.01-0.1	[40,52,54]
Compound	Odour perception	Odour threshold mg/kg*	Reference
Methyl caprylate	Coriander		[52]
Methyl 3-methylbutanoate	Fruity		[53]
Methyl propanoate	Floral/pineapple		[52]
Myrtenal	Nuts/sweet		[52]
Nerolidol	Green fruity, fir, pine, linoleum	0.01-0.1	[40,52]
n-hexanal	Green, sour	0.01-0.1	[40,52]
n-hexyl acetate	Banana/pineapple/cooked apple	0.01-0.1	[40,52]
n-nonyl acetate	Gardenia		[52]
Non-2-en-1-ol	Cooked milk		[52]
Nonanal	Green-pungent		[52]
Octanal	Chemical/green		[52]
Octyl acetate	Perfumed		[52]
Pentanal	Green		[52]
Propanoic acid	Fruity, silage	0.1-1	[40]
Trans-2-hexenal	Sweet	0.01-0.1	[40,52,54]
Trans-hex-2-enol	Green, fruity, burnt	0.1-1	[40]
Trans-hex-3-enol	Chemical		[52]
Trans-nonadien-2,4-al	Tissue		[52]
Trans-nonadien-2,4-al	Tissue		[52]

Flavour impact compounds to the flavour of fresh strawberries have been found to be *cis*-3-hexenal, γ-decalactone, methyl and ethyl 2-methylbutanoate, 2,5-dimethyl-4-hydroxy-3(*2H*)-furanone (DMHF) [46]. For a typical strawberry flavour DMHF and 2,5-dimethyl-4-methoxy-3(*2H*)-furanone (DMMF, Mesifuran) are very important compounds [32, 40, 47-48].

DMHF is water-soluble and easily degraded by elevated temperatures and acidic pH, with better stability observed at +5 °C and pH 4 [49-50]. Descriptions of their odour perceptions are dependent on the concentration and ratio of key aroma compounds. Sulphur containing compounds have been noticed to play an important role in strawberry flavour as well [51]. Alcohols and C_6 aldehydes are mainly responsible for the green and pungent impression [45,52].

In our own Finnish study the profiles of volatile aroma compounds in the headspace (HS) of strawberry varieties were analysed by using gas chromatography-mass spectrometry (GC-MS) applying dynamic purge-and-trap sampling [33]. Frozen samples of the strawberries were gently melted in a microwave oven and homogenised for each analysis. A total of 23 esters, 7 aldehydes, 7 alcohols and 8 ketones were identified from six different strawberry varieties. Difference between the strawberry varieties was significant due to the volatile profiles. Based on SPME sample collection and GC-sniffing analyses methyl butanoate, ethyl butanoate, 2-heptanone, methyl hexanoate, ethyl hexanoate, and linalool were described as compounds of the contributing to odour of strawberry variety 'Senga Sengana'.

In addition to volatile compounds six odour attributes (total odour, sweet, green, fruity, strawberry flavour, off-odour) of strawberries were evaluated with a trained panel (n=14) by applying generic descriptive analysis. Intensities of odour properties were significantly different between the strawberry varieties 'Senga Sengana', 'Jonsok', 'Korona', 'Polka', 'Honeoye', and 'Bounty' (Table 3).

Flavour profile including odours together with sweetness and sourness was compared to chemical composition containing a total of 79 variables such as volatile compounds [33], sugars (fructose, glucose and sucrose), acids (citric and malic acid) soluble solids (°Brix), pH and titratable acidity [20]. Sweetness and strawberry flavour were located at the opposite side relative to sourness and strawberry odour [55]. This indicates that taste may more important flavour component of frozen strawberries than odour, although the odour is also important.

The strongest predictors for strawberry sweetness within varieties were the ratio of Sugar/Acid (β-coefficient = 0.253), sucrose (0.215), sum of fructose, glucose and sucrose (0.200), methyl pentanoate (0.239), methyl butanoate (0.195), and pH (0.134). The correlation between these showed a linear regression $y = 0.96x + 0.12$, with a Root Mean Square error (RMSE) of 0.25.

For fruity-flavour the strongest predictors were sucrose (0.202), methyl pentanoate (0.239), methyl butanoate (0.221), sum of citric and malic acid (-0.241), 2-heptanone (-0.209), and ratio of °Brix and dry matter (-0.151). The correlation between these compounds and fruity-flavour showed a linear regression $y = 0.94x + 0.26$, with RMSE 0.15. Within 'Senga Sengana' samples, the fruity-odour had a strong relationship ($y = 0.81x + 0.34$, RMSE 0.13) with *trans*-2-hexenal (0.900), and green-odour ($y = 0.84x + 0.59$, RMSE 0.20) with magnesium (0.915).

Compounds with a strong variety effect were 3-methyl-2-pentanone, hexanal, methylethyl butanoate, 3-methylbutyl acetate, propyl butanoate, and methyl hexanoate. Of those methylethyl butanoate, 3-methylbutyl acetate, propyl butanoate were missing or at a low level in 'Honeoye'. 'Bounty' lacked 3-methyl-2-pentanone and 3-methylbutyl acetate, 'Korona' 3-methyl-2-pentanone, and 'Polka' 3-methylbutyl acetate. The level of hexanal was very low in 'Senga' and 'Jonsok', but high in the profile of 'Honeoye'.

Table 3. Ranges of variation in intensities of sensory properties (0-10) in strawberry varieties (n=6) with results of ANOVA

Quality factor	Intensity	ANOVA Samples
Sweet odour	2.1-4.6	***
Green odour	1.3-2.6	***
Fruity odour	2.3-4.1	*
Strawberry odour	2.7-4.5	n.s.

Off-odour	1-2.9	**
Fruity flavour	3.5-5.3	***
Strawberry flavour	2.8-5.8	**

ANOVA *= $p<0.05$, ** = $p<0.01$, *** = $p < 0.001$, n.s. = non significant difference.

In general, 'Korona' was evaluated to be sweetest and least sour of the varieties, while 'Honeoye' was the opposite. 'Polka' and 'Korona' were sweet and strawberry-like, while 'Honeoye', 'Jonsok' and 'Senga Sengana' were sourer with a strong off-odour. The year-dependent variation of properties was highest in 'Bounty', which was similar to 'Korona' and 'Polka' in the sunny and warm growing season. In a rainy season 'Bounty' was similar to 'Senga' and 'Jonsok' when chemical composition and sensory properties were compared.

4.3. Sea Buckthorn Odour

During the last decades the composition and health beneficial effects of sea buckthorn have been widely studied due to the special nutritional composition and the health value. However, very few studies have been performed on the sensory properties of the berry. Sea buckthorn berries are known to be intensely sour and astringent with a mild but unique aroma [21,35,56]. Esters are the most numerous compounds that characterise the volatile aroma compound composition in sea buckthorn juice.

The juice headspace has been characterized by esters formed of ethane – pentane, iso- and ante-iso alcohols and butane – pentane, iso- and ante-iso acids. The most abundant esters are 3-methylbutyl hexanoate, 3-methylbutyl 3-methylbutanoate, 3-methylbutyl benzoate, 3-methylbutyl 2-methylbutanoate, ethyl hexanoate and 3-methylbutyl octanoate. Terpenes and aromatic compounds, which generally are typical for fruits and berries in general, are present only in low contents in sea buckthorn [39].

Different origins and times of harvest have shown to have a clear effect on the profiles of volatiles [35]. Varieties 'Oranzhevaya' and 'Chuiskaya' have shown to have high contents of ethyl 3-methylbutanoate as well as 3-methylbutanol, which is low in 'Raisa'. The proportion of ethyl butanoate is higher in 'Oranzhevaya' and 'Pvoshodnaya' in relation to the other varieties. 'Pvoshodnaya' had also high proportions of ethyl hexanoate and ethyl octanoate. Compared to the other samples, 'Avgustinka' was low in ethyl hexanoate and, on the contrary, very high in 3-methylbutyl 3-methylbutanoate.

Although sea buckthorn's smell is mild it is also characteristic and an important factor of the berry offering a wonderful detail to flavour. Based on the orthonasal odour study of sea buckthorn from four different origin there was a significant difference between berry sub species (ssp) [36]. However, sample berries were growing in the same geographical area. A total of 74 volatile compounds were identified and a total of 91 compounds were detected in the headspace of the sea buckthorn berries.

The most numerous compounds found were esters such as ethyl hexanoate, 3-methylbutyl 3-methylbutanoate and ethyl 2-methylbutanoate (Table 4). Higher amount of ethanol was correlating with higher intensity of pungent odour that was related to two varieties of ssp. *mongolica* origin 'Avgustinka' and 'Trofimovskaja'. Propyl 2-

methylbutanoate was correlating with fermented odour and was related to the sample of wild strain ssp. *sinensis*. Based on GC-sniffing aromagram ethanol was described as solvent and pungent like. Ethanol was important descriptor for 'Avgustinka' and 'Trofimovskaja'. Compounds described as mushroom and fertiliser like or fermented were most abundant and also only or most often perceived in wild strain of ssp. *sinensis* origin.

Table 4. Common sea buckthorn aroma compounds with odour perception description analysed with GC-sniffing and range of relative concentrations of most abundant volatile compounds

Compound	Description	Concentration[1]
Ethanol	Solvent, pungent	20-70
Ethyl 2-methylbutanoate	sweet, strawberry	29-326
Ethyl 3-methylbutanoate	sweet, fruity	46-610
Propyl 2-methylbutanoate	sweet, berrylike	0-9
2-methylpropyl 2-methylbutanoate	mushroom, solvent	0-309
2-methylpropyl 3-methylbutanoate	mushroom, fertiliser	0-686
Ethyl hexanoate	fruity, berrylike	50-1693
3-metylbutyl 2-methylpropanoate		0-321
2-methylbutyl 2-methylbutanoate		0-604
3-methylbutyl 3-methylbutanoate	fermented, spoiled, compost	3-1517
Ethyl benzoate	sweet, plastic, artificial	5-278
Ethyl octanoate	coconut, synthetic	9-382
3-methylbutyl hexanoate		1-268
3-methylbutyl benzoate	pungent, sour	2-141

[1]Relative concentrations were calculated dividing the peak area with internal standard (methyl butanoate) peak area and multiplying the ratio with internal standard concentration.

5. Taste Properties of Black Currant, Bilberry and Crowberry

The perception of taste begins when specific non-volatile food components contact receptors in the human mouth. The chemical signals are converted into the electrical signals by receptor cells and transducted to central nervous system. There the information is perceived as sensation and recognized if possible. Sense of taste detects at least sweetness, saltiness, sourness, bitterness, and umami.

In this part of the chapter, the taste properties and chemical profiles of black currant, bilberry and crowberry and their fractions are described briefly. The key chemical properties contributing to taste and astringency of these berries will be discussed. Some other berries are also included and the references are shown later in the text. Although astringency is a chemically induced tactile sensation rather than a taste quality it is included here to orosensory properties together with taste modalities due to its importance in berry flavour.

5.1. Taste Chemistry of the Berries

There are many qualitative and quantitative methods that may be applied to analyses of non-volatile orosensory contributing compounds. The modern methods using liquid chromatography (LC) coupled with mass spectrometry (MS) or 1D/2D-NMR experiments for example are very important tools [57-62]. In these approaches the sample preparation such as special fractionation should be optimized carefully.

In this chapter sugars and organic fruit acids were determined as trimethylsilyl derivatives by gas chromatography coupled with flame ionization detector [20]. Sorbitol and tartaric acid were used as internal standards. Compounds were identified with the help of reference compounds and the previous knowledge of these compounds in berries. Sugar and acid contents were determined from diluted juice and extracts. Anthocyanins, flavonol glycosides and their aglycones and hydroxycinnamic acid derivatives of the berry fractions were analyzed with LC-DAD and LC-MS. For anthocyanin analysis; samples were prepared by extracting the fraction consecutively with acidified methanol and for analysis of other phenolic compounds; extractions were made using ethyl acetate. Additionally, acid hydrolysis was used to verify the aglycon parts of the compounds. The quantitative analyses and preliminary identifications were carried out with the reverse phase LC-DAD with the help reference compounds and UV-vis spectra. The quantifications were carried out using external standards. The corresponding reference compound was used when commercially available and for others the most abundant reference compound in corresponding phenolic compound class was used. The identifications were confirmed with LC-MS in mass range of *m/z* 250–1000. For detailed description of the methods used with black currant, bilberry and crowberry, see original publications [57-59].

5.2. Taste Properties of the Berry Fractions

Black currants, crowberries and bilberries were fractioned to the sensory and chemical analyses in order to determine the key sensory properties of each part of the berry and essential compounds contributing to them. Fractionation and sample preparation for crowberry samples is shown in Figure 1. Berries were first thawed and crushed and then fractioned by juice pressing and ethanol extraction of the press residue (Residue I, Figure 1). Ethanol was evaporated after the extractions and filtration of extracts and the extracts were dissolved to either water or corresponding berry juice. This processing resulted in fractions: juice, press residue, several ethanol extracts and a residue after ethanol extractions (Residue II) and for crowberry, a residue after supercritical fluid extraction (SFE, Residue III). Though the separate extracts are not further discussed in this book chapter (see literature references for more details) the combination of the extracts (Extract, Figure 1) is shown in results. The compositional and sensory analyses were carried out for all the fractions.

Orosensory profiles of the berry fractions were analysed by generic descriptive analyses with trained panels. For all three berries, at least sweetness, sourness, bitterness and astringency was used and other attributes varied according to the berry. The juice fraction was the sweetest in every berry. For black currant it was also the sourest (Figure 2). The press residue fractions were very mild and almost tasteless compared to the juice fractions. The extracts, on the other hand, were significantly the most astringent in all cases and for bilberry and crowberry, the extract was also somewhat bitter. In addition to astringency and the taste attributes, woody, watery and dusty properties were also perceived from the crowberry samples.

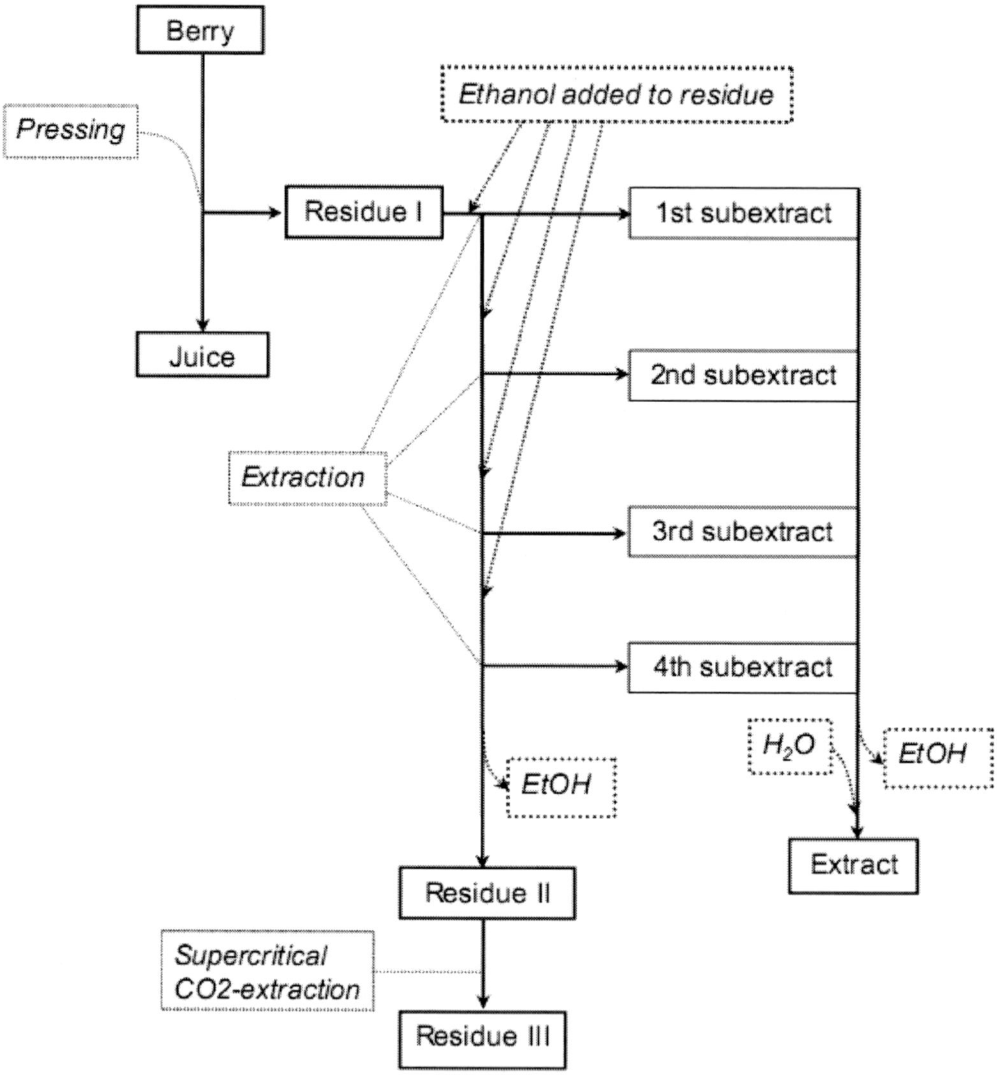

Figure 1. Preparation of crowberry samples. For other berries (bilberry and crowberries) the scheme is similar with some modifications. After extracting the juice by pressing, the phenolic compounds and the rest of the sugars and organic fruit acids were extracted with ethanol and eventually some waxes and other nonpolar soluble compounds were extracted with CO2 (SFE).

As dusty and woody properties were strongest in the extracts these attributes could be similar tactile attributes to astringency showing the range of tactile oral perceptions combined usually just as astringency. The solid residues left from the extraction process were milder and more tasteless than the press residue. For crowberries (Figure 3), the sensory profile of

SFE residue was very similar to ethanol extraction residue as these residues were practically identical. For black currants the different kind of effect of ethanol on the press residue was studied as the first subextract was applied back to the press residue after ethanol removal. The sensory profile of this residue was identical to the press residue. For bilberries, first two subextracts were applied to the juice fraction. This supplemented juice sample did not differ in any sensory attribute from the actual juice fraction (see also Figure 4).

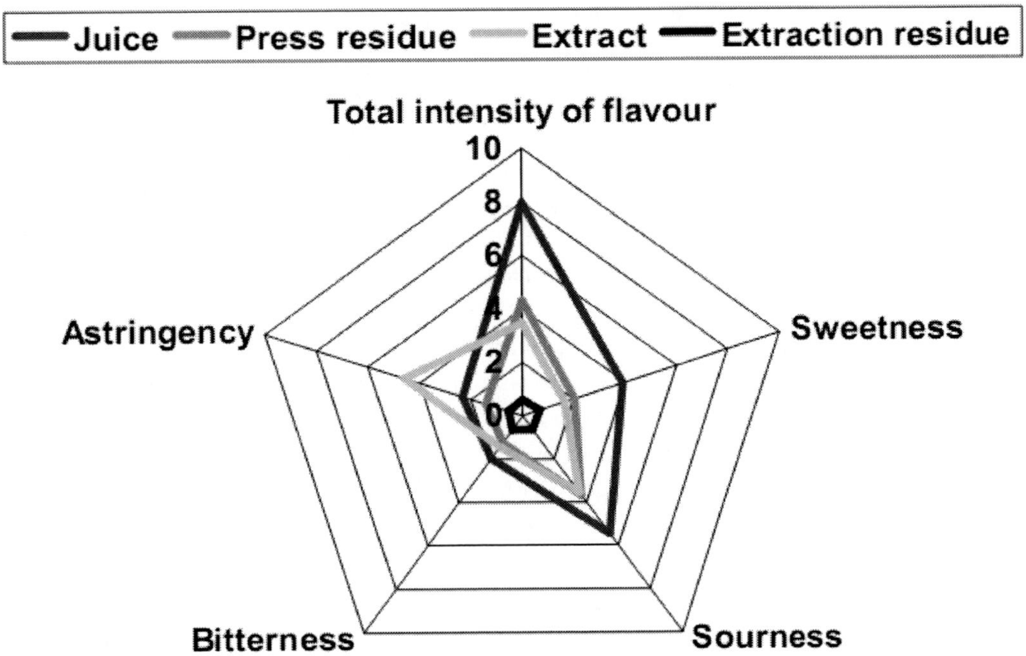

Figure 2. The most abundant sensory attributes (0-10) of the black currant fractions. More samples and attributes are included in the original study. Juice is significantly the sweetest, the sourest and it has the strongest total intensity of flavour. The extract was the most astringent. The press residue was similar to extract with an exception of astringency. The extraction residue was significantly the weakest in all attributes.

5.3. Taste Contributing Berry Compounds

Glucose and fructose were the most abundant sugars in black currant, bilberry and crowberry. Small contents of sucrose as well as other sugars were found also. Citric, malic and quinic acids were the most abundant organic fruit acids. The significant majority of these compounds were located in the juice fractions of the berries as the rest left to the press residue was extracted mainly in the first ethanol extraction step. The sugars contributed very strongly to the sweetness of the juice fractions. In black currant particularly the sugars along with the acids were the most significant contributors to the sensory profile of the juice fraction. In the other two berries the acids similarly contributed to sourness though the juice fractions were not the sourest of the sample fractions. As comparing these three berries, the sugar to acid ratio was the lowest in black currant juice which was sweet and sour, and the highest in crowberry juice which was sweet, but not notably sour. The bilberry juice was in between with relatively sweet and sour characteristics. In the juice of sea buckthorn the acid content contributes to sourness and sweetness is strongly correlating with sugar content and the sugar to acid ratio [21]. In addition to sourness, organic fruit acids, especially malic acid, are known to elicit astringency [21]. Interestingly some sugar compounds seem to have stronger influence on astringency than on sweetness in the sea buckthorn berries [21,63].

The anthocyanins in bilberries and crowberries consisted mostly of galactosides, glucosides and arabinosides of delphidin, cyanidin, malvidin, peonidin, and petunidin with the first two sugar moieties and the first three aglycones being the most abundant. In black currants, there were four major anthocyanins, rutinosides and glucosides of delphidin and cyanidin found along with traces of other minor anthocyanins. The flavonol glycosides in bilberries and crowberries consisted mostly of galactosides, glucosides, xylosides arabinosides of myricetin, quercetin, laricitrin, isorhamnetin and syringetin with the first two sugar moieties and the first two aglycones being the most abundant. In black currants, there were rutinosides, glucosides, malonylglucosides and arabinosides of myricetin, quercetin and kaempferol found. Hydroxycinnamic acids in these berries were mostly derivatives of p-coumaric and caffeic acid. Most of the phenolic compounds were concentrated in the press residues of the berries and were extractable with number of consecutive ethanol extractions.

Phenolic compounds, especially flavonol glycosides and hydroxycinnamic acid derivatives, correlate strongly with astringency of the berry fractions. These compounds are very soluble in ethanol and especially in ethanol-water solutions. The contents of the compounds contributing to astringency along with perceived astringency decline in number of extractions. These compounds may be released from the berry skin structures more effectively with ethanol than with human saliva. The compounds may be bound to the fibre fractions of the skin-rich residue and not be as biologically available in the intestine as they may be after separation.

The Figure 3 shows the interactions between sensory characteristics and chemical variables in crowberry fractions analysed with a multiregression method. Juice, Extract and three residues from Figure 1 were chosen to the PLS2-model.

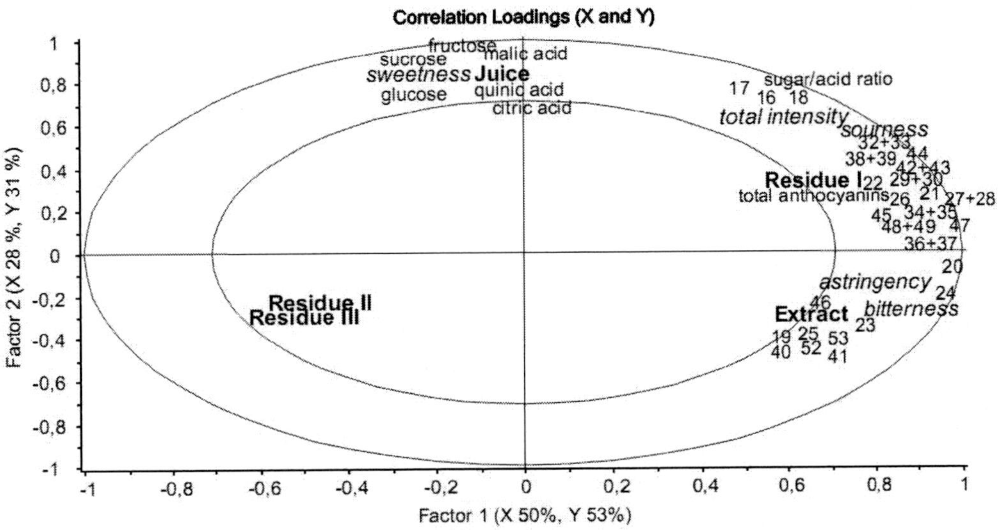

Figure 3. The PLS2 plot of the interactions between the sensory profile and chemical variables in crowberry samples with two components. Five samples included are the same as in Figure 1. Sensory attributes are total intensity of flavour, sweetness, sourness, bitterness and astringency and the rest are excluded. Chemical variables (n = 44) are the sugars, fruit acids, flavonol glycosides and hydroxycinnamic acids found in the samples. Individual anthocyanins are summed here to make variable total anthocyanins. Numbering of the variables is shown in Laaksonen et al. [58].

The regression revealed that 78 % of the chemical properties explained 84 % of variance in sensory properties. Various sugars explained the sweetness of the juice. The sugar/acid ratio correlated to sourness stronger than the individual acid compounds. Phenolic variables around Extract were compounds existing in very small quantities in this sample. These compounds included flavonols in the forms of aglycons and glycosides. Some of these compounds may exist naturally in the berry fractions or they may result in the extraction process. Most of the other flavonol glycosides, found mainly in the press residue (Residue I), were also perceived as astringent and bitter. Two residues (II and III) after extraction processes had very mild profiles and they did not contain significantly any sensory contributing compounds.

Flavonol glycosides, hydroxycinnamic acid derivatives and various other phenolic compounds, such as hydrolysable and condensed tannins, contribute astringency also in red currants [60], black tea [61] and red wine [62]. Detection thresholds of these phenolic compounds can be very low. Similar compounds can be found in various berries and foodstuffs whose sensory and especially astringency contributing compounds have not been studied yet. The astringency in berries may also be conducted by various nitrous compounds in addition to flavonol glycosides [60].

5.4. Pleasantness of Berries

For many people, food flavour has a great impact on food choice, acceptability and eating. Berries are mostly used in juices and jams, and often consumed with added sugar and flavour additives. Natural unprocessed berries may be perceived as unpleasant for many reasons [55]. Strawberry flavour depends on a ratio of sugars and acids and is sensitive to numerous pre- and post-harvesting factors. Both the sea buckthorn and black currant are naturally sour, bitter tasting and highly astringent [21,57]. By combining processed berry fractions, new and more pleasant taste properties can be found whilst adding the nutritionally important compounds in the berry product.

Sugars and acids in the juice fraction can mask the astringency caused by the phenolic compounds in the extracts. By adding phenolic extracts prepared from the press residue to the juice, the contents of phenolic compounds can be significantly increased without significantly altering the sensory properties of the juice [59].

To test the pleasantness and the possible flavour effect of ethanol-extracted phenolic fraction addition to berry juice, two bilberry juices were prepared. The first one was a conventional cold pressed bilberry juice. To the other juice sample the two first extracts of the press residue was added (Figure 1). The ratio of juice and extract was according to yields of these fractions. Ethanol was removed before addition.

Pleasantness of two juices was tested with consumers ($n = 53$, Figure 4). No statistically significant differences were found between the samples in neither odour ($p = 0.592$) nor flavour ($p = 0.058$). However, too high content of extract might decrease the pleasantness of juice. The number of ethanol extracts added will be a critical factor of the juice. Moreover, with supplemented juice a significant difference between odour and flavour ($p = 0.001$) was detected. Odour of the latter sample was more pleasant than its flavour. This finding indicates that non-volatile compounds are important flavour compounds, as well.

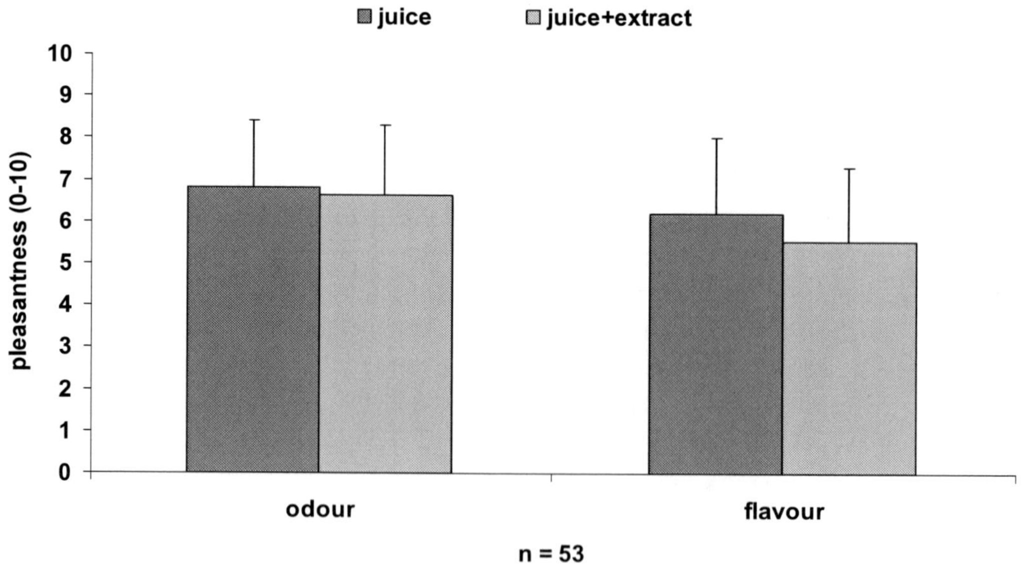

Figure 4. The pleasantness of bilberry juice and the same juice supplemented with phenolic extract from the same berry at the scale of 0 (extremely unpleasant) to 10 (extremely pleasant). The test was

conducted in a public place with no laboratory conditions, so the results are considered as indicative only.

Conclusion

A berry matrix is a complex system with different chemical compounds. The interactions of those compounds and the resulting odour, taste and flavour interactions cause the multidimensional sensation that a person perceives. The compounds may elicit directly or by the secondary interactions or in mixtures to flavour. Berry flavour is contributed by a mixture of volatile and non-volatile compounds. The chemical composition of berries depends on many factors such as genotype and origin of berry. Despite their positive nutritional value, consumers find them often unpleasant because of their strong sensory properties such as odour and taste.

Volatile aroma compounds may affect on ortho- and retronasal odour. Odour of both strawberry and sea buckthorn is characterised by various esters. In strawberry also furanones, aldehydes, terpenes, sulfur compounds and alcohols are important odour active compounds.

Many of the bioactive compounds have been reported to contribute to sensory attributes in berries and other foodstuffs. Sugars and organic fruit acids are mainly found in the juice fractions of berries. The quantities of these compounds and especially the ratio between sugars and acids have an influence on the perceived sourness and sweetness. Other bioactive compounds, such as various phenolic compounds, are mainly found in the skin fractions of berries and these compounds may taste bitter or have natural mouth-drying and astringent properties. The taste properties can be affected or modified by processing the berries, because the concentration of these compounds varies in different parts of the berries and some of these compounds may change or be released during processing. Comprehensive understanding of phytonutrients as taste contributing compounds is required for improving nutrition and to provide tools for nutrition counselling as well as food development.

References

[1] Tahvonen, R.; Hietanen, A.; Sankelo, T.; Korteniemi, V-M.; Laakso, P.; Kallio, H.; Black currant seeds as a nutrient source in breakfast cereals produced by extrusion cooking. *Zeitschrift für Lebensmitteluntersuchung und Forschung,* 1998, *A206*, 360-363.

[2] Tahvonen, R.L.; Schwab, U.S.; Yli-Jokipii, K.M; Mykkänen, H.M.; Kallio, H.P. Black currant seed oil and fish oil supplements differ in their effects on fatty acid profiles of plasma lipids, and concentrations of serum total and lipoprotein lipids, plasma glucose and insulin. *Journal of Nutritional Biochemistry*, 2005, *16*, 353-359.

[3] Yang, B.; Kalimo, K.; Mattila, L.; Kallio, S.; Katajisto, J.; Peltola, O.; Kallio, H. Effect of dietary supplementation with sea buckthorn (*Hippophaë rhamnoides*) seed and pulp oils on atopic dermatitis. *Journal of Nutritional Biochemistry*, 1999, *10*, 622-630.

[4] Yang, B.; Kalimo, K.O.; Tahvonen, R.L.; Mattila, L.M.; Katajisto, J. K., Kallio, H.P. Effect of dietary supplementation with sea buckthorn (*Hippophaë rhamnoides*) seed and pulp oils on the fatty acid composition of skin glycerophospholipids of patients with atopic dermatitis. *Journal of Nutritional Biochemistry*, 2000, *11*, 338-340.

[5] Larmo, P.; Alin J.A.; Salminen, E.K.; Kallio, H.P.; Tahvonen, R. Efficacy of sea buckthorn (*Hippophaë rhamnoides* L.) in prevention and treatment of common cold and other infections: a double-blind, randomized, placebo-controlled trial. *European Journal of Clinical Nutrition,* 2008, *62*, 1123-1130.

[6] Kallio, H.; Yang, B. Sea Buckthorn – unique berry for natural health. *Innovations in Food Technology,* 2002, *15*, 81-82.

[7] Lehtonen, H.-M.; Rantala, M.; Suomela, J.-P.; Viitanen, M.; Kallio, H. Urinary excretion of the main anthocyanin in lingonberry (*Vaccinium vitis-idaea*), cyaniding 3-O-galactoside, and its metabolites. *Journal of Agricultural and Food Chemistry, 2009, 57,* 4447-4451.

[8] Lehtonen, H.-M.; Lehtinen, O.; Suomela, J.-P., Viitanen, M.; Kallio, H. Flavonol glycosides of sea buckthorn (*Hippophaë rhamnoides* ssp. *sinensis*) and lingonberry (*Vaccinium vitis-idaea*) are bioavailable in humans and monoglucuronidated for excretion. *Journal of Agricultural and Food Chemistry,* 2010, *58*, 620-627.

[9] Hakala, M.; Lapveteläinen, A.; Tahvonen, R.; Huopalahti, R.; Kallio, H. Quality factors of Finnish Strawberries. *Acta Horticulturae*, 2002, *567*, 727-730.

[10] Yang, B.; Kallio, H. Composition and physiological effects of sea buckthorn (*Hippophaë*) lipids. *Trends in Food Science & Technology*, 2002, *13*, 160-167.

[11] Kärppä, J.; Kallio, H.; Peltonen, I.; Linko, R. Anthocyanins of crowberry, *Empetrum-nigrum* coll. *Journal of Food Science*, 1984, *49*, 634-636.

[12] Yang, B.; Linko, A.-M.; Adlecreutz, H.; Kallio, H. Secoisolariciresinol and matairesinol of sea buckthorn (*Hippophaë rhamnoides*) berries of different subspecies and harvesting times. *Journal of Agricultural and Food Chemistry,* 2006, *54*, 8065-8070.

[13] Yang, B.; Halttunen, T.; Raimo, O.; Price, K.; Kallio, H. Flavonol glycosides in wild and cultivated berries of three major subspecies of *Hippophaë rhamnoides* and changes during harvesting period. *Food Chemistry*, 2009, *115*, 657-664.

[14] Johansson, A.; Laakso, P.; Kallio, H.; Characterization of seed oils of wild, edible Finnish berries. *Zeitschrift für Lebensmitteluntersuchung und Forschung,* 1997, *A204,* 300-307.

[15] Yang, B; Kallio, H. Fatty acid composition of lipids in sea buckthorn (*Hippophaë rhamnoides* L.) berries of different origins. *Journal of Agricultural and Food Chemistry,* 2001, *49*, 1939-1947.

[16] Kallio, H.; Yang, B.; Peippo, P.; Tahvonen, R.; Pan, R. Triacylglycerols, glycerophospholipids, tocopherols and tocotrienols in berries and seeds of two subspecies (ssp. *sinensis* and ssp. *mongolica*) of sea buckthorn (*Hippophaë rhamnoides*). *Journal of Agricultural and Food Chemistry*, 2002, *50*, 3004-3009.

[17] Yang, B.; Koponen, J.; Tahvonen, R.; Kallio, H. Plant sterols in seeds of two species of *Vaccinium* (*V. myrtillus* and *V. vitis-idaea*) naturally distributed in Finland. *European Food Research and Technology,* 2003, *216*, 34-38.

[18] Yang, B; Kallio, H. Analysis of triacylglycerols of seeds and berries of sea buckthorn of different origins by mass spectrometry and tandem mass spectrometry. *Lipids*, 2006, *41*, 1-12.
[19] Kallio, H.; Nieminen, R.; Tuomasjukka S.; Hakala, M. Cutin composition of five Finnish berries. *Journal of Agricultural and Food Chemistry*, 2006, *54*, 457-462.
[20] Kallio, H.; Hakala, M.; Pelkkikangas, AM.; Lapveteläinen, A. Sugars and Acids of Strawberry Varieties, *European Food Research and Technology*, 2000, *212*, 81-85.
[21] Tiitinen, K.; Hakala, M.; Kallio, H. Quality components of sea buckthorn (*Hippophae rhamnoides*) varieties. *Journal of Agricultural and Food Chemistry,* 2005, *53*, 1692-1699.
[22] Tiitinen, K.; Yang B.; Haraldsson, G.; Jonsdottir S.; Kallio, H. Fast analysis of sugars, fruit acids and vitamin C in sea buckthorn (*Hippophaë rhamnoides* L.*)* varieties. *Journal of Agricultural and Food Chemistry,* 2006, *54,* 2508-2513.
[23] Hakala, M.; Lapveteläinen, A.; Huopalahti, R.; Kallio, H.; Tahvonen, R. Effects of varieties and cultivation conditions on the composition of strawberries. *Journal of Food Composition and Analysis*, 2003, *16,* 67-80.
[24] Kallio, H.P., Yang, B., Peippo, P. Effects of different origins and harvesting time on vitamin C, tocopherols, and tocotrienols in sea buckthorn (*Hippophaë rhamnoides*) berries. *Journal of Agricultural and Food Chemistry,* 2002, *50*, 6136-6142.
[25] Yang, B.; Karlsson, R.; Oksman, P.; Kallio, H. Phytosterols in sea buckthorn (*Hippophaë rhamnoides* L.) berries: identification and effects of different origins and harvesting times. *Journal of Agricultural and Food Chemistry*, 2001, *49*, 5620-5629.
[26] Yang, B; Kallio, H. Effects of harvesting time on triacylglycerols and glycerophospholipids of sea buckthorn (*Hippophaë rhamnoides* L.) berries of different origins. *Journal of Food Composition and Analysis*, 2002, *15*, 143-157.
[27] Zheng, J.; Yang, B.; Tuomasjukka, S.; Ou, S.; Kallio, H. Effects of latitude and weather conditions on contents of sugars, fruit acids, and ascorbic acid in blackcurrant (*Ribes nigrum* L.). *Journal of Agricultural and Food Chemistry,* 2009, *57*, 2977-2987.
[28] Yang, B.; Halttunen, T.; Raimo, O.; Price, K.; Kallio, H. Flavonol glycosides in wild and cultivated berries of three major subspecies of *Hippophaë rhamnoides* and changes during harvesting period. *Food Chemistry*, 2009, *115*, 657-664.
[29] Zheng, J.; Kallio, H.; Yang, B. Effects of latitude and weather conditions on sugars, fruit acids and ascorbic acid in currant (*Ribes* sp.) cultivars. *Journal of the Science of Food and Agriculture*, 2009, *89*, 2011-2023.
[30] Kallio, H.; Development of volatile aroma compounds in arctic bramble, *Rubus arcticus* L. *Journal of Food Science,* 1976, *41*, 563-566.
[31] Kallio, H. Chemical constituents of the volatile aroma compounds in *Rubus arcticus* L. subsp. *stellatus* (Sm.) Boivin, with reference to *Rubus arcticus* L. subsp. *arcticus*. *Reports from the Kevo Subarctic Research Station*, 1975, *12*, 60-65.
[32] Kallio, H. Identification of vacuum steam-distilled aroma compounds in the press juice of arctic bramble, *Rubus arcticus* L. *Journal of Food Science,* 1976, *41*, 555-562.
[33] Hakala, M.; Lapvetelainen, A.; Kallio, H. Volatile compounds of selected Strawberry varieties analyzed by Purge-and-Trap headspace GC-MS, *Journal of Agricultural and Food Chemistry,* 2002, *50*, 1133-1142.

[34] Hakala, M.; Ahro, M.; Kauppinen, J.; Kallio, H. Determination of strawberry volatiles with low resolution gas phase FT-IR analyser. *European Food Research and Technology*, 2001, *212*, 505-510.

[35] Tiitinen, K.; Hakala, M.; Kallio, H. Headspace volatiles from frozen berries of sea buckthorn (*Hippophaë rhamnoides* L.) varieties. *European Food Research and Technology*, 2006, *223*, 455-460.

[36] Lundén, S.; Tiitinen, K.; Kallio, H. Aroma analysis of sea buckthorn berries by sensory evaluation, headspace SPME and GC-olfactometry. In Blank I., Wüst M., Yeretzian, C. Editors. In: Expression of Multidisciplinary Flavour Science. Institut of Chemistry and Biological Chemistry Zürich, University of Applied Sciences, Switzerland, 2010, pp. 490-493.

[37] Forney, C.F.; Kalt, W.; Jordan, M.A. The composition of strawberry aroma is influenced by cultivar, maturity and storage. *HortScience,* 2000, *35*, 1022-1026.

[38] Latrasse, A. Title: Fruits III. In: Maarse H. *Volatile Compounds in Foods and Beverages*. Marcel-Dekker: New York, 1991, pp. 329-387.

[39] Honkanen, E.; Hirvi, T. The flavour of berries. In: Morton ID, MacLeod AJ. In: Food Flavours. Part C: *The Flavour of Fruits*, Elsevier, 1990, pp. 125-193.

[40] Larsen, M.; Poll, L. Odour thresholds of some important aroma compounds in strawberries. *Zeitschrift für Lebensmitteluntersuchung und Forschung*, 1992, *195*, 120-123.

[41] Larsen, M.; Poll, L.; Olsen, C.E. Evaluation of the aroma composition of some strawberry (*Fragaria ananassa* Duch) cultivars by use of odour threshold values. *Zeitschrift für Lebensmitteluntersuchung und Forschung,* 1992, *195*, 536-539.

[42] Ulrich, D.; Hoberg, E.; Rapp, A.; Kecke, S. Analysis of strawberry flavour - discrimination of aroma types by quantification of volatile compounds. *Zeitschrift für Lebensmitteluntersuchung und Forschung A*, 1997, *205*, 218-223.

[43] Ulrich, D.; Krumbein, A.; Rapp, A. Gaschromatographische analyse der aromastoffe von erdbeere, kirche und tomaate nach festphasen-mikroextraktion. *Deutche lebensmittel-Rundschau,* 1997, *93*, 311-316.

[44] Gomes da Silva, M.D.R.; Chaves das Neves, H.J. Differentation of strawberry varieties through Purge-and-Trap HRGC-MS, HRGC-FTIR and principal component analysis. *Journal of High Resolution Chromatography*, 1997, *20*, 275-283.

[45] Gomes da Silva, M.D.R.; Chaves das Neves, H.J. Complementary use of hyphenated purge-and trap gas chromatography techniques and sensory analysis in the aroma profiling of strawberries (*Fragaria ananassa*). *Journal of Agricultural and Food Chemistry*, 1999, *47*, 4568-4573.

[46] Fischer, N.; Hammerschmidt, F.J. A contribution to the analysis of fresh strawberry flavour. *Chemie, Mikrobiologie, Technologie der Lebensmittel*, 1992, *14*, 141-148.

[47] Hirvi, T.; Honkanen, E. The volatiles of two new strawberry cultivars, "Annelie" and "Alaska Pioneer", obtained by backcrossing of cultivated strawberries with wild strawberries, Fragaria vesca, Rügen and Fragaria virginiana. *Zeitschrift für Lebensmitteluntersuchung und Forschung*, 1982, *175*, 113-116.

[48] Sanz, C.; Richardson, D.G.; Perez, A.G. 2,5-dimethyl-4-hydroxy-3(2H)-furanone and Derivatives in Strawberries during ripening, Chapter 24 in *Fruit Flavors.* (Rousseff, R.

& Leahy, M., eds.) American Chemical Society Symposoium Series 596, 1995, Washington DC. pp 268-275.

[49] Hirvi, T.; Honkanen, E.; Pyysalo, T. Stability of 2,5-dimethyl-4-hydroxy-3(2H)furanone and 2,5-dimethyl-4-methoxy-3(2H)furanone in aqueous buffer solutions. *Lebensmittel-Wissenschaft und Technologie*, 1980, *13*, 324-325.

[50] Roscher, R.; Schwap, W.; Schreier, P. Stability of naturally occuring 2,5-dimethyl-4-hydroxy-3[2H]-furanone derivates. *Zeitschrift für Lebensmitteluntersuchung und Forschung*, 1997, *204*, 438-441.

[51] Dirinck, P.J.; De Pooter, H.L.; Willaer, G.A.; Schamp, N.M. Flavor quality of cultivated strawberries: the role of the sulfur compounds. *Journal of Agricultural and Food Chemistry*, 1981, *29*, 316-321.

[52] Perez, A.G.; Rios, J.J.; Sanz, C.; Olias, J.M. Aroma components and free amino acids in strawberry variety Chandler during ripening. *Journal of Agricultural and Food Chemistry*, 1992, *40*, 2232-2235.

[53] Schieberle, P.; Hofmann, T. Evaluation of the character impact odorants in fresh strawberry Juice by quantitative measurements and sensory studies on model mixtures. *Journal of Agricultural and Food Chemistry,* 1997, *45*, 227-232.

[54] Ulrich, D.; Rapp, A.; Hoberg, E. Analyse des Erdbeerearomas - Quantifizierung der flüchtigen komponenten in kulturerdbeervarietäten und der Walderbeere. *Zeitschrift für Lebensmitteluntersuchung und Forschung A*, 1995, *200*, 217-220.

[55] Sandell, M.; Tiitinen, K.; Pohjanheimo, T.; Kallio, H.; Breslin, P.A.S. Why naturally healthy berries may be seen as unpleasant and non-appetitive. In. Takeoka, G.; Ebeler, S.; Kubota, K.; and Tamura, H. Editors, Food Flavour: Chemistry, Sensory Evaluation and Biological Activity. American Chemical Society, Oxford University Press, 2008, pp. 219-228.

[56] Tang, X.; Kälviäinen, N.; Tuorila, H. Sensory and hedonic characteristics of juice of sea buckthorn (*Hippophae rhamnoides* L.) origins and hybrids. *Lebensmittel Wissenschaft und Technologie*, 2001, *34*, 102-110.

[57] Sandell, M.; Laaksonen, O.; Järvinen, R.; Rostiala, N.; Pohjanheimo, T.; Tiitinen, K.; Kallio, H. Orosensory profiles and chemical composition of black currant (*Ribes nigrum*) juice and fractions of press residue, *Journal of Agricultural and Food Chemistry*, 2009, *57*, 3718-3728.

[58] Laaksonen, O.; Sandell, M.; Järvinen, R.; Kallio, H. Orosensory contributing compounds in crowberry (*Empetrum nigrum*) press-byproducts. *Food Chemistry* 2011, *124*, 1514-1524.

[59] Laaksonen, O.; Sandell, M.; Kallio, H. Chemical factors contributing to orosensory profiles of bilberry (*Vaccinium myrtillus*) fractions, *European Food Research and Technology*, 2010, *231*, 271-285.

[60] Schwarz, B.; Hofmann, T. Isolation, structure determination, and sensory activity of mouth-drying and astringent nitrogen-containing phytochemicals isolated from red currants (*Ribes rubrum*). *Journal of Agricultural and Food Chemistry*, 2007, *55*, 1405-1410.

[61] Scharbert, S.; Holzmann, N.; Hofmann, T. Identification of astringent taste compounds in black tea infusions by combining instrumental analysis and human bioresponse. *Journal of Agricultural and Food Chemistry,* 2004, *52*, 2498-2508.

[62] Hufnagel, J.C.; Hofmann, T. Orosensory-directed identification of astringent mouthfeel and bitter-tasting compounds in red wine. *Journal of Agricultural and Food Chemistry*, 2008, *56*, 1376-1386.

[63] Kallio, H.; Lassila, M.; Järvenpää, E.; Haraldsson, G.; Jonsdottir, S.; Yang, B. Inositols and methylinositols in sea buckthorn (*Hippophaë rhamnoides*) berries. *Journal of Chromatography B*, 2009, *877*, 2426-2432.

In: Berries: Properties, Consumption and Nutrition
Editor: Carlo Tuberoso
ISBN 978-1-61470-257-3

Chapter VI

European Elderberry (*Sambucus Nigra* L.) and American Elderberry (*Sambucus Canadensis* L.): Botanical, Chemical and Health Properties of Flowers, Berries and Their Products

Valentina Schmitzer*, Robert Veberic‡ and Franci Stampar£
University of Ljubljana, Biotechnical Faculty,
Department of Agronomy, Ljubljana, Slovenia

Abstract

A full evaluation of elderberry botany, production, orchard establishment and technology together with chemical composition of flowers, berries and elder products is presented. The uses of American and European Elderberry are discussed and medical reports on both elder flowers and berries highlighted. The antioxidant, antimicrobial, anti-inflammatory and cancer-chemo preventive properties of elderberry products are reported. Chemical composition of elderberry consists of primary metabolites (organic acids, sugars), secondary metabolites (phenols) and several other constituents (vitamins A and C, cytokines). Elder flowers are distinguished by their intensive, pleasant odor and serve as a basis for industrially produced soft drinks and extracts. They are a rich source of potential bioactive flavonoids and phenolic acids; quercetin-3-rutinoside (rutin), quercetin-3-glucoside (isoquercitrin), kaempferol-3-rutinoside, isorhamnetin-3-rutinoside and isorhamnetin-3-glucoside were identified among flavonoids and among derivates of

* E-mail: valentina.schmitzer@bf.uni-lj.si. Tel: +386 13203000. Fax. +386 14231088.
‡ E-mail: robert.veberic@bf.uni-lj.si.
£ E-mail: franci.stampar@bf.uni-lj.si.

phenolic acids, caffeic and *p*-coumaric acid were identified. Flavonol glycosides rutin, kaempferol-3-rutinoside and isorhamnetin-3-rutinoside are the major flavonoids in elder flowers, present in much higher concentrations than in elder fruit. Elder flowers exhibit a much stronger neutralizing activity of free radicals compared to elderberry fruit, which is characterized by high organic acids levels, particularly citric acid, and the most abundant sugars in berries, fructose and glucose. These make the ripe berries ideal for processing to juices, candy and concentrates. Among phenolic compounds in elder berries, anthocyanins, quercetins and other polyphenolic flavonoids are of great interest due to their health-beneficial properties. Cyanidin-3-glucoside and cyanidine-3-sambubioside are the prevalent anthocyanins in elder berries, characterizing their purple color and particularly important for natural pigment industry. Other anthocyanins, such as cyanidin-3-sambubioside-5-glucoside, cyanidin-3,5-diglucoside and cyanidin-3-rutinoside are only presented in minor concentrations. In the group of quercetins, quercetin, rutin and quercetin 3-glucoside were detected; with rutin the predominant one. In elderberry extracts and wine, a high content of both primary and secondary metabolites has also been reported. Anthocyanins, as well as other flavonoids, exhibit antioxidant, immune-stimulating, antibacterial, antialergic and antiviral properties; therefore, their consumption may contribute to prevention of several degenerative diseases such as cardiovascular disease, cancer, inflammatory disease and diabetes.

Introduction

Berries are rich sources of primary and secondary metabolites, the latter particularly important as they provide a number of beneficial functions for human health such as antioxidant protection and therapeutic benefits including reduced risk of coronary heart disease, reduced risk of stroke, anticarcinogenic activity, improved visual acuity, and improved cognitive behavior [1-3]. Small fruits containing anthocyanins and other polyphenols, particularly strawberry, raspberry, blueberry, cranberry, and currants, have received much attention; however, some species such as elderberry, are still fairly unknown.

Elderberry flowers and fruit are now predominately used for various processed products and many species and cultivars with high concentrations of organic acids, anthocyanins and other phenolics have been bred for commercial growing. Historically, elderberries have been used medicinally by many indigenous cultures. Native Americans even used the hollow stems and bark of the American elderberry to make toys and musical instruments. The name Elder, is probably derived from the Anglo-Saxon word *aeld*, meaning fire. Old names like Holler, Hylder, Hyllantree, and the German word Holunder all refer to an ancient vegetation goddess and elder-tree was even considered sacred. Therefore, elderberry was often planted around the house and on the farm grounds. Since elders never seemed to get struck by lightning, having it grow near the house was believed to protect the house as well. However, in Christianity, the sacred elder tree became a tree of witches and the old stories were soon distorted. The Church portrayed elder as a tree of sorrow because Judas supposedly hung himself from one after betraying Jesus. Even the cross upon which Jesus was crucified was said to have been made of elder wood. According to Christian mythology this was the reason why elders never since could grow up straight and even to this day barely have the strength to support themselves.

Elderberry cultivars are now planted for ornamental purposes, elderflower extracts are used for beverage and food flavoring [4], and elderberry berries are globally utilized as a medicine or a source of dietary supplement [5-6]. The purple-black fruits of elderberries (*Sambucus* spp. L.) are one of the richest sources of anthocyanic pigments and phenolic compounds among small fruits and have strong antioxidant capacity [6-7]. High amounts of anthocyanins, especially cyanidin 3-sambubioside and cyanidin 3-glucoside are important constituents of elderberry fruit and make them ideal for processing to elderberry juices, extracts and alcoholic beverages such as elderberry wine.

Species Distribution, Habitat and Botanical Properties

Elderberry (*Sambucus*) genus was previously classified in the honeysuckle family (Caprifoliaceae) but due to new genetic research and reclassification [8] it now belongs to moschatel family (Adoxaceae). Plants from this family are mostly woody perennials and include vines, shrubs, and small trees with orange to black berries. Fruit characteristics such as number of berries in umbels, the size and color of berries as well as branching patterns are found to be particularly important for the classification of individual species [9].

The *Sambucus* genus consists of 5 to 30 species, native mostly to the Northern hemisphere, although they have become naturalized throughout much of the temperate and subtropical regions. Because their fruit are highly desirable to birds, elderberry rapidly colonizes moist and sunny areas along railways, roadways, forest edges, and fence lines [6]. In most parts of Europe, black or common elder (*Sambucus nigra* L.), also called black elderberry, elder, elderberry, common elder, elder bush and European elder, is the most widespread species, whereas in North America American elderberry (*Sambucus canadensis* L.), also called common elder, sweet elder, pie elder, elder-blow and blackberry elder, is the prevailing species. The American and European elderberry are closely related and are combined as two subspecies of *S. nigra* [10]. Other species and varieties belonging to the *Sambucus* genus are grouped in five complexes: (1) *S. nigra* complex comprising of *S. australis*, *S. canadensis*, *S. cerulea*, *S. javanica*, *S. lanceolata*, *S. nigra*, *S. palmenis*, *S. peruviana*, *S. simpsonii* and *S. velutina;* (2) *S. melanocarpa* as an intermediate between *S. nigra* and *S. racemosa* group; (3) *S. racemosa* complex comprising of *S. calicarpa*, *S. chinensis*, *S. latipinna*, *S. microbotrys*, *S. pubens*, *S. racemosa* , *S. sieboldiana*, *S. tigranii* and *S. williamsii*, (4) *S.australasica* and *S. gaudichaudiana*; and (5) *S. adnata* and *S. ebulus*. Lesser known species of the *Sambucus* genus native to North and South Americas are *S. melanocarpa*, *S. neomexicana*, *S. Mexicana*, *S. velutina* and *S. cerulea* [11]. The most widely spread species are *S. nigra* and *S. canadensis*.

Sambucus Nigra

Sambucus nigra is a European species with an oceanic to sub oceanic, cool-temperate and west Mediterranean range. The species is common in western and central Europe as well as in North Africa, Scandinavia and Great Britain. Its naturalized distribution area reaches 63° N latitude in western Norway (with scattered naturalized shrubs up to at least 68 ° N) and approximately 55° N in Lithuania [12]. The populations in the Atlas Mountains of Morocco, Algeria and Tunisia have been introduced as well as that on the Azores. *S. nigra* is present in the northern and western part of the Iberian peninsula, in Sicily and mainland Greece but is absent from Crete. It occurs sporadically in western and eastern Turkey, particularly in the northern coastal strip. The eastern limit of its distribution is approximately 55° E. In mountainous regions, *S. nigra* cannot be found in the higher altitudes, above 1500 m in the Alps, 900 m in the Tatra mountains, 2200 m in Morocco and 1200 m in Caucasus. Its precise limits as a native shrub are difficult to establish, because in some places *S. nigra* populates only areas near houses and roads [13].

S. nigra is associated with moderately to highly eutrophic and disturbed soils, for example in floodplains, coastal scrub or along forest margins and in forest gaps, or anthropogenically in hedgerows, abandoned gardens, around farm houses and on post-industrial wasteland. *Sambucus nigra* is less frequently found within forests, but it cannot survive under deep shade [12]. In central Europe *S. nigra* is not a typical forest plant, because the most important habitat factors are high light availability and nutrient-rich, neutral to basic soils. It very easily colonizes both natural and man-made forests or shrublands, and in many locations the species has an anthropogenic origin. In its introduced range, *S. nigra* occurs mainly in anthropogenic habitats, *e.g.* parks and gardens, near enclosures and countryside houses. In cities it is often found in abandoned places, unmanaged parks, for example in old, disused dumping-grounds, deserted allotments, forest margins, near streets and roads.

Sambucus nigra is a shrub or small tree up to 10 m high, with brownish-grey bark and white pith. Strong erect shoots grow from the base and branches are often arching. Leaves are 20 cm in length, with 5-7 leaflets. Leaflets are 3-9 cm long, ovate, pointy, serrate, and rarely pubescent beneath. Typically they are dark green, although ornamental varieties and selections have been identified that are variegated, lime green and purple and are popular plants for landscaping [6]. Stipules are absent or very small. Inflorescence is flat topped, 10-20 cm in diameter, with 5 primary rays. Corolla is approximately 5 mm in diameter; flowers are hermaphrodite and cream white with cream anthers. Individual fruit is a 3-8 mm black drupe and contains 3-5 seeds [13]. Collectively hundreds of fruits produce very large clusters. Rubbing the leaf produces a strong odor. *S. nigra* reproduces by seeds and also vegetative. Most shrubs produce copious amounts of fruit and viable seed every year. *S. nigra* usually flowers in its third or fourth year, rarely in its second. Flowering is generally in June and July and flowers have a strong odor, which may deter some visitors, but attracts others such as beetles, particularly longhorn beetles and flies, which pollinate the flowers. Fruits ripen in mid to late summer (August or September) and birds are considered the main dispersal agents of *S. nigra* seeds, which either regurgitate or defecate the seeds after ingesting the fruit [12].

Sambucus Canadensis

Most of the botany, plant morphology and fruit development are very similar between *S. nigra* and *S. canadensis* species, however American elderberry tends to spread more aggressively by underground rhizomes and is usually multi-trunked. European elderberry, on the other hand, is a single-trunked or few-trunked large shrub or small tree.

American elderberries (*S. canadensis*) are erect, stoloniferous, long-lived, perennial shrubs native to eastern regions of North America. *S. canadensis* is spread east of the Rocky Mountains in the United States and Canada. It ranges from Nova Scotia south to Florida and west to Manitoba and Texas [14]. It is commonly found throughout the mountain, piedmont, and coastal plain regions of the Southeast as it tolerates a wide variety of climatic conditions, withstanding winter temperatures of -40 degrees C in the northernmost part of its range to summer temperatures of more than 38 degrees C in the southern portion. The species occurs in a variety of habitats from low bottomlands to high mountain elevations [15].

American elder is most often found on open or semi-open sites with fertile, moist soils, such as stream edges, fencerows, old fields, pastures, disturbed sites, swamps, bogs, and roadsides; however, it also occurs in alluvial forests and upland woods [14]. It is a common species of southern bottomland hardwood forests, where it grows in seasonally to intermittently flooded forests and in transition zones grading from wetland to upland sites. *S. canadensis* thrives in fertile soils but will grow in sandy and bottomland soils, heavy clays, peats, and muck. It is adapted to a wide variety of soil-moisture combinations but generally prefers moist, well-drained sites [16]. American elder prefers full sun but may occur on sites with partial shade during the day.

American elder is a deciduous flowering shrub that normally grows 2 to 4 m tall, but in favorable conditions it can reach the height of 9 m. The plant is stoloniferous and thicket-forming, with many tightly clustered stems arising from the base [16]. The lateral roots form a fibrous, shallow system and upright stems spread vigorously forming an elliptical to round shape.

Main stems are thinly woody, with large white pith. Bark is light brown, yellowish brown, or grayish brown and dotted with prominent cork-like lenticels [14]. Smaller lateral branches have dark green bark and are nearly herbaceous, usually dying back in the winter [15]. Buds are medium-sized, conical and somewhat depressed. The opposite, pinnately compound leaves have 5 to 11 (usually 7) bright- to medium-green with lanceolate to ovate 10 to 30 cm long leaflets. The margins are finely toothed, and the lower leaflets are occasionally divided into 3 segments [14]. Leaflets are rounded to wedge-shaped at the base and tapered to the pointed tips, 6 to 15 cm long and 2.5 to 6 cm wide [16].

The upper leaf surface is lustrous and smooth; the lower surface is paler and barely pubescent. Petioles are 3 to 10 cm long and may be naked or pubescent. The showy white flowers and dark purple fruits, both borne in umbrella-shaped clusters, are outstanding seasonal features of American elder. The 6 mm, star-shaped flowers are creamy to white and clustered in terminal convex or flattened cymes 5 to 25 cm in diameter [14,16].

Stalked glands may be present in the forks of the cymes. The plants bloom in early summer (June to August), bearing hermaphrodite flowers on large cymes produced laterally on perennial canes and terminally on new canes. Individual cymes can have hundreds of mature fruit, botanically described as berries, which ripen from late summer to fall, depending on location. Individual berries are small (8 mm in diameter), with 4 oblong, tan to yellowish seeds.

Elderberry Uses and Production

There are several positive socio-economic benefits of growing elderberry, because of its diverse uses. In Europe, it is cultivated for flower and berry production as well as ornamental purposes. The flowers of *S. nigra* are used for the preparation of drinks and medicines; elderberry-flower wine is very popular in England. Elderberry berries are mainly used for food colorants and components in pharmaceuticals, processed to concentrates, syrups, jellies, ice-cream, and juices; frequently they are consumed in preserves and alcoholic beverages such as elderberry wine. The flowers, fruits, leaves, bark and roots of *S. nigra* are thus often utilized for medical purposes. For example, dried fruits, flowers and cortex have been used as diaphoretic and diuretic medicines. Tea from *S. nigra* flowers is used against colds, flu, and high temperature. *Sambucus nigra* bark and fruits are potent in the treatment of respiratory problems such as hay fever and asthma. Berries are rich in vitamins and polyphenols and are best used to ward of various winter illnesses. The leaves contain cyanogenic glycosides from which hydrogen cyanide is released by enzyme action. Although European elderberry is not generally considered poisonous, isolated cases of animal and human poisoning have been reported after eating bark, leaves, berries, roots and stems. Extracts from *S. nigra* are used in horticulture as a repellent against insects as they have an unpleasant odor. *Sambucus nigra* has also been planted for erosion control. It is not used as timber due to its small dimensions and soft wood properties. However, because of its whiteness, close grain, good cutting and polishing properties, the wood is suitable for making pegs and other small wooden items such as musical instruments and toys [12].

Similarly, *Sambucus canadensis* has been used for a variety of purposes: the dark, juicy berries for making wines, jellies and pies; the flowers for flavoring candies and jellies; the bark for making a black dye; and the leaves, bark and flowers for making a variety of homemade medicinal remedies [16]. Although the cooked ripe fruit is edible, raw or unripe berries and other plant parts are somewhat toxic with a laxative effect. American elderberry is also a good plant species to use for wildlife habitat improvement and is considered one of the best low, summer-fruiting shrubs for wildlife. Easily established, it can be planted singly or in numbers to form thickets and hedges and can be used in a variety of habitat settings.

Commercial elderberry production is scattered across Austria, Germany, Denmark, and Hungary in Europe (*S. nigra* cultivars), and in central Chile (*S. canadensis* cultivars). Historically, the production of American elderberry was concentrated in Oregon in the USA, but production has rapidly decreased in the past few decades. In the last 50 years only a few producers in the USA managed to establish small orchards generally for local processing into pies, jams, jellies, and particularly wines. Elderberry wine production in the USA and Canada probably started with the arrival of the first European settlers who brought this tradition from their homeland. Since the early 1990s, elderberry production is slowly increasing in Canada with orchards being established in Ontario, Quebec, Nova Scotia, New Brunswick and Newfoundland [17]. In some parts of the world (Midwestern USA), wild harvested flowers and fruit is also an important aspect of elderberry processing. The majority of the *S. nigra* cultivars have been developed in Denmark ('Allesø', 'Korsør', 'Sambu', 'Sampo') but the origin of the most popular cultivar 'Haschberg' can be traced to Klosterneuburg, Austria. *Sambucus canadensis* cultivars have been developed decades ago at the New York

Agricultural Experiment Station and at Agriculture and Agri-Food Canada in Nova Scotia ('Adams I', 'Adams II', 'Nova', 'York', 'Johns') [10].

For commercial harvest, the whole umbel or fruit cluster is picked and the entire crop either processed to flower extract or into juices and purees, when fruit is harvested. Flowers are harvested in early summer (mid June) and berries when fully ripe, reaching a purple black color in late summer and are harvested over a 2 week period. In European countries there is a practice to hand-pick approximately one third of the umbels for flowers so that the rest of the fruit crop increases in size and also attains a better chemical composition. Elderberry fruit is mainly picked by hand, although mechanical harvesting is a possibility. A few umbels are borne in the first year; however, plants reach full production in the third or fourth year after planting. After the fruit is harvested, it must be transported to the processing plant as soon as possible to prevent internal heating in the containers or preferably frozen immediately. Fruit yields from a commercial orchard of 6 to 12 tons per hectare have been reported [18].

Propagation, Orchard Establishement and Cultivation Technology

European and American elderberry can be propagated by seed, seedlings, or cuttings, all of which are commercially available [16]. Fruits and cuttings can also be easily removed from wild plants without severe damage to the plant; however, virus free material should be ensured for commercial orchards [15]. Stem cuttings from vigorous 1-year-old canes may be taken from spring through fall. They should be approximately 25 to 46 cm long and include 3 sets of opposite buds. Cuttings taken in mid-summer and treated with 0.5% indolebutyric acid powder will root readily, but fall cuttings should be placed in peat moss, kept at 4.4 degrees C through the winter, and transplanted outside in the spring [19]. Rooted stolons can be severed from the parent plants in early spring or late fall and, if possible, left in place to establish new root systems. When removed, fragile roots of the new plants should be wrapped in plastic or burlap until replanting.

Elder is easily grown from seeds; however, propagation by seeds does not insure uniformed plants for production orchards, thus it is usually only applied for ornamental purposes. Seeds can be collected as soon as the fruit is ripe, stored or immediately planted by crushing the fruit and drying it or by macerating the seeds with water to remove the pulp before drying [20]. Seeds should be planted 6 mm deep at a rate of 35 seeds per 30-cm intervals in the spring, or in the late fall if well mulched. Larger seedlings should be transplanted as soon as possible after they are obtained, either in the fall or spring. Late fall or early winter are the best planting times since the plants are dormant, and some root growth may occur during the winter [14]. Roots of bare-root seedlings should be soaked in water for a couple of hours prior to planting.

Because elderberries do not bloom until late June, it is not necessary to select a site with excellent air flow, as is the case with most other fruit crops, such as apple and pear. However, late frosts tend to damage young shoots and locations with heavy winds should also be avoided. Higher altitudes (over 600 m) are also not suitable for elderberry production because of uneven fruit ripening and flower drop due to lower temperatures and high humidity levels.

Otherwise, the plants will grow in any humus rich soil (3-4%), from sandy to loamy, with pH levels of about 5.5 to 6.5. Planting should be done in early spring and prior to planting the site should be plowed, well tilled, and soil amended with organic matter similarly to apple orchards. Fertilizer needs are dependent on the quantity of nutrients previously available in the soil. If the humus level in soil is too low (lower than 2 %), organic matter should be incorporated. The usual planting distance is 4 m apart in the row with rows 5-6 m apart. Preferably two year old plants should be planted in orchards, because pruning is easier and plants can already be commercially harvested in the third or fourth year after planting. After the planting, elderberry branches should be pruned back to 2 buds, and can either be trained as a bush or small tree. The latter training system is prevalent in Europe, in the USA elderberry is mostly pruned back every year as a bush. In the second year after planting, branches are thinned out during the winter; up to 7 are left to form a compact canopy and later 15 to 20 strong branches should be maintained. Healthy, vigorous elderberry plants send up a number of new canes each year and these new shoots attain full height in one season. New canes do not have side shoots (laterals) the first year, but often bear single, large, late-ripening clusters on their terminals. The most fruitful canes are those in their second year, when they produce several lateral branches. Fruit clusters are borne terminally on the wood of the current season's growth. The older trunks of elderberries lose vigor and become weak after two or three years. Little pruning is required. All dead, broken and weak canes should be cutoff before growth starts in the spring. An equal number of 1-, 2- and 3-year-old canes may be left; canes older than 3 years should all be removed to encourage the emergence of new, more fruitful canes. Although, elderberry is winter hardy and rarely dies because of winter injury, small lateral twigs near the tops of canes often freeze back. Bushes will live for 30 years or more but it is not the general practice to keep them that long [18].

Birds can be a serious problem in commercial orchards. In larger plantings, the percentage loss may be less and the destruction less noticeable. Placing nets over the bushes is the only effective control measure for birds. Small plantings should not be located near wooded areas where birds can hide [15]. Other problematic pests include leaf borers, mites, mice, voles and cane borers. These can cause considerable damage to branches. However, the damage is usually not serious enough to justify spraying. When the top of a cane is broken off by wind or during harvest, the adult borer lays its eggs in the exposed pith. The larvae hatch and bore down to the bottom of the cane causing the cane to die. Burning the infested canes can discourage the multiplication of the insect and helps greatly in its control. Mildew on the leaves and berries just before harvest can be a problem, especially if the weather is cool during ripening and if the bushes are planted to closely where air circulation is poor. When mildew is serious, a fungicide spray could control it. Tiny eriophyid mites, visible only under the microscope, sometimes attack the leaves and cause yellow bands which resemble the symptoms of a mottle virus. These can be controlled by dormant sprays but their damage is not usually extensive. Diseases and insects are not generally serious on elderberries and sprays usually are not applied [18].

As elderberry roots are formed very close to the surface caution should be put with mechanical tillage for weed removal. Usually it is best to apply contact herbicides for weed control in the row and mulch the remaining site as often as possible. This often also helps to prevent voles from inhabiting the orchard and supplies elderberry bushes with additional nitrogen. Mineral fertilizers should be used in small doses from March to June, and when flowering is abundant additional nitrogen can be added later in the season to encourage new vigorous growth for the next year.

Chemical Composition of Elderberry Flowers, Fruit, and Products

Elderberry Flowers and Their Products

Elderberry flowers are distinguished by their intensive, pleasant odor and serve as a basis for industrially produced soft drinks and also as extracts to increase the nutritional value of different foods and diets. Elderflowers are a rich source of potential bioactive flavonoids and phenolic acids (Table 1). Christensen *et al.* [4] reported six flavonol glycosides and eleven phenolic acids in fresh elderflowers and their extracts. Among flavonoids, quercetin-3-rutinoside (rutin), quercetin-3-glucoside (isoquercitrin), kaempferol-3-rutinoside, isorhamnetin-3-rutinoside, isorhamnetin-3-glucoside and quercetin-3-6-acetylglycoside were identified; and among phenolic acids derivates of quinic acid containing caffeic or *p*-coumaric acid moieties were determined. Similar results were also obtained when analyzing elderflower extracts. Flavonol glycosides rutin, kaempferol-3-rutinoside and isorhamnetin-3-rutinoside are the major flavonoids in elderflowers contributing as much as 90% to the total flavonoids content. The major phenolic acids in elderberry flowers are 5-caffeoylquinnic acid and 1,5-di-caffeoylquinnic acid comprising over 70% of the total phenolic acid content. As much as 21.0 mg per g dry weight of rutin is reported in elderflowers [4]. Opposed to the chemical composition of elderberry fruit, which is especially rich in anthocyanins, flowers do not contain any pigments from this group. The concentration of flavonoids, however, is greatest in elderberry flowers [5] and according to their research, elderflowers exhibit a much stronger neutralizing activity of free radicals compared to elderberry fruit and DPPH values between 91.95 and 94.15 are reported.

Products such as cough syrups ad infusions made from elderberry flowers are quite common, and safe taken in moderate doses; however, for bests results, it is recommended that only 30% (m/m) elder flowers are to be used in teas and infusions in mixtures with other plant materials [21].The consumption of tea infusion is among the most commonly used ways of elderflower antioxidant's intake; the prevalent phytocemicals being quercetin-rutinoside (rutin) and other flavonols, chlorogenic acid, caffeic acid and flavan-3-ols (catechins). The reported electrochemical activity (EA) of elderflower infusion is equivalent to 21 g ascorbic acid equivalents (AAE) per kg dry flowers and the content of rutin in the infusion 10.9 g per kg of dry flower weight. This compound is mostly responsible for the distinct yellow color of the infusion. Free radical scavenging capacity, using the DPPH assay, revealed a 5.2% antiradical activity of L-ascorbic acid [21].

Elder flower syrup has a somewhat different composition with compounds from the group of phenolic acids (protocatechulic acid and derivates of caffeic acid) and flavan-3-ols (catechins) are most abundant. When compared to elder flower infusion, the EA was only about 42% [21]. However, EA of elder flower syrups depends greatly on the technology used and the content of elder flower and other ingredients in the maceration process. For example, the addition of citric acid adjusting the pH level to 3.1 very much affects the polyphenoloxidase (PPO) activity and affectively decreases subsequent browning of the syrup. Traditionally prepared syrups from fresh flowers (flower heads soaked in cold water, addition of citric acid – lemons, and sucrose) posses much less EA and are very pale compared to commercially available syrups, where other flower extracts (such as hibiscus and apple concentrate) have been added or prepared from dried elderflowers or extracts.

Table 1. Compounds in berries and flowers of *Sambucus nigra* L. and *Sambucus canadensis* L

	Sambucus nigra L.	*Sambucus canadensis* L.
berries	*Sugars* (fructose, glucose, sucrose) *Organic acids* (citric, malic, shikimic, fumaric acid) *Flavonoids* (quercetin-3-*O*-rutinoside, quercetin-3-*O*-glucoside, kaempferol-3-*O*-rutinoside, isorhamnetin-3-*O*-rutinoside, isorhamnetin-3-*O*-glucoside) *Phenolic acids* (neochlorogenic acid, chlorogenic acid, cryptochlorogenic acid) *Anthocyanins* (cyanidin-3-*O*-sambubioside-5-*O*-glucoside, cyanidin-3,5-*O*-diglucoside, cyanidin-3-*O*-sambubioside, cyanidin-3-*O*-glucoside,cyanidin-3-*O*-rutinoside, cyanidin-3-*O*-rhamnoglucoside, cyanidin-3-*O*-xyloglucoside, pelargonidin-3-*O*-glucoside, delphinidin-3-*O*-rutinoside, pelargonidin-3-*O*-sambubioside) *Proanthocyanidins* (dimers, trimers and tetramers) *Vitamins* (A, E)	*Sugars* (fructose, glucose, sucrose) *Organic acids* (citric, malic, shikimic, fumaric acid) *Flavonoids* (quercetin-3-*O*-rutinoside, quercetin-3-*O*-glucoside, epigallocatechin, quercetin monoglucoside, kaempferol-3-*O*-rutinoside, isorhamnetin-3-*O*-rutinoside, isorhamnetin-3-*O*-glucoside) *Phenolic acids* (neochlorogenic acid, chlorogenic acid, cryptochlorogenic acid) *Anthocyanins* (yanidin-3-*O*-sambubioside-5-*O*-glucoside, cyanidin-3,5-*O*-diglucoside, cyanidin-3-*O*-sambubioside, cyanidin-3-*O*-glucoside, cyanidin-3-*O*-(6-*O*-*E*-*p*-coumaroyl-2-*O*-*β*-D-xylopyranosyl), cyanidin-3-*O*-(6-*O*-*Z*-*p*-coumaroyl-2-*O*-*β*-D-xylopyranosyl)-*β*-glucopyranoside-5-*O*-*β*-D-glucopyranoside, cyanidin-3-*O*-(6-*O*-*E*-*p*-coumaroyl-2-*O*-*β*-D-xylopyranosyl)-*β*-D-glucopyranoside, -3-*O*-rutinoside)
flowers	*Flavonoids* (quercetin-3-rutinoside, quercetin-3-glucoside, kaempferol-3-rutinoside, isorhamnetin-3-rutinoside, isorhamnetin-3-glucoside, quercetin-3-6-acetylglycoside *Phenolic acids* (5-caffeoylquinnic acid, 1,5-di-caffeoylquinnic acid)	*No data reported to the present day*

Elderberry Fruit and Their Products

The fruit of *Sambucus nigra* and *Sambucus canadensis* contains several constituents responsible for its pharmacological activity (Table 1). Among these are the flavonoids quercetin and rutin, anthocyanins identified as cyanidin-3-*O*-glucoside and cyanidin-3-*O*-sambubioside [7], the hemagglutinin protein Sambucus nigra agglutinin III (SNA-III) [22], cyanogenic glycosides including sambunigrin, [23] viburnic acid, and vitamins A and C [24].

The juice pressed from elder berries contains many primary metabolites: various sugars and organic acids. High concentrations of organic acids are important in processing, since, unlike sugars, they cannot be added to the final product. Among secondary metabolites, elderberry juice is predominantly characterized by high amounts of anthocyanins. These are a class of flavonoids responsible for the attractive orange to blue color of flowers, as well as an important fruit quality indicator, since they greatly influence fruit appearance and flavor [6].They have gained an increasing interest as functional compounds in food colorants and as potent agents against oxidative stress, reducing oxidative damage to the human body. Anthocyanins, as well as other flavonoids – like quercetins, exhibit antioxidant, anticarcinogenic, immune-stimulating, antibacterial, antialergic and antiviral properties; therefore, their consumption may contribute to prevention of several degenerative diseases such as cardiovascular disease, cancer, inflammatory disease and diabetes [5, 25]. These compounds are well known free radical scavengers, reported as potential chemo-preventive agents.

Elder berry chemical composition has been thoroughly explored and compounds from the groups of primary and secondary metabolites determined [7].The former group consists of various sugars and organic acids. The most abundant sugars in black elderberry fruit are fructose and glucose, sucrose is detected only in small amounts [7]. The total sugar content in elderberry fruit averages from 68.53 to 104.16 g per kg fresh weight (FW) and is, like in other fruit, such as sweet cherry [26] and peach [27], strongly dependant on cultivar. Elderberry fruit contains moderate amounts of sugars compared to apple, which contains 115-183 g per kg total sugars [28] and significantly lower amounts of total sugars than sweet cherry, which averagely contains 150-230 g per kg [26]. The content level of sugars in elderberry fruit is comparable to sour cherry fruit (*Prunus cerasus* L.), which contain approx. 90 g per kg total sugars and are also mainly used in processing [29]. The amount of sugar in elderberry fruit, however, is not the focal chemical compound for technological processing, as fructose and sucrose can easily be added to the final products (i.e. juices, concentrates, spreads and beverages).

Among organic acids, four have been identified in elder berries: citric acid, malic acid, shikimic acid and fumaric acid [7]. Citric acid is the most abundant organic acid, followed by malic acid and minor concentrations of shikimic and fumaric acid. The concentration of citric acid in the fruit of black elderberry is reported in range from 3.11 g per kg to 4.81 g per kg FW [7]. Compared to apple, which contains between 0.07-0.52 g per kg FW citric acid [28], sweet cherry, which contains between 0.11-0.54 g per kg FW citric acid [26] and sour cherry, which contains between 0.08-0.14 g per kg FW citric acid [29], elderberry fruit is exceptionally rich in this organic acid. The content of citric acid in fruit is a particularly important parameter and although elder berries contain lower amounts of total organic acids than apple, which on average contains between 6.00 and 14.00 g per kg FW organic acids [28] and sweet cherry, which on average contains between 3.50 and 8.20 g per kg FW organic acids [26], it is widely used for processing purposes due to the high levels of citric acid.

Berries are particularly rich in flavonoids compounds, including anthocyanidins and proanthocyanidins as well as flavonols. The most important polyphenols in elderberry fruit are thought anthocyanins, being responsible for the colour [21]. Total monomeric anthocyanin content of different *S. nigra* cultivars is reported in range from 170 to 343 mg cyanidin-3-*O*-glucoside per 100 g and for *S. canadensis* in range from 106 to 444 mg cyanidin-3-*O*-glucoside per 100 g [6]. Much higher values of total monomeric anthocyanin content were determined in elder berries in a study of Kaack [30], where values ranged from 518 to 1028 mg cyanidin-3-*O*-glucoside per 100 g.

High performance liquid chromatography analysis of European elder (*Sambucus nigra*) fruit revealed the presence of four main anthocyanins: cyanidin-3-*O*-sambubioside-5-*O*-glucoside, cyanidin-3,5-*O*-diglucoside, cyanidin-3-*O*-sambubioside, cyanidin-3-*O*-glucoside, cyanidin-3-*O*-rutinoside, cyanidin-3-*O*-rhamnoglucoside and cyanidin-3-*O*-xyloglucoside have also been reported [7,25]. Lee and Finn [6] reported the presence of non-cyanidin-based pelargonidin-3-*O*-glucoside and delphinidin-3-*O*-rutinoside in *S. nigra* berries and Wu *et al.* [31] also pelargonidin-3-*O*-sambubioside, although these were only present in trace amounts. According to Wu *et al.* [31] and Veberic *et al.* [7] the two prevalent anthocyanins in *S. nigra* are cyanidin-3-*O*-glucoside and cyanidin-3-*O*-sambubioside, with the major anthocyanin cyanidin-3-*O*-sambubioside, accounting for more than half of all determined anthocyanins, approximately. In comparison to sweet cherry, which contains, on average, 100-120 mg total anthocyanins per 100 g FW [26] elderberry fruit has significantly higher anthocyanin content as it reaches levels between 602.90 and 1265.30 mg per100 g FW [7]. While berries of *S. nigra* contain primarily four anthocyanins, berries of *S. canadensis* contain seven [25]. In addition to cyanidin-3-*O*-sambubioside-5-*O*-glucoside, cyanidin-3,5-*O*-diglucoside, cyanidin-3-*O*-sambubioside and cyanidin-3-*O*-glucoside they also accumulate more stable acylated anthocyanins cyanidin-3-*O*-(6-*O*-*E*-*p*-coumaroyl-2-*O*-*β*-D-xylopyranosyl), cyanidin-3-*O*-(6-*O*-*Z*-*p*-coumaroyl-2-*O*-*β*-D-xylopyranosyl)-*β*-glucopyranoside-5-*O*-*β*-D-glucopyranoside, and cyanidin-3-*O*-(6-*O*-*E*-*p*-coumaroyl-2-*O*-*β*-D-xylopyranosyl)-*β*-D-glucopyranoside [25]. Lee and Finn [6] determined the presence of petunidin-3-*O*-rutinoside in berries of *S. canadensis* present only in trace amounts.

Both *S. nigra* and *S. canadensis* contain many polyphenolic compounds; among those cinnamic acids (neochlorogenic acid, chlorogenic acid, and cryptochlorogenic acid) and flavonol-glycosides (quercetin-3-*O*-rutinoside, quercetin-3-*O*-glucoside, kaempferol-3-*O*-rutinoside, isorhamnetin-3-*O*-rutinoside and isorhamnetin-3-*O*-glucoside have been identified [6]. The main quercetin in berries is quercetin-3-*O*-rutinoside (rutin), with values ranging from 35.6 mg per 100 g FW to 52.0 mg per 100 g FW in berries of *S. nigra* [7]. Similar values (15.0 to 41.9 mg per 100 g FW) are reported for *S. canadensis* berries [6]. The other two quercetins are present in considerably lower amounts, especially the aglycone quercetin; the concentration of this was approximately 1/10 of the amount of rutin. Total quercetins are reported in range from 51.9 mg per100 g FW to 73.4 mg per 100 g FW [7], total cinnamic acids in range from 28.7 to 42.8 mg per 100 g FW and total polyphenols in range from 85.7 to

140.3 mg per 100 g FW [6]. A series of proanthocyanidins (dimers, trimers and tetramer) as well as gallocatechin, and other flavonols have been reported in *S. nigra* berries [21,25]. There is a slight difference in polyphenolic composition of *S. canadensis* berries; mainly they contain quercetin based glycosides. Specifically, rutin, epigallocatechin, and quercetin monoglucoside [25] as well as neochlorogenic and chlorogenic acid [6] are the predominant constituents.

S. nigra and *S. canadensis* fruit have higher antioxidant capacity than vitamin C or E and are thus capable of enhancing immune system response through elevated production of cytokines [25]. Dawidowitz *et al.* [5] report the antioxidant activity (calculated by the DPPH method) of elder berries in range from 50.3 to 67.7, mainly attributed to the presence of flavonols and anthocyanins. Thus, their antioxidant capacity ranks high when compared to other well known small fruit, such as cranberry [21]. Using the ORAC method, Wu *et al.* [31] showed that especially *S. canadensis* berries posses a much higher potential than cranberry and blueberry, two fruits praised for their high antioxidant potential.

Among elderberry products, elderberry juice, spreads and wine are most widely marketable. Elderberry juice pressed from *S. nigra* berries are characterized by the two major anthocyanins (cyanidin-3-*O*-sambubioside and cyanidin-3-*O*-glucoside) as well as high levels of catechins and phenolic acids such as chlorogenic acid, neochlorogenic acid, rutin and other flavonols [21,32]. The average content of cyanidin-3-*O*-sambubioside in elder berry juice pressed from different *S. nigra* cultivars is 379 mg per 100 ml, 331 mg per 100 ml cyanidin-3-*O*-glucoside, 81.7 mg per 100 ml cyanidin-3-*O*-sambubioside-5-*O*-glucoside and 24.9 mg per 100 ml cyanidin-3,5-*O*-diglucoside [32]. Fruit juice pressed from fresh or frozen elder berries has a concentration of soluble solids above 13% w/w, indicating a satisfactory content of sugars, and titratable acidity of between 0.6 and 1.7 [32], an important parameter for a balanced taste. Comparing the beneficial effects of fresh fruit with processed ones, it should be kept in mind that especially anthocyanin stability is affected by numerous factors during processing and an almost total destruction of these pigments as well as chlorogenic acid is reported during production of elderberry spread [21].

During the elderberry fruit wine making process, significant changes take place in the composition and content of polyphenolic compounds resulting from fruit disintegration as well as fermentation and aging. Alcoholic fermentation of elderberry fruit yields an intensely purple-red colored elderberry wine with a high content of anthocyanic pigments and total phenolic content similar to red wines [33]. The beneficial compounds present in elderberry juice, have also been determined in elderberry wine. The compositional analysis of organic acids revealed malic and citric acids the predominant organic acids in fruit wine from *S. nigra* berries [33]. In elderberry wine, numerous phenolic compounds are present; among those Schmitzer *et al.* [33] identified chlorogenic acid and neochlorogenic acid, quercetin-3-*O*-rutinoside, quercetin-3-*O*-glucoside, kaempferol-3-*O*-rutinoside and five cyanidin based anthocyanins. Anthocyanins were the predominant polyphenols in elderberry must and wine. Cyanidin-3-*O*-sambubioside is the major anthocyanin in elderberry must; however, in elderberry wine cyanidin-3-*O*-glucoside is detected in highest concentrations [33]. During elderberry wine making process, significant transformations in phenolics take place and the composition of anthocyanic pigments is altered. Vinification results in a minor decrease of anthocyanin content but, formation of new, more stable, polymeric pigments has been reported [33]. Quercetin-3-*O*-rutinoside is the most abundant quercetin followed by quercetin-3-glucoside, which is comparable to the compositional analysis of elderberry fruit as well as elderberry juice. Similar to compositional analysis of elderberry juice, neochlorogenic acid and chlorogenic acid have been detected in elderberry must and wine; the latter was significantly higher in elderberry wine compared to must and aged wine [33].

As a result of chemical reactions of monomeric and dimeric phenolics during processing from musts to wine as well as aging, many polymeric compounds are formed causing differences in both total phenolic content (TPC) and antioxidative potential (AP). Both parameters are significantly higher in elderberry wine compared to elderberry must [33]. TPC of elderberry wine is reported to be 2004.13 mg GAE per L, comparable to TPC measured in different red wines, which on average contain 2000 mg GAE L [34]. AP of elderberry must is reported to be 8.18 mM trolox per L and increases significantly in elderberry wine to 9.95 mM trolox per L [33]. Elderberry wine is therefore an appealing alcoholic beverage not only because of its intense red coloration but mostly due to its high total phenolic content. It could be used as a potential additive to other alcoholic beverages, with inadequate coloration.

Clinical Studies on Potential Helth Effects of Elderberry

Elder Flowers

In folk medicine, *Sambucus nigra* flower was traditionally suggested as a remedy for diabetes [35]. Researchers in Northern Ireland conducted an in vitro study to evaluate the effect on blood sugar. In the two-armed study, aqueous extract of elder flower significantly increased glucose uptake, glucose oxidation, and glycogenesis in rat abdominal muscle. Elder flower extract incubated with rat pancreatic cells also had a dose-dependent stimulatory effect on insulin secretion. The researchers concluded elder flowers contain water-soluble constituents capable of direct stimulation of insulin secretion and glucose metabolism [36]. Further clinical studies are required before elderberry can be recommended for use in diabetes.

Elder Berries

As mentioned before, the fruit of *Sambucus nigra* and *Sambucus canadensis* contains several constituents responsible for pharmacological activity. Among these are the flavonoids quercetin and rutin, anthocyanins identified as cyanidin-3-glucoside and cyanidin-3-sambubioside [7], the hemagglutinin protein *Sambucus nigra* agglutinin III (SNA-III) [22], cyanogenic glycosides including sambunigrin, [23] viburnic acid, and vitamins A and C [24]. Due to limited research, the pharmacokinetics of many constituents of elderberry is not completely understood. Available research has focused on the absorption and urinary excretion of the anthocyanin constituents. Historically, researchers were uncertain whether anthocyanins were absorbed unless they were first hydrolyzed in the gastrointestinal tract.

Recently, however, several small pharmacokinetic studies of elderberry extract in healthy volunteers demonstrated elder berry anthocyanins are indeed absorbed and excreted in an intact form. Within four hours of consuming 12 g elderberry extract containing 720 mg total anthocyanins, the two major anthocyanins in elderberry extract were identified in the urine of four elderly women [37]. A similar study involving 16 healthy volunteers confirmed the presence of the same two anthocyanins in the urine of study subjects after oral administration of elderberry extract [38]. One study investigated the absorption of elderberry anthocyanins in a single male subject given 25 g elderberry extract (1.5 g total anthocyanins); high-performance liquid chromatography (HPLC) analysis detected two anthocyanin peaks in his plasma collected 30 minutes after consuming elderberry extract [39], and this was later confirmed in a study by Milbury *et al.* [40].

While there are several mechanisms responsible for the beneficial effects of *Sambucus nigra* and *S. canadensis* and extracts of their berries, perhaps the most important and best studied are the antiviral effects. A powerful antioxidant activity *in vitro* has been demonstrated and Youdim *et al.* [41] have reported that elderberry anthocyanins can be taken by endothelial cells, which are subsequently effectively protected against oxidative stress. Sambucol®, a syrup containing 38-percent standardized extract of elder berries, was developed and studies have shown it to neutralize and reduce the infectivity of influenza viruses A and B [42], HIV strains and clinical isolates [43], and Herpes simplex virus type 1 (HSV-1) strains and clinical isolates. It probably does so in the same manner as with influenza viruses, via neutralization of the virus resulting in reduced infectivity.

Elderberry extracts also have immune-modulating activity in healthy individuals as well as in those with viral infections or other diseases characterized by immunosuppression. Production of certain cytokines leads to activation of phagocytes and facilitates their movement to inflamed tissues [44]. Elder berries also contain several anthocyanin flavonoids known to possess significant antioxidant properties. Research has demonstrated that even low-level concentrations of elderberry anthocyanins can efficiently regenerate alpha-tocopherol from alpha-tocopheroxyl radicals in models of copper-mediated LDL oxidation [45]. Since it has been observed that anthocyanin glycosides are indeed absorbed in humans, it is likely that supplementing with elderberry extracts containing anthocyanins provides significant antioxidant benefit in increased protection against oxidative stress.

Numerous disease conditions are characterized by oxidative stress, including cardiovascular disease, cancer, neurodegenerative disease, peripheral vascular disease, autoimmune diseases, and multiple sclerosis. Bioactivity relevant to inhibition of both the initiation and promotion stages of carcinogenesis was detected in fruit extracts from *S. nigra* and *S. canadensis* [25]. The ability of elderberry extract to provide antioxidant protection via inhibition of LDL-oxidation and scavenging of free radicals makes it a potentially valuable tool in the treatment of disease resulting from oxidative stress [45].

Thus, we can conclude that elderberry, its extracts and products can be regarded as potent medicinal additives in the future as many traditional applications have been proven with clinical and in-vitro studies. Recent findings promote the use of elderberry mostly due to its high antioxidative status and favorable phenolic profile for novel pharmacological studies and later on for clinical applications.

References

[1] Prior, R.L. Absorption and metabolism of anthocyanins: Potential health effects. In: Meskin MS, Bidlack WR, Davies AJ, Levis DS, Randolph RK, editors. *Phytochemicals: Mechanisms of action*. Boca Raton: CRC Press; 2003.

[2] Zafra-Stone, S.; Yasmin, T.; Bagchi, M.; Chatterjee, A.; Vinson, J.A.; Bagchi, D. Berry anthocyanins as novel antioxidants in human health and disease prevention. *Moecular Nutrition and Food Research*, 2007, *51*, 675-83.

[3] Ozgen, M.; Scheerens, J.C.; Reese, R.N.; Miller, R.A. Total phenolic, anthocyanin contents and antioxidant capacity of selected elderberry (*Sambucus canadensis* L.) accessions. *Pharmacognosy Magazine*, 2010, *6*, 198-203.

[4] Christensen, L.P.; Knaack, K.; Frette, X.C. Selection of elderberry (*Sambucus nigra* L.) genotypes best suited for the preparation of elderflower extracts rich in flavonoids and phenolic acids. *European Food Research and Technology*, 2007, *227*, 293-305.

[5] Dawidowicz, A.L.; Wianowska, D.; Baraniak, B. The antioxidant properties of alcoholic extracts from *Sambucus nigra* L. (antioxidative properties of extracts). *Food Science and Technology*, 2006, *39*, 308-315.

[6] Lee, J.; Finn, C.E. Anthocyanins and other polyphenolics in American elderberry (*Sambucus canadensis*) and European elderberry (*S. nigra*) cultivars. *Journal of the Science of Food and Agriculture,* 2007, *87*, 2665-2675.

[7] Veberic, R.; Jakopic, J.; Stampar, F.; Schmitzer, V. European elderberry (*Sambucus nigra* L.) rich in sugars, oganic acids, anthocyanins and selected polyphenols. *Food Chemistry*, 2009, *114*, 511-515.

[8] Donoghue, M.J.; Bell, C.D.; Winkworth, R.C. The evolution of reproductive characters in dipsacales. *International Journal of Plant Science*, 2003, 164, 453-464.

[9] Jordheim, M.; Giske, N.H.; Andersen, Ø.M. Anthocyanins in Caprifoliaceae. Biochemical *Systematics and Ecology*, 2007, *35*, 153-159.

[10] Finn, C.E.; Thomas, A.L.; Byers, P.L.; Serçe, S. Evaluation of American (*Sambucus canadensis*) and European (*S. nigra*) elderberry genotypes grown in diverse environments and implications for cultivar development. *Hortscience*, 2008, *43*, 1385-1391.

[11] Kearney, T.H.; Peebles, R.H. *Arizona Flora*. Berkeley, California: University of California Press, 1960.

[12] Atkinson, M.D.; Atkinson, E. *Sambucus nigra* L. Biological Flora of the British Isles, *Journal of Ecology*, 2002, *90*, 895-923.

[13] Tutin, Y.G.; Heywood, V.H.; Burges, N.A.; Moore, D.M.; Valentine, D.H.; Walters, S.M.; Webb, D.A. *Flora Europaea*, Vol. 4. Cambridge: Cambridge University Press, 1976.

[14] Foote, L.E.; Jones, S.B. *Native Shrubs and Woody Vines of the Southeast: Landscaping Uses and Identification*. Portland, Oregon: Timber Press, 1989.

[15] DeGraaf, R.M.; Witman, GM. *Trees, Shrubs, and Vines for Attracting Birds*. Amherst: University Massachusetts Press, 1979.

[16] Vines, R.A. *Trees, Shrubs, and Vines of the Southwest*. Austin: University of Texas Press, 1960.

[17] Charlebois, D. Elderberry as a medicinal plant. In: Janick J, Whipkey A, editors. *Issues in new crops and new uses*. Alexandria, VA: ASHS Press, 2007.

[18] Roger, D.W. *Elderberry Culture in New York State*. New York: New York's Food and Life Sciences Bulletin 91, 1981.

[19] Bir, R.E. *Growing and Propagating Showy Native Woody Plants*. Chapel Hill: University of North Carolina Press, 1992.

[20] Young, J.A.; Young, C.G. *Collecting, Processing and Germinating Seeds of Wildland Plants*. Portland, Oregon: Timber Press, 1986.

[21] Cejpek, K.; Malouušková, I.; Konečný, M.; Velíšek J. Antioxidant activity in various prepared elderberry foods and supplements. *Czech Journal of Food Science*, 2009, *27*, 45-48.

[22] Mach, L.; Scherf, W.; Ammann, M.; Poetschl, J.; Bertsch, W.; Marz, L.; Glossl, J. Purification and partial characterization of a novel lectin from elder (*Sambucus nigra* L.) fruit. *Biochemical Journ al*, 1991, *278*, 667-671.

[23] Buhrmester, R.A.; Ebingerla, J.E.; Seigler, D.S. Sambunigrin and cyanogenic variability in populations of *Sambucus canadensis* L. (Caprifoliaceae). *Biochemical Systematics and Ecology*, 2000, *28*, 689-695.

[24] Duke, J.A. *Handbook of Medicinal Herbs*. Boca Raton: CRC Press, 1985.

[25] Thole, J.M.; Kraft, T.F.B.; Sueiro, L.A.; Kang, Y.-H.; Gills, J.J.; Cuendet, M.; Pezzuto, J.M.; Seigler, D.S.; Lila, M.A. A comparative evaluation of the anticancer properties of European and American elderberry fruits. *Journal of Medicinal Food*, 2006, *9*, 498-504.

[26] Usenik, V.; Fabcic, J.; Stampar, F. Sugars, organic acids, phenolic composition and antioxidant activity of sweet cherry (*Prunus avium* L.). *Food Chemistry*, 2008, *107*, 185-192.

[27] Colaric, M.; Veberic, R.; Stampar, F.; Hudina M. Evaluation of peach and nectarine fruit quality and correlations between sensory and chemical attributes. *Journal of Science of Food and Agriculture*, 2005, *85*, 2611-2616.

[28] Hofer, M.; Grill, D.; Hecke, K.; Herbinger, K.; Keppel, H.; Monschein, S.; Stampar, F.; Toplak, H.; Veberic, R. Inhaltsstoffe alter Apfelsorten unter diätetischem Aspekt – Schwerpunkt Diabetes. *Jurnal des Ernährungsmedizin*, 2005, *7*, 30-33.

[29] Bonerz, D.; Würth, K.; Dietrich, H. Analytical characterization and the impact of ageing in anthocyanin composition and degradation in juices from five sour cherry cultivars. *European Food Research and Technology*, 2006, *224*, 355-364.

[30] Kaack, K. 'Sampo' and 'Samdal', elderberry cultivars for juice concentrate. *Fruit Varieties Journal*, 1997, *51*, 28-31.

[31] Wu, X.; Gu, L.; Prior, R.L.; Mckay, S. Characterization of anthocyanins and procyanidins in some cultivars of *Ribes*, *Aronia* and *Sambucus* and their antioxidant capacity. *Journal of Agriculture and Food Chemistry*, 2004, *52*, 7846-7856.

[32] Kaack, K.; Fretté, X.C.; Christensen, L.P.; Landbo, A.-K.; Meyer, A.S. Selection of elderberry genotypes best suited for the preparation of juice. *European Food and Research Technology*, 2008, *226*, 843-855.

[33] Schmitzer, V.; Veberic, R.; Slatnar, A.; Stampar, F. Elderberry (*Sambucus nigra* L.) Wine: A Product Rich in Health Promoting Compounds. *Journal of Agricultural and Food Chemistry*, 2010, *58*, 10143-10146.

[34] Minussi, R.C.; Rossi, M.; Bologna, L.; Cordi, L.; Rotilio, D.; Pastore, G.M.; Duran, N. Phenolic compounds and total antioxidant potential of commercial wines. *Food Chemistry*, 2003, *82*, 409-416.

[35] Atkinson, M. *Herbs for your health*. New York: Dalesman Books, 1979.

[36] Grey, A.M.; Abdel-Wahab, Y.H.; Flatt, P.R. The traditional plant treatment, *Sambucus nigra* (elder), exhibits insulin-like and insulin-releasing actions in vitro. *Journal of Nutrition*, 2000, *130*, 15-20.

[37] Wu, X.; Cao, G.; Prior, R.L. Absorption and metabolism of anthocyanins in elderly women after consumption of elderberry or blueberry. *Journal of Nutrition*, 2002, *132*, 1865-1871.

[38] Mulleder, U.; Murkovic, M.; Pfannhauser, W. Urinary excretion of cyanidin glycosides. *Journal of Biochemical and Biophysical Methods*, 2002, *53*, 61-66.

[39] Cao, G.; Prior, R.L. Anthocyanins are detected in human plasma after oral administration of an elderberry extract. *Clinical Chemistry*, 1999, *45*, 574-576.

[40] Milbury, P.E.; Cao, G.; Prior, R.L; Blumberg, J. Bioavailability of elderberry anthocyanins. *Mechanisms of Aging and Development*, 2002, *123*, 997-1006.

[41] Youdim, K.A.; Martin, A.; Joseph, J.A. Incorporation of elderberry anthocyanins by endothelial cells increases protection by oxidative stress. *Free Radical Biology and Medicine*, 2000, *29*, 51-60.

[42] Zakay-Rones, Z.; Thorn, E.; Wollan, T.; Wadstein, J. Randomized study of the efficacy and safety of oral elderberry extract in the treatment of influenza A and B virus infections. *Journal of International Medical Research*, 2004, *32*, 132-140.

[43] Sahpira-Nahor, O.; Zakay-Rones, Z.; Mumcuoglu, M. The effects of Sambucol® on HIV infection in vitro. *Annual Israel Congress of Microbiology*, February 6-7, 1995.

[44] Janeway, C.A.; Travers, P.; Walport, M.; Shlomchik, M.J. *Immuno Biology 5: The Immune System in Health and Disease*. New York: Garland Publishing, 2001.

[45] Abuja, P.M.; Murkovic, M.; Pfannhauser, W. Antioxidant and prooxidant activities of elderberry (*Sambucus nigra*) extract in low-density lipoprotein oxidation. *Journal of Agricultural and Food Chemistry*, 1998, *46*, 4091-4096.

In: Berries: Properties, Consumption and Nutrition
Editor: Carlo Tuberoso
ISBN 978-1-61470-257-3

Chapter VII

Myrtle (*Myrtus communis* L.) Berries: Composition and Properties

***Carlo I. G. Tuberoso*[*a] *and Christina D. Orrú*[b]**
[a]Department of Toxicology, University of Cagliari, Cagliari, Italy
[b]Laboratory of Persistent Viral Diseases, Rocky Mountain Laboratories, National Institute of Allergy and Infectious Diseases, National Institutes of Health, Hamilton, MT, USA

Abstract

Myrtle (*Myrtus communis* L.) berries are very popular fruits in the Mediterranean area. They are used for food aromatization and for the preparation of characteristic alcoholic products such as liqueur, eau-de-vie and wine. The berries are spherical in shape, dark red to violet in color, and contain organic acids, carbohydrates, phenolic compounds, volatiles, lipids, anions and cations. Their distinctive flavor and color are due to their volatiles and polyphenols content, respectively. The main compounds in myrtle berries' volatile fraction are α-pinene, limonene and 1,8-cineole. The phenolic compounds fraction is characterized by gallic acid, flavonoids and anthocyans that represent the most abundant phytochemicals in myrtle berries. The anthocyanin profile shows five anthocyanin glucosides and four anthocyanin arabinosides with malvidin-3-*O*-glucoside, delphinidin-3-*O*-glucoside, and petunidin-3-*O*-glucoside as major peaks. Flavonoid profile is characterized by myricetin-3-*O*-galactoside, myricetin-3-*O*-rhamnoside, myricetin and quercetin. Myricetin and gallic acid derivatives are thought to be the most efficient molecules in inhibiting free radical and lipid peroxidation. Myrtle berry extracts prepared using solvents with different polarity (water, ethanol, and ethyl acetate) were analyzed using several in vitro tests to investigate their antioxidant properties. The strongest antiradical and antioxidant activities (measured with DPPH and FRAP tests, respectively) were found in ethanol and ethyl acetate extracts. These same

* Department of Toxicology, University of Cagliari, Via Ospedale 72, 09124 Cagliari, Italy, E-mail: tuberoso@unica.it.

extracts also showed the highest content of phenolic compounds. The ethyl acetate extract had the strongest protective effect in assays of thermal (140°C) cholesterol degradation and Cu^{2+}-mediated LDL oxidation, inhibiting the reduction of polyunsaturated fatty acids and cholesterol, and the increase of their oxidative products. These results suggest that besides the well-established food use, myrtle berries could be used in dietary supplement preparation or as food additives. Therefore, because of their multiple possible uses, a cultivar selection programme has been recently started with the aim of providing berries with the best nutritional properties for industrial use.

Introduction

Myrtle (*Myrtus communis* L, Mirtaceae), is an evergreen shrub or small tree endemic to the Mediterranean area that can also be found in several other regions all over the world. It has been cited in the Bible and in many ancient medicinal plant books, such as the *De Materia Medica* of Dioscorides. The essential oil obtained by hydrodistillation of myrtle leaves and, sometimes, flowers and berries has been used for its antimicrobial, tonic, and balsamic properties, and it is currently used in the flavor and fragrance industry. Extracts from leaves and berries are used to make cosmetics and toilettes products like shampoo and skin care products. Myrtle berries are mostly utilized in some areas of the Mediterranean for food aromatization, and to prepare alcoholic products such as liqueur, eau-de-vie and wine [1,2].

Botanical Description

The myrtle shrub is one to three meters tall, grows spontaneously along the coast and in the internal hill regions of the Mediterranean area, and it is widely spread in the islands, where it is one of the most common species [1,2]. This plant is able to adapt to a variety of climates and has a remarkable resistance to pests and diseases. Myrtle leaves are coriaceous and ovate shaped with a straight edge. Flowers bloom in summer and have a star-like shape, with five (or more) white petals and sepals, and a large number of stamens. In the Mediterranean area the fruits mature in November-December and the berry production can be up to 4 kg per plant. Myrtle berries are spherical in shape, dark red to violet in color, with a balsamic and fragrant aroma and an astringent, bitter and spicy taste. Myrtle berry's characteristics vary significantly according to the phenotype and year of production, but the average values are: width 0.5-1.3 cm, length 0.8-1.5 cm, fresh weight 0.2-0.5 g, water content 65-70%; number of seeds per berry 4-16 (seeds amount to 13-24%, w/w of the fresh berry) [3-5]. Their main use in the food industry is as flavoring of beverages, sweets and jams. Sometimes, plants bearing only white berries can be found. These white berries are very similar in size, shape and chemical composition to the red-violet ones, but they lack the pigments (anthocyanins). During the past few years a cultivar selection programme has been carried out to provide berries to the industry with the best technological and nutritional properties. Cultivation of myrtle is rather easy, nonetheless at the moment harvesting represents the most expensive step of berries production. Currently, the goal is to develop a mechanized system to harvest the berries to significantly reduce the cost of harvesting.

Myrtle Berries Chemical Composition

Myrtle berries contain all the main chemical classes: organic acids (gluconic acid, malic acid, citric acid, shikimic acid, and quinic acid), carbohydrates, volatiles (monoterpenes, alcohols, esters, ethers, sesquiterpenes, oxides), amino acids, phenolic compounds (gallic acid derivatives, anthocyanins and flavonoids, tannins, etc.), lipids (oleic acid, linoleic acid, palmitic acid, and linolenic acid), anions (Cl^-, PO_4^{3-}, SO_4^{2-}) and cations (K^+, Mg^{2+}, Na^+, Ca^{2+}) (Table 1) [5-14].

These compounds contribute to the distinctive sensory properties of myrtle berries. For instance, the berries are not usually eaten fresh because of the astringent-bitter taste due to tannins, while volatiles and polyphenols compounds are responsible for the typical flavor and color of myrtle berries.

Table 1. Chemical profile of myrtle berries.

Class	Compounds
Organic acids	gluconic acid, malic acid, citric acid, quinic acid, shikimic acid
Fatty acids	carboxylic acids with chain length ranging from C_{20} to C_{30}, represented mainly by linoleic acid, palmitic acid, oleic acid, linolenic acid
Phenolic compounds	gallic acid, 3,4-dihydroxybenzoic acid, epi-gallocatechin, ellagic acid, (+) catechin, (-) epicatechin-3-*O*-gallate, (-) epigallocatechin, (-) epigallocatechin-3-*O*-gallate *Anthocyanins*: mono glucosides and arabinosides of malvidin, delphinidin, peonidyn, petunidin, and cyanidin *Flavonoids*: myricetin, myricetin-3-*O*-galactoside, myricetin-3-*O*-rhamnoside, myricetin-3-*O*-arabinoside, myricetin-3-(6''-*O*-galloyl galactoside), quercetin, quercetin-3-*O*-glucoside, quercetin-3-*O*-rhamnoside, kaempferol
Volatile compounds	α-thujene, α-pinene, β-pinene, myrcene, α-phellandrene, δ-3-carene, α-terpinene, p-cymene, limonene, 1,8-cineole, γ-terpinene, terpinolene, linalool, terpinen-4-ol, α-terpineol, linalyl acetate, myrtenyl acetate, terpenyl acetate, neryl acetate, geranyl acetate, methyleugenol, β-caryophyllene, α-humulene, allo-aromadendrene, β-selinene, germacrene B, spathulenole, caryophyllene oxide
Aminoacids	aspartic acid, glutamic acid, hystidine, lysine, phenylalanine, valine, alanine, proline
Other	oleanolic acid, ursolic acid, α-tocopherol, myrtucommulone
Inorganic compounds	*Anions*: Cl^-, PO_4^{3-}, SO_4^{2-} *Cations*: K^+, Mg^{2+}, Na^+, Ca^{2+}

Source: [5-14].

Volatiles compounds. The essential oil yield from myrtle berries is very low, approximately 0.02-0.03 mL/100 g dried weight. Typically, berries' essential oil composition is very similar to that of the leaves coming from the same plant. Interestingly, a significant chemical variability in essential oils' composition obtained from different plants exists. Literature data show that α-pinene, limonene, 1,8-cineole, myrtenyl acetate, linalool and linalyl acetate are the most abundant compounds, but sometimes one or more of them can be missing [16]. For instance, myrtle volatiles from Morocco, ex-Yugoslavia, Spain, Albania, and Croatia contain variable levels of myrtenyl acetate. Essential oils obtained from Sardinian and Corsican myrtle berries belong to a different chemotype, contain α-pinene, 1,8-cineole, limonene, and are characterized by the presence of just traces or complete lack of myrtenol and myrtenyl acetate [13,15]. Figure 1 shows a typical GC-MS chromatogram on DB-5 column of an essential oil from Sardinian myrtle berries, characterized by an elevated content in monoterpenes (65.7-89.1% of the total). However, a remarkable variability among the compounds present can be noticed: α-pinene (18.2-38.9%), limonene (3.7-44.5%), 1,8-cineole (5.8-24.8%), geranyl acetate (0.2-13.0%), linalool (0.4-14.7%), p-cymene (0.1-10.3%), δ-3-carene (0.0-6.1%), terpinolene (0.0-5.9%), γ-terpinene (0.5-5.8%), terpenyl acetate (0.1-5.4%). Myrtle berries contain some level of sesquiterpenes, representing 5.0% of the entire oil at the most, with β-caryophyllene, caryophyllene oxide, germacrene B, and spathulenol being the most abundant.

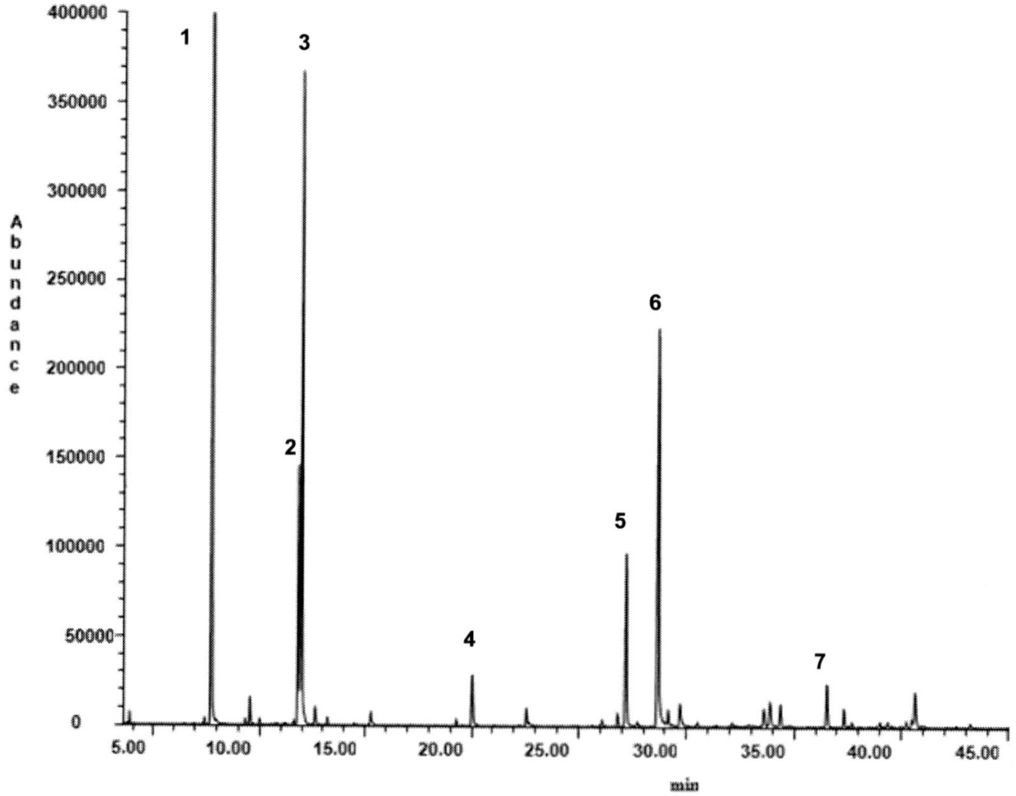

Figure 1. TIC (Total Ion Current) of the essential oil from myrtle berries. 1) α-pinene, 2) limonene, 3) 1,8-cineole, 4) α-terpineol, 5) terpenyl acetate, 6) geranyl acetate 7) caryophyllene oxide. Volatile compounds eluted from a DB-5MS column with operative condition described by Tuberoso *et al.* [13].

Phenolic compounds. The phenolic fraction analyzed by HPLC-DAD, HPLC-MS and MS/MS showed the presence of gallic acid derivatives (gallic acid, 3,4-dihydroxybenzoic acid), flavonoids and anthocyans as the major polyphenolic compounds in myrtle berries [7,10,14]. The anthocyanin profile indicates the presence of five anthocyanidins (malvidin, delphinidin, peonidin, petunidin, and cyanidin) in both their glucosides and arabinosides derivatives. No aglycones and diglycosides were found. Malvidin-3-*O*-glucoside is the most abundant compound, followed by delphinidin-3-*O*-glucoside, and petunidin-3-*O*-glucoside (Figure 2).

Flavonoid profile is characterized by myricetin-3-*O*-galactoside, myricetin-3-*O*-rhamnoside, myricetin and quercetin, but also derivatives like myricetin-3-(6''-*O*-galloyl galactoside) can be found. So far no major variability has been observed in the phenolic fraction of berries from different geographical areas, although an interesting difference in anthocyanin glucosides and arabinosides percentage can be related to the geographical origin of the plant [12].

Phenolic compounds are responsible for many aspects of berries' properties. Sensory properties are influenced by the presence of tannins (taste) and anthocyanins (color). Flavonoids have interesting biological activities. Myricetin-3-*O*-galactoside and myricetin-3-*O*-rhamnoside are potent free radical and lipid peroxidation inhibitors and have antigenotoxic and antimutagenic properties [15]. Remarkably, depending on the polarity of the extraction solvents used, these phytochemicals can be selectively extracted from berries allowing to target the desired active component.

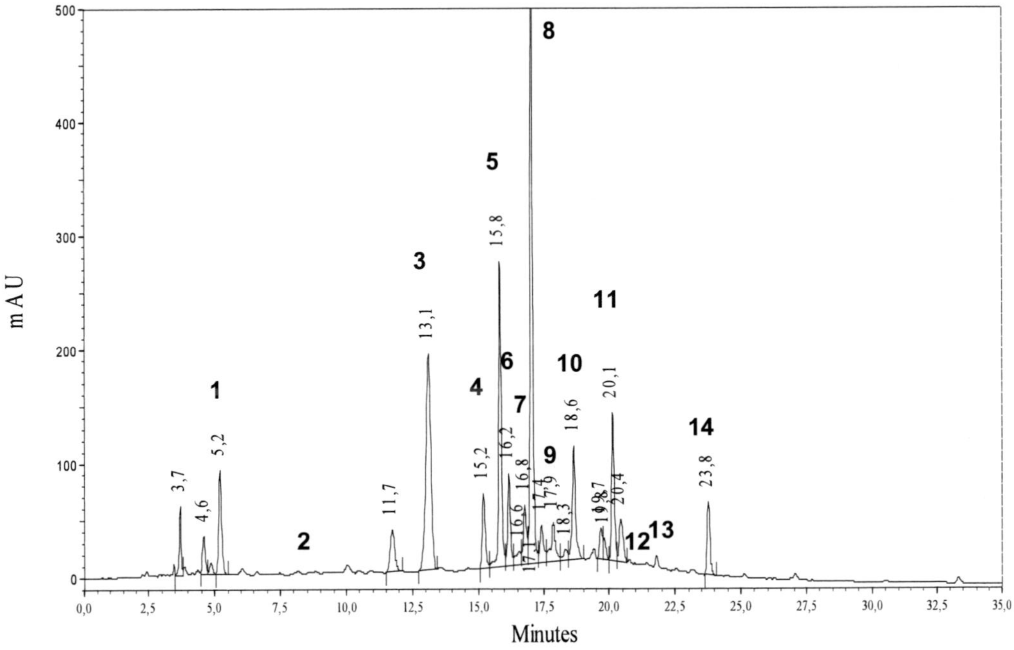

Figure 2. HPLC-DAD (λ=280nm) chromatogram of myrtle berries alcoholic extract [7]. 1) gallic acid, 2) 3,4-dihydroxybenzoic acid, 3) delphinidin-3-*O*-glucoside, 4) cyanidin-3-*O*-glucoside, 5) petunidin-3-*O*-glucoside, 6) delphinidin-3-*O*-arabinoside, 7) peonidin-3-*O*-glucoside, 8) malvidin-3-*O*-glucoside, 9)

malvidin-3-*O*-arabinoside, 10) myricetin-3-*O*-galactoside, 11) myricetin-3-*O*-ramnoside, 12) ellagic acid, 13) myricetin-3-*O*-arabinoside, 14) myricetin.

Myrtle Liqueur

Among the various alcoholic beverages obtained from myrtle berries, Sardinian myrtle liqueur has shown a constant market growth. The liqueur "*Mirto di Sardegna*" has been legally recognized by the European Union as "spirit drinks with geographical designations". Briefly, this liqueur is traditionally obtained by hydro-alcoholic extraction of the violet-colored mature berries at room temperature for 4-5 weeks. Next, the extract is diluted in water and sugar until the alcoholic grade is adjusted to 28-32 % v/v and the sugar content ranges between 20 and 30% w/v [2]. A minimum of 150 g of berries should be used to make a liter of liqueur. No aromatic or preservative substances are added. Furthermore, the so-called "white myrtle" liqueur is made by alcoholic extraction of myrtle leaves, but its market share represents only 10% of total sales.

Industrially produced myrtle liquors require longer maceration periods and adequate technological procedures to extract all the phytochemicals and obtain a liqueur with stable flavor and color. Several berry processing techniques have been suggested to improve extraction efficiency for the production of myrtle liqueur. The use of more berries, ultrasonic extraction, the use of enzymes to improve either the color or the aroma, and nitrogen atmosphere saturation to improve the stability against the oxidative degradation that occurs during extraction were tried [18]. Moreover, since myrtle berries are seasonal, strategies to prolong the availability of berries and the stability their extracts have been proposed. Postharvest treatments like freezing (-20°C) and cold storage after treatment in water or soy lecithin at different temperatures have been tried with no conclusive evidence of improved storage duration. The goal is to obtain a balance between the cost of the procedures and the results obtained. Among the technological processes used by the industry, the nitrogen-modified atmosphere was the most suitable technique. The liqueur maintained a higher level of anthocyanins, had better color parameters (CIE L*a*b*) and superior organoleptic characteristics compared to the traditionally stored liquors. Although the use of nitrogen is expensive, this practice is quite widespread in the food industry, and it could be applied to myrtle liqueur production.

Myrtle liqueur's peculiar flavor and color are strongly associated with its contents of volatiles and polyphenols respectively. A comparison of the volatiles fraction of myrtle alcoholic extract percentage with the essential oil from the same berries has shown a similar compound pattern, with high levels of α-pinene, 1,8-cineole and limonene [13,17]. The flavor of ethanolic extracts and liqueurs depends on the presence of both terpenes and ethyl esters of fatty acids, mainly ethyl palmitate, ethyl linoleate, ethyl linolenate, and ethyl stearate. Thus, the spicy flavor of terpenes is softened by the gentle smell of new-formed esters. Anthocyanins are responsible for the purple color and, during the liqueur's ageing, they disappear slowly, creating polymeric forms of the polyphenolic compounds. Consequently, myrtle berries alcoholic extracts turn from red-purple to tawny color, in a similar way to red wine's ageing.

Biological Activities

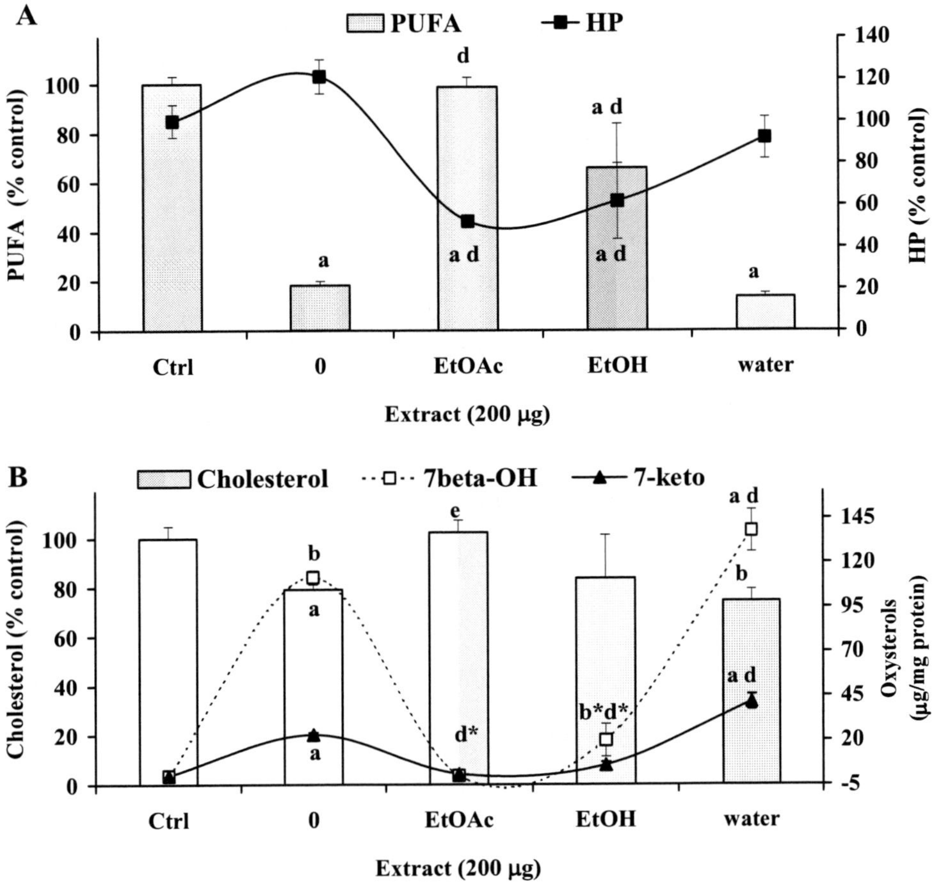

Figure 3. Total values of the polyunsaturated fatty acids (PUFA: arachidonic acid 20:4, eicosapentaenoic acid 20:5 n-3, eicosatrienoic acid 20:3, and docosahexaenoic acid 22:6 n-3), conjugated dienes fatty acids hydroperoxides (HP), cholesterol and oxysterols (7β-OH and 7-keto) measured in control (Ctrl), and during LDL oxidation at 37°C for 2 h with 5 μM $CuSO_4$, in the absence (oxidised control, 0), and in the presence of 200 μg of the EtOAc, EtOH, and water extracts [7].

The study of the chemical composition of Sardinian myrtle liqueur gave some interesting hints that help to identify and avoid frauds. The presence of myrtenyl acetate indicates the use of non local berries. The presence of acylated anthocyanins, not naturally present in myrtle berries, can indicate fraudulent addiction of red grape extracts. Also, a study of the organic acid fraction can be helpful: presence of tartaric acid (absent in myrtle berries) suggest the addition of grape extracts and unusually high levels of gluconic acid can indicate prolonged liqueur storage or the use of old berries to make the liquor.

Myrtle berries extracted with solvents at different polarities have shown several interesting biological properties. Inhibitory activities against food-borne pathogens and spoilage bacteria [19] and ulcer-protective effects [20] have been reported. Water, methanol, ethanol, and ethyl acetate extracts were tested with different in vitro assays to investigate their antioxidant properties [7-21]. A significant positive correlation exists between antiradical/antioxidant activities and content of phenolic compounds. Therefore, the most potent activities can be found in solvents that preferentially extract polyphenols, like methanol, ethanol and ethyl acetate. Typical screening assays like DPPH and FRAP tests showed potent antiradical and antioxidant activities in ethanol and ethyl acetate extracts [7].

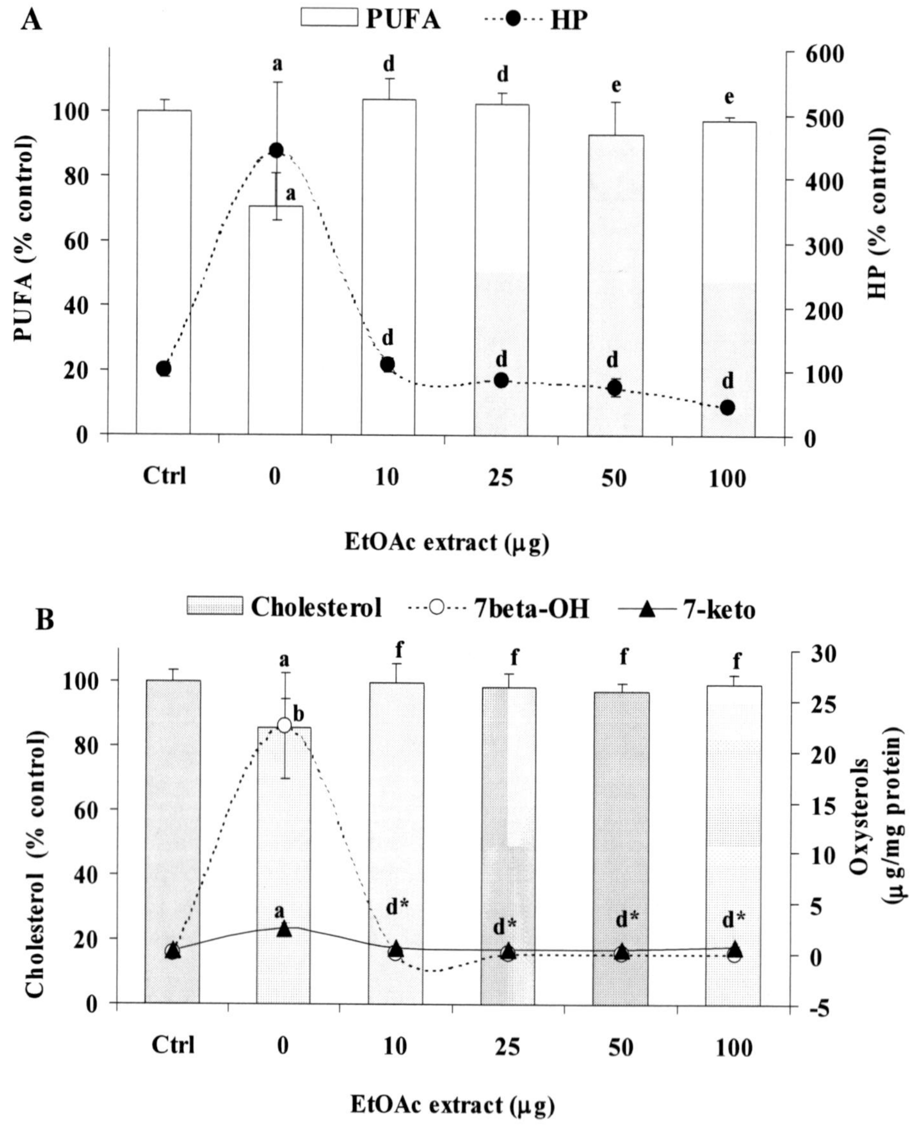

Figure 4. Total values of the PUFA, HP, cholesterol and oxysterols measured in control (Ctrl) and during LDL oxidation at 37° C for 2 h with 5 μM $CuSO_4$, in the absence (oxidised control, 0), and in the presence of different amounts (10–100 μg) of the EtOAc extract [7].

Similar results were obtained with antioxidant assays that use biological models, such as protection on cholesterol and LDL oxidation. The berries extracts were assayed for their ability to protect cholesterol against oxidative, solvent-free, degradation at high temperature (140°C), for 1 or 2 h. Under these conditions, the ethanol and ethyl acetate extracts were active, but the ethyl acetate extract showed the best protecting activity. The same results were obtained when testing the ability to protect LDL against copper-induced oxidation at 37°C (Figure 3).

Figure 4 shows the values of polyunsaturated fatty acids, hydroperoxides (Fig. 4A), cholesterol, 7β-OH, and 7-keto (Fig. 4B), measured for control LDL, and during Cu^{2+} induced oxidation in the absence or in the presence of different amounts (10–100 μg) of ethyl acetate extracts. The ethyl acetate extract showed a substantial total protection, when compared to the oxidized control, with all doses tested for PUFA and cholesterol, with values of HP and oxysterols similar to the control [7]. The antioxidant activity observed in ethyl acetate extract may depend on the higher lipophilicity of this system, and consequently on the reduced polarity of the extracted compounds. The ethyl acetate extract is the richest in flavonol aglycones (myricetin) and contains high levels of gallic acid derivatives. These compounds are thought to be the most potent molecules in inhibiting free radical and lipid peroxidation. The intriguing antioxidant properties of the ethanolic extract might depend on the high levels of myricetin-3-*O*-galactoside and myricetin-3-*O*-rhamnoside, molecules that are very potent in inhibiting free radical and lipid peroxidation [15].

Interestingly, phenolic compounds and their biological properties are still present in the extracts used for food production. Several studies report high levels of antioxidant and antiradical activities also in the myrtle liqueur [22,23], and these activities correlate with the amount of phenolic compounds present. These properties give a special nutritional value to the myrtle liqueur, similar to that of red wine.

Conclusions

The results here reported suggest that, besides traditional food use, myrtle berries could be widely employed in many other fields, such as the nutraceutical sector. In fact, proprieties of *in toto* extracts obtained from myrtle berries make this fruit suitable to be used in the preparation of dietary supplements. The food industry can benefit from natural additives with antioxidant and preservative properties derived from myrtle berries. Purified fractions and single molecules extracted from the phenolic fraction have potential pharmaceutical use in drug preparation. Thus, the versatility of *Myrtus communis* berries employment is a powerful tool for the economic development of areas with limited resources.

References

[1] Atzei, A.D. Le piante nella tradizione popolare della Sardegna. Carlo Delfino ed. Sassari, Italy, 2003, 319-324.

[2] AA. VV. Caratterizzazione del liquore Mirto di Sardegna Tradizionale. Aspetti storici, geografici, tecnico economici-gestionali e chimico-merceologici; Ed. Confindustria della Sardegna, Cagliari, Italy, 1998.

[3] Tuberoso, C.I.G.; Melis, M.; Angioni, A.; Pala, M.; Cabras, P. Myrtle hydroalcoholic extracts obtained from different selections of *Myrtus communis* L. *Food Chemistry*, 2007, *101*, 806-811.

[4] Mulas, M.; Cani, M.R.; Brigaglia, N. Characters useful to cultivation in spontaneous populations of *Myrtus communis* L. Symposium on Plant Biotechnology as a tool for the exploitation of mountain lands. *Acta Horticulturae*, 1998, *457*, 271-278.

[5] Aydin, C.; Ozcan, M. M. Determination of nutritional and physical properties of myrtle (*Myrtus communis* L.) fruits growing wild in Turkey. *Journal of Food Engineering*, 2007, *79*, 453-458.

[6] F.M. Piras, M.F. Dettori, A. Magnani. ToF-SIMS PCA analysis of *Myrtus communis* L. *Applied Surface Science*, 2009, *255*, 7805–7811.

[7] Tuberoso, C.I.G.; Rosa, A.; Bifulco, E.; Melis, M.P.; Atzeri, A.; Pirisi, F.M.; Dessì, M. A. Chemical composition and antioxidant activities of *Myrtus communis* L. berries extracts. *Food Chemistry*, 2010, *123*, 1242-1251.

[8] Franco, M.A.; Versini, G.; Mattivi, F.; Dalla Serra, A.; Vacca, V.; Manca, G. Analytical characterization of myrtle berries, partially processed products and commercially available liqueurs. *Journal of Commodity Science*, 2002, *41*, 143-267.

[9] Wannes, W.A.; Mhamdi, B.; Sriti, J.; Marzouk, B. Glycerolipid and fatty acid distribution in pericarp, seed and whole fruit oils of *Myrtus communis* var. *italica*. *Industrial Crops and Products*, 2010, *31*, 77-83.

[10] Barboni, T.; Cannac, M.; Massi, L; Perez-Ramirez, Y.; Chiaramonti, N. Variability of polyphenol compounds in *Myrtus communis* L. (Myrtaceae) berries from Corsica. *Molecules*, 2010, *15*, 7849-7860.

[11] Cakir, A. Essential oil and fatty acid composition of the fruits of *Hippophae rhamnoides* L. (Sea Buckthorn) and *Myrtus communis* L. from Turkey. *Biochemical Systematics and Ecology*, 2004, *32*, 809–816.

[12] Montoro, P.; Tuberoso, C.I.G.; Perrone, A.; Piacente, S.; Cabras, P.; Pizza C. Characterisation by liquid chromatography-electrospray tandem mass spectrometry of anthocyanins in extracts of *Myrtus communis* L. berries used for the preparation of myrtle liqueur. *Journal of Chromatography A*, 2006, *1112*, 232-240.

[13] Tuberoso, C.I.G.; Barra, A.; Angioni, A.; Sarritzu, E.; Pirisi, F.M. Chemical composition of volatiles in Sardinian myrtle (*Myrtus communis* L.) alcoholic extracts and essential oils. *Journal of Agricultural and Food Chemistry*, 2006, *54*, 1420-1426.

[14] Montoro, P.; Tuberoso, C.I.G.; Piacente, S.; Perrone, A.; De Feo, V.; Cabras, P.; Pizza C. Stability and antioxidant activity of polyphenols in extracts of *Myrtus communis* L. berries used for the preparation of myrtle liqueur. *Journal of Pharmaceutical and Biomedical Analysis*, 2006, *41*, 1614-1619.

[15] Hayder, N.; Bouhlel, I.; Skandrani, I.; Kadri, M.; Steiman, R.; Guiraud, P.; Mariotte, A.-M.; Ghedira, K.; Dijoux-Franca, M.-G.; Chekir-Ghedira L.. In vitro antioxidant and antigenotoxic potentials of myricetin-3-O-galactoside and myricetin-3-O-rhamnoside from Myrtus communis: Modulation of expression of genes involved in cell defence system using cDNA microarray. *Toxicology in Vitro*, 2008, *22*, 567–581.

[16] Pereira, P.C.; Cebola, M.J.; Bernardo-Gil, M.G. Evolution of the yields and composition of essential oil from Portuguese myrtle (*Myrtus communis* L.) through the vegetative cycle. *Molecules*, 2009, *14*, 3094-3105.

[17] Barboni, T.; Venturini, N.; Paolini, J.; Desjobert, J.-M.; Chiaramonti, N.; Costa, J. Characterisation of volatiles and polyphenols for quality assessment of alcoholic beverages prepared from Corsican *Myrtus communis* berries. *Food Chemistry*, 2010, *122*, 1304–1312.

[18] Tuberoso, C.I.G.; Barra, A.; Cabras, P. Effect of different technological processes on the chemical composition of myrtle (*Myrtus communis* L.) alcoholic extracts. *European Food Research and Technology*, 2008, *226*, 801-808.

[19] Amensour, M.; Bouhdid, S.; Fernández-López, J.; Idaomar, M.; Skali-Senhaji, N.; Abrini, J. Antibacterial activity of extracts of *Myrtus communis* against food-borne pathogenic and spoilage bacteria. *International Journal of Food Properties*, 2010, *13*, 1215-1224.

[20] Sumbul, S.; Ahmad, M.A.; Asif, M.; Saud, I.; Akhtar M. Evaluation of *Myrtus communis* Linn. berries (common myrtle) in experimental ulcer models in rats. *Human & Experimental Toxicology*, 2010, *29*, 935-944.

[21] Amensour M.; Sendrah, E; Abrini, J; Bouhdid, S; Perez-Alvarez, J.A.; Fernandez-Lopez, J. Total phenolic content and antioxidant activity of myrtle (*Myrtus communis*) extracts. *Natural Product Communications*, 2009, *4*, 819-824.

[22] Alamanni, M.C.; Cossu, M. Radical scavenging activity and antioxidant activity of liquors of myrtle (*Myrtus communis* L.) berries and leaves. *Italian Journal of Food Science*, 2004, *16*, 197-208.

[23] Vacca, V.; Piga, A.; Del Caro, A.; Fenu, P.A.M.; Agabbio M. Changes in phenolic compounds, colour and antioxidant activity in industrial red myrtle liqueurs during storage. *Nahrung/Food*, 2003, *47*, 442-447.

In: Berries: Properties, Consumption and Nutrition
Editor: Carlo Tuberoso
ISBN 978-1-61470-257-3

Chapter VIII

Colombian Bilberry (*Vaccinium Meridionale* Swartz): Chemical Composition, Antioxidant Activity, Anthocyanin and Non-Anthocyanin Phenolic Composition as Compared to Other *Vaccinium* Species

Gloria Astrid Garzón[*]
Departamento de Química,
Universidad Nacional de Colombia, Bogotá, Colombia

Abstract

Vaccinium meridionale Swartz is a wild shrub belonging to the family of Mirtaceae and native to the country of Colombia. The fruit which is called mortiño or agraz is a bilberry, 5 -10 mm in diameter, with many small seeds and a sour and tart character. Berries are eaten fresh or processed into dried fruit, sauces, jellies, yogurt bases, wine and jams. The consumption and potential for export of *V. meridionale* is increasing due to the known nutraceutical properties of bilberries (*Vaccinium myrtillus* L.), including management of visual disorders and protection against cancer, age-related neurodegenerative conditions, and inflammatory responses. These nutraceutical properties are strongly associated with the content and profile of anthocyanins and non-anthocyanin polyphenols, which are also partially responsible for the high antioxidant activity of bilberries. Given the supporting information on the potential nutraceutical properties of bilberry, it is of interest to characterize the wild *Vaccinium* species that grow in Colombia. Accordingly, available information on the chemical composition, total

[*] Departamento de Química, Universidad Nacional de Colombia, AA 14490 Bogotá, Colombia, E-mail: agarzonmo@unal.edu.co.

anthocyanin and phenolic contents, anthocyanin profile, non-anthocyanin phenolic profile, and antioxidant activity of Colombian bilberry is summarized, discussed and compared with reports for other well-characterized *Vaccinium* species. The reported anthocyanin content of *V. meridionale* ranges between 201 ± 10 and 329.0 ± 28.0 mg cyanidin 3-glucoside equivalents/100 g FW while the total phenolic content varies between 609.0 ± 39.0 and 758.6 ± 62.3 mg gallic acid equivalent/100 g FW. Unlike other bilberries, Colombian bilberries contain only cyanidin and delphinidin. Cyanidin 3-galactoside is the major anthocyanin representing 43% of the total peak area. Non-anthocyanin phenolics include hydroxycinnamic acids and flavonols and the most abundant compound is chlorogenic acid. Berries of *V. meridionale* show high antioxidant activity. The reported ABTS radical scavenging activity is within 45.5 ± 2.3 - 86.9 ± 4.4 µmol Trolox equivalents/g FW. This radical scavenging activity is close to that one of blueberries, which constitute one of the richest reported antioxidants. Similarly, the ferric reducing antioxidant potential (FRAP) (87.0 ± 17.8 µmol Trolox equivalents/g FW or 116.0 ± 23.7 µmol ferric iron reduced/g FW) is close to that one of *V. myrtillus.* Overall, results from available studies show that the anthocyanin composition of Colombian wild bilberry can be differentiated from other bilberries by their unique pattern. Moreover, *V. meridionale* berries are an excellent source of dietary phytochemicals such as anthocyanins and polyphenolics, being comparable to *V. myrtillus*. Consequently, there is potential for the use of *V. meridionale* as a source of phytochemicals in the nutraceutical and functional food market.

Introduction

The *Vaccinium* genus belongs to the Ericaceae family and comprises more than 150 species including bilberries, some of which have been domesticated in the USA and Canada. Unlike North American domesticated species, *Vaccinium meridionale* Swartz is a wild shrub native to Andean South America, where it grows on open mountain slopes between 2200 and 3400 m above sea level. The fruit is a bilberry, 5-10 mm in diameter, with many small seeds and a sour and tart character. The color varies from green to dark purple during ripening.

In the country of Colombia bilberries, also called mortiño berries or agraz, are collected from wild bushes and sold fresh in the local markets during two ripening seasons; one between April and May and the other between September and December. The fruit is also processed into dried fruit, sauces, jellies, yogurt bases, wine, and jams.

Bilberries are of current interest due to their high content of anthocyanins, non-anthocyanin phenolics and antioxidant activity, which are related to protective effects against diseases including cancer [1], management of visual disorders [2], age-related neurodegenerative diseases, inflammatory responses, and diverse degenerative diseases [3].

European and North American bilberries have been characterized as having high concentrations of flavonoids with potential use for the food, nutraceutical, and pharmaceutical industries [4,5]. Characterized phenolic compounds include gallic and ellagic acids, ellagitannins, flavan-3-ols, proanthocyanidins, flavonol glycosides, hydroxycinnamic acids and anthocyanins, [6]. Stilbenes have been also found [7]. Total phenolic contents and antioxidant capacities have been determined and depend on variety, maturity, and location [8].

Considering the supporting information on the potential nutraceutical properties of bilberry, it is of interest to characterize the wild *Vaccinium* species that grow in Colombia. This chapter summarizes findings on chemical composition, total anthocyanin and phenolic contents, anthocyanin profile, polyphenolic profile, and antioxidant activity of Colombian bilberry (*V. meridionale* Swartz) as compared to the reported compositions for other well-characterized *Vaccinium* species.

Chemical Composition

Three authors have documented the chemical composition of Colombian bilberry. The average titratable acidity of the fruit found by Garzón *et al.* [9] was 1.35 ± 0.20, which is close to the value of *V. myrtillus* (1.52) found by Prior *et al.* [8]. Garzón *et al.* [9] also determined a pH of 2.85 ± 0.16 while Ligarreto [10] reported a pH value ranging between 2.2 and 2.7. According to Garzón *et al.* [9], the total soluble solids content was 7.00 ± 0.01 which was a lower value than the one reported by Ligarreto [10] (12.6-15.2), but in accordance to the value of 7.00 reported by Vasco *et al.* [11] for mortiño berries (*V. floribundum*) from Ecuador and lower than the value for *V. myrtillus* (10) [8]. Garzón *et al.* [9] concluded that the high titratable acidity of *V. meridionale* along with its low total soluble solids content seems to be the explanation for the low sugar/acid ratio (5.27 ± 0.70) of this fruit, which is lower than that one of *V. myrtillus* (6.60) reported by Prior *et al.* [8].

According to Vallejo [12], the moisture content of Colombian bilberry ranged from 84.2-85.6 %, which is higher than the value found by Vasco *et al.* [11] for *V. floribundum* from Ecuador (81.0 ± 2.0 %).

Conversely, the dietary fiber content (2-51- 2.56 %), was lower than the one found for mortiño berries from Ecuador as reported by the same authors (7.6 ± 2.2 %).

The ascorbic acid content of *V. meridionale* found by Garzón *et al.* [9] is 8.10 ± 1.50 mg/100 g FW. This content is 8 fold higher than the one reported by Prior *et al.* [8] for *V. myrtillius* (1.3 mg/100 g FW), but it is within the range of some *V. corymbosum* and *V. ashei* cultivars (6.2-14.6 mg/100 g FW) reported by the same author and close to the content in *V. floribundum* (9.0 mg/100 g FW) as reported by Vasco *et al.* [11].

Antioxidant Activity

Reports from Ligarreto [10] and Garzón *et al.* [9] show that Colombian bilberry has high antioxidant activity as indicated by the ABTS and FRAP assays. The ABTS radical scavenging activity found by Ligarreto [10] was about twice fold the one reported by Garzón *et al.* [9]. Analysis by the first author indicates that the antioxidant activity of Colombian bilberries is 86.9 ± 4.35 μmol Trolox equivalents/g FW while the second author found a value of 45.5 ± 2.3 μmol Trolox equivalents/g FW. This radical scavenging activity is close to that of *V. floribundum* from Ecuador (47.9 μmol Trolox equivalents/g FW) [11] and comparable to that one of blueberries (45.9 μmol Trolox equivalents/g), which constitutes one of the richest reported antioxidants [13].

The contribution of ascorbic acid to the total antioxidant capacity of complex mixtures of antioxidants can be calculated from the ABTS assay [14]. Ascorbic acid has a molar activity equal to that of Trolox; thus, since the ascorbic acid content of Colombian bilberry corresponds to a concentration of 0.94 μmol Trolox equivalents/g FW, it represents only 2.1% of the total observed Trolox equivalent antioxidant capacity (45.5 μmol TEAC/g) [9].

Although the anthocyanin and non-anthocyanin phenolic contents and composition *V. meridionale* was somewhat different from that of *V. myrtillus* from the northern United States, *V. meridionale* provided similar iron reducing capacity. Investigations by Garzón *et al.* [9] showed that the FRAP value was 87.0 ± 17.8 μmol Trolox equivalents/g FW or 116.0 ± 23.7 μmol ferric iron reduced/g FW. Moyer *et al.* [15] found 94.9 μmol ferric iron reduced/g FW for *V. myrtillus* harvested in the Pacific Northwest United States.

The ABTS method measures the ability of the antioxidant to quench radicals (probably by an electron transfer reaction) while the FRAP assay measures the potential of an antioxidant to reduce the yellow ferric-TPTZ complex to a blue ferrous-TPTZ complex by electron-donating substances under acidic conditions.

According to the results obtained by the authors, Colombian bilberry is a good electron donor as its extract was able to quench $ABTS^{\cdot +}$ radicals and reduce the ferric complex to a ferrous complex. The high ABTS and FRAP values of *V. meridionale* extract along with its low content of ascorbic acid, suggest that phenolic compounds are the main contributors to the high antioxidant activity of this fruit.

Anthocyanins and Totalphenolics Content

The anthocyanin concentration in Colombian bilberries has been reported by two authors. In 2009 Ligarreto [10] found 201 ± 10 mg cyanidin 3-glucoside/100 g FW while Garzón *et al.* [9] reported 329 ± 28 mg cyanidin 3-glucoside/100 g FW. This last value is within the range (300-698 mg cyanidin 3-glucoside/100 g) reported for *V. myrtillus* native to parts of Europe and northern regions of Asia [16], comparable to the anthocyanin concentration (300 mg cyanidin 3-glucoside/100 g) found by Prior *et al.* [8] for bilberry from northern United States and by Vasco *et al.* [11] for *V. floribundum* form Ecuador (345 mg cyanidin 3-glucoside/100 g). Regarding the total phenolic content, Ligarreto [10] reported a lower content (609 ± 39 mg gallic acid equivalents/100 g FW) than Garzón *et al.* [9] (758.6 ± 62.3 mg gallic acid equivalents/100 g FW).

These values are lower than that one of *V. floribundum* form Ecuador (882 mg gallic acid equivalents/100 mg FW) [11] and high compared to that one of other *Vaccinium* species. Prior *et al.* [8] reported 525 mg gallic acid equivalents/100 g FW for North American *V. myrtillus* and a range between 190-473 mg gallic acid equivalents/100 g FW for several cultivars of *V. corymbosum, V. ashei* and *V. angustifolium*. It has been reported that plant phenolics show qualitative and quantitative variation at different genetic levels (between and within species and clones) [17] and between different physiological and developmental stages [18]. Phenolics also vary in response to environmental factors, such as light intensity and nutrient availability [19].

All these factors may contribute to the differences in anthocyanin and phenolic content between *V. meridionale* and other *Vaccinium* species previously studied.

Anthocyanins and Non-Anthocyanin Phenolics Composition

The first investigation on the anthocyanin and non-anthocyanin phenolics composition in Colombian bilberries was done in 2010 by Garzón *et al.* [9]. The profiles were determined by HPLC-DAD/MS/MS. Five anthocyanins were identified as shown on Figure 1. Peaks 1, 2, 3 and 5 represented 99% of the total area while peak 4 accounted for 1%. Cyanidin-based anthocyanins represented 77% of the total anthocyanin content, which is lower than the content found in *V. floribundum* from Ecuador (88 % of the total anthocyanin content) [11]. Cyanidin 3-galactoside was the major anthocyanin representing 43% of the total peak area while cyanidin 3-glucoside and cyanidin 3-arabinoside were also found and the two remaining peaks were dephinidin-based anthocyanins.

Mass spectral data of the anthocyanins in Colombian bilberry (Table 1) showed that peak 1 revealed a molecular ion at *m/z* 465 and a major fragment at *m/z* 303, corresponding to a delphinidin derivative. The neutral loss of 162 mass units matched one molecule of hexose. As a result, peak 1 was tentatively identified as delphinidin 3-hexoside.

Peaks 2 and 4 revealed a molecular ion at *m/z* 449 and a fragment ion at *m/z* 287 produced by the loss of a hexose unit. This, along with authentic standards confirmed the HPLC-DAD identification of these peaks as cyanidin 3-galactoside and cyanidin 3-glucoside, respectively.

Peaks 3 and 5 produced molecular ions at *m/z* 435 and 419 and major fragments at *m/z* 303 and 287, which corresponds to the anthocyanidins delphinidin and cyanidin, respectively, after the loss of a pentoside. The fragmentation pattern, retention time and UV-Vis spectra of peak 5 matched that of the cyanidin 3-arabinoside standard. Accordingly, peak 3 was tentatively identified as a delphinidin 3-pentoside and peak 5 was labeled as cyanidin 3-arabinoside. The anthocyanin fragmentation pattern of molecular ions matched with those of previous studies in mortiño berries from Ecuador [11].

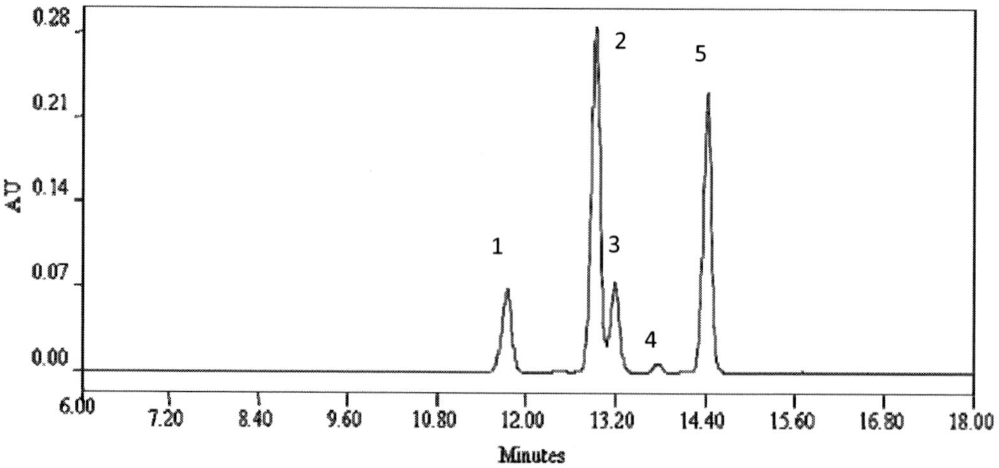

Figure 1. HPLC profile of anthocyanins in Colombian bilberry (*V. merdionale*) detected at 512 nm. 1) delphinidin 3-hexoside; 2) cyanidin 3-galactoside; 3) delphinidin 3-pentoside, 4) cyanidin 3-glucoside; 5) cyanidin 3-arabinoside.

Table 1. Chromatographic and spectroscopic characteristics of anthocyanins detected in *V. meridionale* Swartz listed according their retention time (Rt)

Peak n°	Peak area* (%)	λmax	Rt (min)	Molecular ion M^+ *m/z*	Fragment ions in MS/MS *m/z*	Tentative peak assignment
1	12	523	11.5	465	303	Delphinidin-3-hexoside
2	43	518	12.8	449	287	Cyanidin-3-galactoside
3	11	525	13.0	435	303	Delphinidin-3-pentoside
4	1	512	13.6	449	287	Cyanidin-3-glucoside
5	33	518	14.3	419	287	Cyanidin-3-arabinoside

* HPLC-DAD.

In general, bilberry has been reported as a source of cyanidin, delphinidin, peonidin, petunidin and malvidin galactosides, with delphinidin and cyanidin glucosides and arabinosides as the most abundant anthocyanins [20]. In contrast, Colombian bilberry contained only cyanidin and delphinidin glycosides, which is in accordance to the anthocyanin composition found in Andean blueberry from Ecuador [11].

Non-anthocyanin phenolics found in *V. meridionale* included hydroxycinnamic acids and flavonols (Table 2).

Table 2. Chromatographic and spectroscopic characteristics of non-anthocynin phenolics detected in *V. meridionale* Swartz listed according their retention time (Rt)

Peak n°	Peak area (%)	λmax	Rt min	Molecular ion $[M-H]^-$ *m/z*	Fragment ions in MS/MS *m/z*	Tentative peak assignment
1	67.9	326,242,290	9.8	353	191, 135,161,179	Caffeoylquinic acid isomer 1
2	3.0	326,242,290	10.3	353	191, 135,161,179	Caffeoylquinic acid

						isomer 2
3	2.9	328,242,290	16.2	367	135,179,161,191	Caffeoyl methyl quinate
4	5.6	328,242,290	17.4	433	161,135,179	Caffeic acid derivative
5	0.5	328,242,290	22.4	475	161,135,179	Caffeic acid derivative isomer 1
6	1.9	328,242,290	23.1	475	161,135,179	Caffeic acid derivative isomer 2
7	3.9	345, 255	18.4	463	300/301, 271,255,179,151	Quercetin hexoside
8	0.7	345, 256	19.7	433	257, 300/301, 271	Quercetin pentoside
9	0.8	357, 256	20.1	433	300/301,271,255	Quercetin pentoside
10	2.2	353, 255	20.6	433	300/301,271,255	Quercetin pentoside
11	4.5	345, 255	21.0	447	300/301,271,255	Quercetin rhamnoside
12	6.1	349, 256	24.1	591	300/301,447,489,529	Quercetin hydroxylmethylglutaryl-α-rhamnoside

* HPLC-DAD.

Six hydroxycinnamic acids were detected (Figure 2A) and quantified at 320 nm in equivalents of chlorogenic acid. Peaks 1, 2 and 3 represented 73.8% of the total nonanthocynin-phenolic peak area and were tentatively identified as members of the chlorogenic acid family.

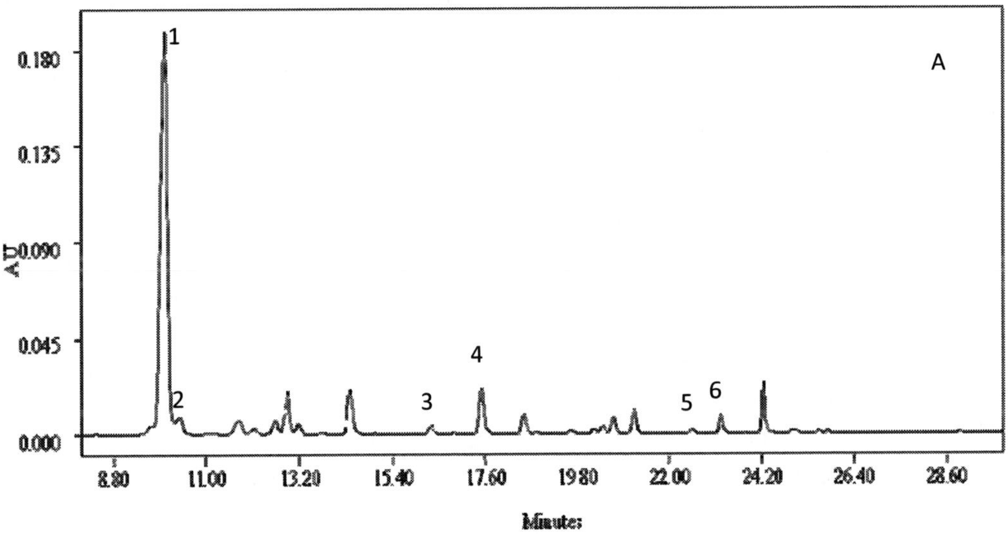

Figure 2. HPLC profiles of nonanthocyanin phenolics in wild bilberry (*V. merdionale*) at 320 nm (A) and 355 nm (B). 1) caffeoylquinic acid isomer 1; 2) caffeoylquinic acid isomer 2; 3) caffeoyl methyl quinate; 4) caffeic acid derivative; 5) caffeic acid derivative; 6) caffeic acid derivative. 7) quercetin hexoside; 8) quercetin pentoside; 9) quercetin pentoside; 10) quercetin pentoside; 11) quercetin rhamnoside; 12) quercetin hydroxylmethylglutaryl-α-rhamnoside. Unlabeled peaks are anthocyanins.

Peaks 1 and 2 had identical UV spectra and MS/MS fragmentation as the 3-caffeoylquinic acid standard, but peak 2 eluted 0.5 min later. HPLC-MS/MS in the negative mode revealed a molecular ion at *m/z* 353 for both peaks corresponding to a molecular formula $C_{16}H_{18}O_9$. The molecular ion was fragmented into four major fragments at *m/z* 191, 135, 161 and 179. Previous publications report that the fragment at *m/z* 191 corresponds to the loss of a hydrogen from quinic acid, fragment at *m/z* 179 corresponds to the [caffeoyl - $H^+]^-$ ion and the ion at *m/z* 135 corresponds to its decarboxylation product [caffeoyl - CO_2 - $H^+]^-$ [21]. The fragment at *m/z* 161 probably reveals the product of [caffeoyl – H_2O- $H^+]^-$. Accordingly, peaks 1 and 2 were identified as caffeoylquinic acid isomers.

Peak 3 represented 2.9% of the total nonanthocyanin-phenolic peak area. It produced a molecular ion at *m/z* 367 in accord with the $C_{17}H_{20}O_9$ and four major fragments at *m/z* 135, 179, 161, and 191. Shakya & Navarre [22] found the same fragmentation pattern in potato phenolics. The parent mass corresponds to caffeoyl methyl quinate while the fragments at *m/z* 135, 179, and 191 are derivatives of caffeic acid as reported by Clifford *at al.* [21].

Peaks 4, 5 and 6 were tentatively identified as caffeic acid derivatives since their molecular ions had the same UV-Vis spectra and MS/MS fragmentation as the caffeic acid standard (*m/z* 161, 135 and 179). However, while peak 4 yielded a molecular ion at *m/z* 433, peaks 5 and 6 gave a molecular ion at *m/z* 475, which suggests that these two compounds were isomers.

The total amount of hydroxycinnamic acids detected in *V. meridionale* was 99.2 ± 6.7 mg/100 g FW (Table 3), which is comparable to the amount of this compound Europeran bilberries (113-231 mg/100 g) [23] and higher than the amount in Andean blueberry form Ecuador (33.7 mg/100 g FW) [11]. Chlorogenic acid accounted for 86.1 mg of the total hydroxycinnamic acids. This amount was 5-fold the amount of that of *V. floribundum* (17 mg/100 g FW) as reported by the same authors.

There were six major flavonols identified (Figure 2B). All peaks and the standards quercetin 3-rhamnoglucoside or rutin generated the aglycone quercetin as fragment with *m/z* 300 (homolytic cleavage) and *m/z* 301(heterolytic cleavage) [24].

Peak 7 revealed a molecular ion at *m/z* 463 corresponding to the $C_{21}H_{20}O_{12}$ formula of quercetin hexoside. Fragmentation of the molecular ion provided six fragment ions at *m/z* 300, 301, 271, 255, 179, and 151, which matched the fragmentation pattern of the rutin standard. The ion at *m/z* 301 is typical of the quercetin aglycon after a neutral loss of 162 amu corresponding to a hexose.

Peaks 8, 9 and 10 yielded a molecular ion at *m/z* 433 in accordance with the formula weight of quercetin-pentosides. Molecular ion from peak 8 fragmented into three ions at *m/z* 301, corresponding to the loss of 132 amu from a pentosyl residue, *m/z* 257 and *m/z* 271. Peaks 9 and 10 were considered isomers as they revealed identical UV spectra and fragment ions at *m/z* 301, 271 and 255.

Peaks 11 and 12 were tentatively identified as quercetin rhamnoside and quercetin hydroxylmethylglutaryl-α-rhamnoside, respectively. This identification was done based on comparison to the identical fragmentation spectra for *Vaccinium vitis-idaea* L. as reported [24]. Peak 11 revealed a molecular ion at *m/z* 447 and MS/MS ions *m/z* 301 due to the neutral loss of 146 amu, which is indicative of a deoxyhexosyl residue (such as rhamnose), as well as product ions of *m/z* 271 and 255. Peak 12 presented a molecular ion at *m/z* 591 and fragment ions at m/z 300/301, 447, 489, and 529.

Table 3. Hydroxycinnamic acids and flavonols in *V. meridionale*

Phenolic Compound	Content[a] (mg/100 g FW)
Hydroxicinnamic acids	*Chlorogenic acid equivalents*
Chlorogenic isomer 1	82.4 ± 3.2
Chlorogenic isomer 2	3.7 ± 0.5
Caffeoyl methyl quinate	3.4 ± 2.4
Caffeic acid derivative	6.7 ± 1.1
Caffeic acid derivative isomer 1	0.7 ± 0.1
Caffeic acid derivative isomer 2	2.3 ± 0.4
Total	99.2 ± 6.7
Flavonols	*Rutin equivalents*
Quercentin hexoside	9.0 ± 0.2
Quercentin pentoside	1.5 ± 0.3
Quercentin pentoside	1.9 ± 0.1
Quercentin pentoside	5.2 ± 1.1
quercetin rhamnoside	10.0 ± 2.6
Quercetin hydroxylmethylglutaryl-α-rhamnoside	14.0 ± 2.7
Total	41.9 ± 4.9
Total nonanthocynin phenolics	141.2 ± 11.9

[a] Results are expressed as mean ± SD (n = 3).

Quercetin glycosides represented 100% of the total flavonoids in *V. meridionale* (41.9 ± 4.9 mg/100 g FW). Bilberries from Finland contain a lower amount of flavonoids (11.2 mg flavonoids/100 g FW) and only 72 % or 8.1 mg /100 g of this total is represented by quercetin while the remaining amount is represented by myricetin [20]. Similarly, *V. floribundum* from Ecuador contains lower amount of flavonoids as compared to *V. meridionale.* In this case, 93 % of total flavonoids (37.5 mg/100 g FW) is represented by quercetin and 7% by myricetin.

In general, the *Vaccinium* family is characteristic for the presence of quercetin glycosides and hydroxycinnamic acids. *V. myrtillus* specifically contains caffeic/ferulic acids, hexoses, deoxy hexoses and pentoses of quercetin as the most abundant flavonols, along with myricetin glycosides [20]. The variation in the content and composition of phenolics within the *Vaccinium* varieties used as comparison may be dependent on the growth environment and genotype [25]. It has been reported that quercetin, cyanidin 3-glucosides and hydroxycinnamic acids are metabolized as a defense response against intense solar radiation [26], which is common in tropical locations like Colombia. This may explain the difference in phenolic content and composition profile between bilberry form northern latitudes versus Colombian bilberry.

Conclusion

This summary shows that the berries of *V. meridionale* can be differentiated from other bilberries by their unique anthocyanin pattern e.g., by the high proportions of both delphinidin and cyanidin. In addition, the authors showed evidence of *V. meridionale* berries being a good source of dietary phytochemicals such as anthocyanins and polyphenolics, being comparable to *V. myrtillus*. As a result, there might be potential of the use of *V. meridionale* as source of natural antioxidants, natural colorants, and an ingredient of functional foods.

References

[1] Zhao, C.; Giusti, M.M.; Malik, M.; Moyer, M.P.; Magnuson, B.A. Effects of commercial anthocyanin-rich extracts on colonic cancer and nontumorigenic colonic cell growth. *Journal of Agricultural and Food Chemistry*, 2004, *52*, 6122–6128.

[2] Canter, P. H.; Ernst, E. Anthocyanosides of *Vacinnium myrtillus* (bilberry) for night visions a systematic review of placebo controlled trials. *Survey of ophthalmoloy*, 2004, *49*, 38-50.

[3] Bao, L.; Yao, X.S.; Yau, C.C.; Tsi, D.; Chia, C.S.; Nagai, H.; Kurihara, H. Protective effects of bilberry (*Vaccinium myrtillus* L.) extract on restraint stress-induced liver damage in mice. *Journal of Agricultural and Food Chemistry*, 2008, *56*, 7803–7807.

[4] Bagchi, D.; Roy, S.; Patel, V.; He, G.L.; Khanna, S.; Ojha, N.; Phillips, C.; Ghosh, S.; Bagchi, M.; Sen, C.K. Safety and wholebody antioxidant potential of a novel anthocyanin-rich formulation of edible berries. *Molecular ad. Cellular Biochemistry*, 2006, 281, 197–209.

[5] Ohr, L.M. Brain food. *Food Technology*, 2005, *59*, 69-70.

[6] Taruscio, T.G.; Barney, D.L.; Exon, J. Content and profile of flavanoid and phenolic acid compounds in conjunction with the antioxidant capacity for a variety of northwest *Vaccinium* berries. *Journal of Agricultural and Food Chemistry*, 2004, *52,* 3169–3176.

[7] Rimando, A.M.; Kalt, W.; Magee, J. B.; Dewey, J.; Ballington, J.R. Resveratrol, pterostilbene, and piceatannol in *Vaccinium* berries. *Journal of Agricultural and Food Chemistry,* 2004, *52*, 4713–4719.

[8] Prior, R.L.; Cao, G.; Martin, A.; Sofic, E.; McEwen, J.; O'Brien, C. Antioxidant capacity as influenced by total phenolic and anthocyanin content, maturity and variety of *Vaccinium* Species. *Journal of Agricultural and Food Chemistry,* 1998, *46*, 2686-2693.

[9] Garzón, G.A.; Narváez, C.; Riedl K.M.; Schwartz S.J. Chemical composition, anthocyanins, non-anthocyanin phenolics and antioxidant activity of wild bilberry (*Vaccinium merdionale*) from Colombia. *Food Chemistry*, 2010, *122*, 980–986.

[10] Ligarreto, G.A. *Perspectivas del cultivo de agraz o mortiño (Vaccinium merdionale Swartz) en la zona altoandina de Colombia.* 1st ed. Bogotá: Gente Nueva Editorial; 2009.

[11] Vasco, C.; Riihinen, K.; Ruales, J.; Kamal-Eldin, A. Chemical composition and phenolic compound profile of mortiño (*Vaccinium floribundum* Kunth). *Journal of Agricultural and Food Chemistry*, 2009, *57*, 8274–8281.

[12] Vallejo, D.A. Fomento al mortiño (*Vaccinium meridionale*) como especie promisoria del Parque Regional Arví. Memoria Institucional, Corantioquia, Medellín. 2000.

[13] Kaur, C.K.; Kapoor, H.C. Antioxidants in fruits and vegetables - the millennium's health. *International Journal of Food Science and Technology*, 2001, *36*, 703-725.

[14] Deighton, N.; Brennan, R.; Finn, C.; Davies, H.V. Antioxidant properties of domesticated and wild Rubus species. *Journal of the Science of Food and Agriculture*, 2000, *80*, 1307-1313.

[15] Moyer, R.A.; Hummer, K.E.; Finn, C.E.; Frei B.; Wrolstad, R.E. Anthocyanins, phenolics, and antioxidant capacity in diverse small fruits: Vaccinium, Rubus and Ribes. *Journal of Agricultural and Food Chemisty*, 2002, *50*, 519–525.

[16] Mazza, G.; Miniati, E. *Anthocyanins in fruits, vegetables and grains*. Boca Raton, FL: CRC Press, Inc. 1993.

[17] Hakulinen, J.; Julkunen-Titto, R.; Tahvanainen, J. Does nitrogen fertilization have an impact on the trade-off between willow growth and defensive secondary metabolism? *Trees–Structure and Function*, 1995, 9, 235–240.

[18] Kause, A.; Ossipov, V.; Haukioja, E.; Lempa, K.; Hanhimäki, S.; Ossipova, S. Multiplicity of biochemical factors determining quality of growing leaves. *Oecologia,* 1999, *120*, 102–112.

[19] Herms, D.A.; Mattson, W.J. The dilemma of plants: to grow or defend. *Quarterly Review of Biology*, 1992, 67, 283–335.

[20] Määttä-Riihinen, K.R.; Kamal-Eldin, A.; Mattila, P.H.; González-Paramás, A.M.; Törrönen, R. Distribution and contents of phenolic compounds in eighteen Scandinavian berry species. *Journal of Agricultural and Food Chemistry*, 2004, *52,* 4477-4486.

[21] Clifford, M.N.; Johnston, K. L.; Knight, S.; Kuhnert, N. Hierarchical scheme for LC-MS^n identification of chlorogenic acids. *Journal of Agricultural and Food Chemistry,* 2003, *51*, 2900-2911.

[22] Shakya, R.; Navarre, D.A. Rapid screening of ascorbic acid, glycoalkaloids, and phenolics in potato using high-performance liquid chromatography. *Journal of Agricultural and Food Chemistry,* 2006, *54*, 5253-5260.

[23] Kähkönen, M. P.; Hopla, A.I.; Heinonen, M. Berry phenolics and their antioxidant activity. *Journal of Agricultural and Food Chemistry*, 2001, *49*, 4076-4082.

[24] Hokkanen, J.; Mattila, S.; Jaakola, L.J.; Pirttila, A.M.; Tolonen, A. Identification of phenolic compounds from lingonberry (*Vaccinium vitis-idaea* L.), bilberry (*Vaccinium myrtillus* L.) and hybrid bilberry (*Vaccinium* x *intermedium Ruthe* L.) leaves. *Journal of Agricultural and Food Chemistry*, 2009, *57*, 9437-9447.

[25] Lätti, A.K.; Riihinen, K.R.; Kainulainen, P.S. Analysis of anthocyanin variation in wild populations of bilberry (*Vaccinium myrtillus* L.) in Finland. *Journal of Agricultural and Food Chemisty,* 2008, *56,* 190-196.

[26] Jaakola, L.; Määttä-Riihinen, K.S.; Karenlampi, S.; Hohtola, A. Activation of flavonoid biosynthesis by solar radiation in bilberry (*Vaccinium myrtillus* L.) leaves. *Planta,* 2004, *218,* 721-728.

In: Berries: Properties, Consumption and Nutrition
Editor: Carlo Tuberoso

ISBN 978-1-61470-257-3

Chapter IX

Updating Allergies to Berries of Genera *Morus, Vaccinium* and *Fragaria*

***Natividad Sebastià*[a], *José M. Soriano*[a], *Pedro Pérez-Bermúdez*[*b] and *Isabel Gavidia*[b]**

[a]Department of Preventive Medicine,
[b]Department of Plant Biology,
Faculty of Pharmacy, University of Valencia, Burjasso, Spain

Abstract

To date, reports on allergenicity of berries are still scarce. Allergies to berries have been mainly associated with similar disorders provoked by fruits that contain proteins that are homologous to those considered to be major fruit allergens: profilins, homologous to Bet v 1 (major birch pollen allergen) and plant nonspecific lipid transfer proteins (ns-LTPs). However, the main factors involved in allergies to fruits have not been well determined due to high variability in the allergen-protein contents of fruits, which are dependent on cultivar, harvest and production systems. It has been observed that clinical reactivity is highly dependent on a variety of factors such as exposure frequency and individual responses to allergens. It is also necessary to determine the actual clinical relevance of *in vitro* assays and to clarify the possible correlation among the results obtained from *in vitro* assays, skin prick tests and oral challenge. Recent research works performed at the molecular level allow the isolation and characterization of those proteins identified as major allergens for allergies to fruits, which is key information for future immunotherapy.

In this chapter we discuss various clinical reports on allergies to *Morus, Vaccinium* and *Fragaria* berries which help clarify the causes and main symptoms associated with this hypersensitive disorder of the immune system.

* Department of Plant Biology, Faculty of Pharmacy, University of Valencia. Av. Vicent A. Estelles s/n. 46100-Burjassot, Spain, E-mail: perezb@uv.es

Introduction

Reactions to foods include local mouth irritation, angioedema, urticaria, asthma, nausea, vomiting, diarrhea, rhinitis, or anaphylaxis. The European Academy of Allergy and Clinical Immunology [1] proposed a mechanistic classification of food allergies: i) *adverse food reactions* are defined as any aberrant reaction after the ingestion of a food or food additive which may be the result of toxic or nontoxic food reactions, ii) *toxic reaction*s can occur in anyone, provided a sufficient dose is ingested (eg, histamine in scombroid fish poisoning), iii) *nontoxic reactions* depend on individual susceptibilities and may be the result of immune mechanisms (allergy or hypersensitivity) or nonimmune mechanisms (intolerance), iv) *IgE-mediated food allergies* have been most clearly delineated, but non-IgE-mediated immune reactions, especially of the gastrointestinal tract, are increasingly recognized, v) *food intolerances* probably account for the majority of adverse food reactions and may be caused by the food's pharmacologic properties (eg; headaches from tyramine in aged cheeses and jitteriness from caffeine in coffee or soft drinks), or by the host's unique susceptibilities, such as metabolic disorders (eg; lactase deficiency) or idiosyncratic responses.

Nowadays, the prevalence of food allergy is around 3% of the adult population and 6-8% in young children [2]. A large number of plant food allergens has so far been identified [3] and most of them can have a cross-reactivity between plant foods and pollens, or different plant sources (eg; fruits and latex) [4]. These allergens can be assigned to only 31 different protein families, where the majority is included in a few types of seed storage or plant defense proteins [5]. These allergens can be grouped into three types of the panallergen family constituted by profilins, homologous to Bet v 1 (major birch pollen allergen) and plant nonspecific lipid transfer proteins (ns-LTPs) [6].

Profilins are the proteins involved in the regulation of the actin cytoskeleton which are ubiquitous allergens. They have been identified in many plant foods as responsible for cross-reactivity with pollens [7]. In fact, human IgE-recognizing pollen profilins are highly cross-reactive to profilins in cherry, pear, apple, celery, soybean, peanut, hazelnut, tomato and bell pepper [8].

There is a group of defense proteins homologous to Bet v 1 which behave as major allergens in patients from northern and central Europe with an allergy to vegetables associated with birch pollen allergy [6].

Nonspecific lipid transfer proteins (ns-LTPs) are divided into families according to their molecular masses; 9-kDa ns-LTP1 and 7-kDa ns-LTP2. ns-LTP1 allergens have a basic pI, a conserved cysteine residue and form a multigenic family whose genes are spatially and temporally regulated [9, 10]. They have been identified as major allergens in fruits from the Rosaceae family. However, given their ubiquitous character, they are widely distributed in other plant organs. These proteins are resistant to heat denaturation and proteolysis by digestive enzymes [11], hence, their importance as phytoallergens. Currently, an increasing number of LTP-homologous proteins with more than 80% similarity has been identified in several plant foods, particularly in stone fruits, but also in blueberry and raspberry containing the LTP homologous protein [8].

Fruits of the genera *Morus, Vaccinium* and *Fragaria* are among the berry fruits with promising health benefits thanks to their high polyphenol antioxidants content, phytochemicals, currently under active research for possible benefits to the cardiovascular system and immune system among others, and as anti-cancer agents [12-14]. Whether reports on the allergenicity of small fruits relates them to a general low allergenicity, small amounts consumed or the restricted time frame of consumption, still remains to be answered [15]. The aim of this chapter is to review, for the first time, the bibliography about allergies produced by species of these three plant genera.

ALLERGY to *Morus* spp

Mulberry (*Morus* spp.) is a genus comprising several species of deciduous trees whose fruits are commonly eaten in southern Europe. Cases of respiratory allergy involving mulberry pollen and contact urticaria have been reported. In the last few years subjects with a severe systemic reaction have been described in the literature, but allergens from mulberry have only been very recently isolated.

Species of the genus *Morus* have been associated in the literature with other fruit allergies as a result of a cross-reactivity allergy. Thus, cross-reactivity has been detected between figs and mulberries, fruits which are respectively produced by species of the genera *Ficus* and *Morus*, which are closely related genera of the family Moraceae. Caiaffa *et al.* [16] described three cases of associated fig (*F. carica)* and mulberry allergies in patients with multiple sensitizations to food allergens (mostly fruit) and airborne allergens. The authors suggested that hypersensitivity to figs and mulberries might be result of allergen cross-reactivity rather than mere coincidence. In the same year, Focke *et al.* [17] considered that figs/mulberries association since they are closely related fruits but, according their point of view, fig allergy does not seem to be jointly tied up with sensitization to mulberry. This group also suggested that allergic reactions to fresh or dried figs can occur as a result of primary sensitization to airborne allergens of the ornamental species *Ficus benjamina*.

Hemmer *et al.* [18] demonstrated that sensitization to *Morus* species, in addition to being related to cross-reactivity allergy with other fruits, arises as primary sensitization to birch pollen. The objective of these researches works was to study the potential cross-reactivity between fig and taxonomically-related fruits (mulberry and jackfruit) with Bet v 1, the major birch pollen allergen.

These authors observed that among 85 patients with isolated birch pollen allergy, 91% had a positive skin test to mulberry. The complete IgE binding to Moraceae PR-10 proteins by recombinant Bet v 1 supported their hypothesis as to the close relationship between birch pollen allergy and sensitization to Moraceae fruits, which represent clinically relevant birch pollen-associated foods.

The first allergen from *Morus* has been isolated and characterized very recently by Ciardiello *et al.* [19]. This allergen does not belong to the family of allergens that is homologous to Bet v 1 since it is a cross-reactive nonspecific lipid transfer protein 1 called Mulberry ns-LTP (Mor n 3). This allergen has 91 residues producing a molecular mass of 9.25 kDa. Figure 1 shows the sequence of amino acids as they occur in this ns-LTP.

10	20	30
ITCGQVSSSL	APCINYLRAG	GVVPANCCNG
40	50	60
VRSLNNAAKT	TADRQAACNC	LKSAFNSIKG
70	80	90
LNLNLAAGLP	GKCGVSVPYK	ISPSTDCKSVK

Figure 1. Peptide sequence of allergen Mor n 3 (UniProt P85894), a nonspecific lipid-transfer protein 1, isolated by Ciardiello et al. [19] from *Morus nigra*.

ALLERGY to *Vaccinium* spp

The first described case of allergy to lingonberry (*Vaccinium vitis-idaea*) was carried out by Barrios *et al.* [20] and Matheu *et al.* [21] with an atopic 25-year-old woman with a history of mite allergic rhinitis, but no food allergies or prior anaphylaxis. The patient entered a restaurant and then ingested meatballs, baked potatoes and lingonberry jam. During the meal, itching and wheals developed around her mouth, and these symptoms were resolved without treatment. Furthermore, this woman later tolerated both beef and potatoes. Skin prick testing by prick-prick method with fresh lingonberry obtained a mean wheal diameter of 5 mm (Saline 0 mm; Histamine 7 mm) and a mean flare diameter of 20 mm. The skin prick tests performed with the foodstuffs involved in the episode produced no reaction. The following tool used was the ingestion of lingonberry jam several days later. She immediately noticed intense itching on her mouth, tongue and throat, and wheals around her mouth. An extract of lingonberry (protein concentration: 0.6 mgr/mL) was analyzed by PAGE. After informed consent, serum was obtained. The IgE-ELISA was positive and the western blot revealed IgE in the patient's serum that bound to 53 kDa, 35 kDa and 27 kDa bands. Gebhardt *et al.* [22] reported, for the first time, in a 21-year-old German nonatopic woman with severe IgE-mediated immediate-type reactions to blueberry (*Vaccinium* spp. not specified in the work). The patient developed flush, itching, facial swelling and shortness of breath on two occasions a few minutes after ingestion of blueberry pancakes and blueberry jam. The allergenic structure responsible for these disorders was much lower in the molecular mass than those found in the lingonberry allergy. An allergen was identified as a nonspecific lipid-transfer protein (ns-LTP) of ca. 10 kDa.

ALLERGY to *Fragaria* spp

Allergy to strawberry has been reported in the literature over the last three decades. Kajosaari [23] indicated that this allergy is common in Finnish children aged 1 to 6 years, whereas Eriksson [24] observed an association between birch pollen and strawberry when studying 600 Swedish pollen allergic patients. Kim and Hussain [25] detected the presence of cross-reacting epitopes or independent sensitization between latex and these berries. In Norway, Eggesbø *et al.* [26] studied the cumulative incidences of parentally perceived adverse reactions to food in 3623 children younger than 2 years of age. Their results reflected that fruits, milk and vegetables accounted for nearly two thirds of all reported reactions. The highest cumulative incidence of adverse reactions was to fruit, at 20.4% by the age of two, with citrus fruits and strawberry as the most common food items in this group.

Besides adverse reactions, strawberry was also included in a case of true multifood allergy in Italy in a 4-year-old child [27], where a wide variety of food was included. The study reported by Eriksson *et al.* [28] described the different hypersensitivity to several foodstuffs among 1139 patients from Sweden, Denmark, Estonia, Lithuania and Russia. In all these countries, children, more often than adults, showed symptoms of allergic reaction to several foods: strawberries together with citrus fruits, tomato, milk, egg and fish were reported to be the most frequent causes of hypersensitivity. Of nonEuropean regions, Rodríguez-Ortiz *et al.* [29] detected in Mexico that, most common allergic reactions reported for foods concerned strawberries, besides dairy products, eggs, seafood, beans, soy, chili, mango and cacao.

Until only a few years ago, however, no single strawberry allergen had been identified and characterized until two strawberry allergens were suggested by two different groups. First, Karamloo *et al.* [30] detected the presence of new allergens in strawberry with a high homology to the discovered Bet v 6 allergen (molecular mass of 30-35 kDa). In this research, they found that a strawberry protein extract yielded a 50% inhibition of IgE binding in an enzyme allergosorbent test (EAST) using a recombinant Pyr c 5 allergen, a Bet v 6 homolog, as a solid phase antigen. The authors found that phenylcoumaran benzylic ether reductases (PCBER) and isoflavone reductases (IFR) may represent a new family of pollen-related food allergens that occur not only in typical birch-pollen-related foods, but also in rarely allergenic fruits and vegetables such as orange, strawberry, persimmon or zucchini.

Second, Karlsson *et al.* [31] carried out an investigation in Sweden including eight patients selected on a case history suggestive of strawberry allergy according to their symptoms after ingesting the fruit. Furthermore, these patients were diagnosed with allergic symptoms against other allergen sources, such as birch, apple and timothy. This study accomplished the isolation and characterization of the allergen, a protein called Fra a 1, which is a homolog of birch pollen allergen Bet v 1. The amino acid sequence of the isolated strawberry allergen is depicted in Figure 2.

10	20	30
AFVLDADNLI	PKKITFGEGS	QYGYVKVEGD
40	50	60
ALSDTLEKID	YETKLVSAPS	SSTIIKTTSK
70	80	90
YHTKGDVEIK	EEHVKAGKEK	AAHLFKLIEG
100		
YLKDHPSEYN		

Figure 2. Peptide sequence of allergen Fra a1 (UniProt Q5ULZ 4) isolated from Fragaria ananassa.

It is interesting to note that, the authors included a personal communication of Salentijn in their report, who suggested a 9 kDa ns-LTP as a possible strawberry allergen, which presents a 74% homology with an apple ns-LTP (Mal d 3). On the basis that hypersensitivity to strawberry is a commonly reported but poorly investigated phenomenon, Zuidmeer *et al.* [32] extended the study on strawberry to identify allergenic proteins in the Mediterranean area, and to also express and characterize recombinant strawberry ns-LTP. They screened a strawberry cDNA library and discovered that this fruit contains genes homologous to Bet v 1, Bet v 6, profilin and ns-LTP. In this study the authors characterized a recombinant strawberry LTP called rFra a 3, which had less allergenic potency than peach and apple LTP and did not seem to be clinically relevant.

On the other hand, Alm *et al.* [33] carried out a comparison of six red and three white varieties of strawberries, and reported that the white fruits presented low levels of the allergen. They also discovered that environmental conditions play an important role in the expression levels of a subset of the strawberry proteome, particularly the enzymes regulating red color formation in ripe fruits. Working on this subject, Muñoz *et al.* [34] demonstrated that the expression of the Fra a 1 allergen, a homolog of Bet v 1, is directly linked to flavonoid biosynthesis by performing an essential biological function in pigment formation in strawberry fruit. White fruits of the mutant strawberry genotype, which are tolerated by allergic individuals, are devoid of Fra a.

References

[1] Bruijnzeel-Koomen, C.; Ortolani, C.; Aas, K.; Bindslev-Jensen, C.; Björkstén, B.; Moneret-Vautrin, D.; Wüthrich, B. Adverse reactions to food. *Allergy*, 1995, *50*, 623-35.

[2] Burks, W.; Ballmer-Weber, B.K. Food allergy. *Molecular Nutrition & Food Research*, 2006, *50*, 595-603.

[3] Breiteneder, H.; Radauer, C. A classification of plant food allergens. *Journal of Allergy and Clinical Immunology*, 2004, *113*, 821-830.

[4] Van Ree, R. Clinical importance of cross-reactivity in food allergy. *Current Opinion in Allergy and Clinical Immunology*, 2004, *4*, 235-240.

[5] Chapman, M.D.; Pomes, A.; Breiteneder, H.; Ferreira, F. Nomenclature and structural biology of allergens. *Journal of Allergy and Clinical Immunology*, 2007, *119*, 414-420.

[6] Fernández-Rivas, M. Cross-reactivity between fruit and vegetables. *Allergologia et immunopathologia*, 2003, *3*, 141-146.

[7] Hofmann, A.; Burks, A.W. Pollen food syndrome: update on the allergens. Review. *Current Allergy and Asthma Reports*, 2008, *8*, 413-417.

[8] Marzban, G.; Mansfeld, A.; Hemmerb, W.; Stoyanova, E.; Katinger, H.; da Câmara Machado, M.L. Fruit cross-reactive allergens: A theme of uprising interest for consumers' health. *BioFactors,* 2005, *23*, 235-241.

[9] Kader, J.C. Lipid-transfer proteins in plants. *Annual Review of Plant Physiology and Plant Molecular Biology*, 1996, *47*, 627-654.

[10] Dubreil, L.; Gaborit, T.; Bouchet, B.; Gallant, D.J.; Broekaert, W.F.; Quillien, L.; Marion, D. Spatial and temporal distribution of the major isoforms of puroindolines (puroindoline-a and puroindoline-b) and non-specific lipid transfer protein (ns-LTP1) of Triticum aestivum seeds. Relationships with their in vitro antifungal properties. *Plant Science*, 1998, *138*, 121–135.

[11] Rougé, P.; Borges, J.P.; Culerrier, R.; Brulé, C.; Didier, A.; Barre, A. Lipid transfer proteins as relevant fruit allergens. *Revue Française d'Allergologie*, 2009, *49*, 58–61.

[12] Prior, R.L.; Cao, G.; Martin, A.; Sofic, E.; McEwen, J.; O'Brien, C.; Lischner, N.; Ehlenfeldt, M.; Kalt, W.; Krewer, G.; Mainland, C.M. Antioxidant capacity as influenced by total phenolic and anthocyanin content, maturity, and variety of *Vaccinium* species. *Journal of Agricultural and Food Chemistry*, 1998, *46*, 2686–2693.

[13] Andallu, B.; Mahalakshmi, S.; Vinay Kumar, A.V. *In vitro* antioxidant activity of mulberry (*Morus indica* L.) leaf extract. *Journal of Pharmacy and Chemistry*, 2008, *2*, 89-93.

[14] Paredes-López, O.; Cervantes-Ceja, M.L.; Vigna-Pérez, M.; Hernández-Pérez, T. Berries: Improving human health and healthy aging, and promoting quality Life-a review. *Plant Foods for Human Nutrition* (*formerly Qualitas Plantarum*), 2010, *3*, 299-308.

[15] Battino, M.; Beekwilder, J.; Denoyes-Rothan, B.; Laimer, M.; McDougall, G.J.; Mezzetti, B. Bioactive compounds in berries relevant to human health. *Nutrition Reviews*, 2009, *67*, S145-150.

[16] Caiaffa, M.F.; Cataldo, V.M.; Tursi, A.; Macchia, L. Fig and mulberry cross-allergy. *Annals of Allergy, Asthma and Immunology*, 2003, *5*, 493-495.

[17] Focke, M.; Hemmer, W.; Wöhrl, S.; Götz, M.; Jarisch, R. Cross-reactivity between *Ficus benjamina* latex and fig fruit in patients with clinical fig allergy. *Clinical & Experimental Allergy*, 2003, *7*, 971–977.

[18] Hemmer, W.; Focke, M.; Marzban, G.; Swoboda, I.; Jarisch, R.; Laimer, M. Identification of Bet v 1-related allergens in fig and other *Moraceae* fruits. *Clinical & Experimental Allergy*, 2010, *4*, 679–687.

[19] Ciardiello, M.A.; Palazzo, P.; Bernardi, M.L.; Carratore, V.; Giangrieco, I.; Longo, V.; Melis, M.; Tamburrini, M.; Zennaro, D.; Mari, A.; Colombo, P. Biochemical, immunological and clinical characterization of a cross-reactive nonspecific lipid transfer protein 1 from mulberry. *Allergy*, 2010, *65*, 597-605.

[20] Barrios, Y.; Matheu, V.; de la Parte, B.; Fernández, M.; Zubeldia, J.M.; Baeza, M.L. Lingonberry Allergy. *Journal of Allergy and Clinical Immunology*, 2004, *113*, S315.

[21] Matheu, V.; Baeza, M.L.; Zubeldia, J.M.; Barrios, Y. Allergy to lingonberry: A case report. *Clinical and Molecular Allergy*, 2004, *2*, 1-3.

[22] Gebhardt, C.; Vieths, S.; Gubesch, M.; Averbeck, M.; Simon, J.C.; Treudler, R. 10 kDa lipid transfer protein: the main allergenic structure in a German patient with anaphylaxis to blueberry. *Allergy*, 2009, *64*, 498-9.

[23] Kajosaari, M. Food allergy in Finnish children aged 1 to 6 years. *Acta Paediatrica Scandinavica*, 1982, *71*, 815-819.

[24] Eriksson, N.E. Clustering of foodstuffs in food hypersensitivity. An inquiry study in pollen allergic patients. *Allergologia et immunopathologia*, 1984, *12*, 28-32.

[25] Kim, K.T; Hussain, H. Prevalence of food allergy in 137 latex-allergic patients. *Allergy and Asthma Proceedings*, 1999, *20*, 95-97.

[26] Eggesbø, M.; Halvorsen, R.; Tambs, K.; Botten, G. Prevalence of parentally perceived adverse reactions to food in young children. *Pediatric Allergy and Immunology*, 1999, *10*, 122-132.

[27] Pajno, G.B.; Passalacqua, G; La Grutta, S; Vita, D.; Feliciotto, R.; Parmiani, S.; Barberio, G. True multifood allergy in a 4-year-old child: a case study. *Allergologia et immunopathologia*, 2002, *30*, 338-341.

[28] Eriksson, N.E.; Möller, C.; Werner, S.; Magnusson, J.; Bengtsson, U.; Zolubas, M. Self-reported food hypersensitivity in Sweden, Denmark, Estonia, Lithuania, and Russia. *Journal of Investigational Allergology and Clinical Immunology*, 2004, *14*, 70-79.

[29] Rodríguez-Ortiz, P.G.; Muñoz-Mendoza, D.; Arias-Cruz, A.; González-Díaz, S.N.; Herrera-Castro, D.; Vidaurri-Ojeda, A.C. Epidemiological characteristics of patients with food allergy assisted at Regional Center of Allergies and Clinical Immunology of Monterrey. *Revista Alergia México*, 2009, *56*, 185-191.

[30] Karamloo, F.; Wangorsch, A.; Kasahara, H.; Davin, L.B.; Haustein, D.; Lewis, N.G.; Vieths, S. Phenylcoumaran benzylic ether and isoflavonoid reductases are a new class of cross-reactive allergens in birch pollen, fruits and vegetables. *European Journal of Biochemistry*, 2001, *268*, 5310-5320.

[31] Karlsson, A.L.; Alm, R.; Ekstrand, B.; Fjelkner-Modig, S.; Schiött, A.; Bengtsson, U.; Björk, L.; Hjernø, K.; Roepstorff, P.; Emanuelsson, C.S. Bet v 1 homologues in strawberry identified as IgE-binding proteins and presumptive allergens. *Allergy*, 2004, *59*, 1277-1284.

[32] Zuidmeer, L.; Salentijn, E.; Rivas, M.F.; Mancebo, E.G.; Asero, R.; Matos, C.I.; Pelgrom, K.T.; Gilissen, L.J.; Van Ree, R. The role of profilin and lipid transfer protein in strawberry allergy in the Mediterranean area. *Clinical & Experimental Allergy*, 2006, *36*, 666-675.

[33] Alm, R.; Ekefjärd, A.; Krogh, M.; Häkkinen, J.; Emanuelsson, C. Proteomic variation is as large within as between strawberry varieties. *Journal of Proteome Research*, 2007, *6*, 3011-3020.

[34] Muñoz, C.; Hoffmann, T.; Escobar, N.M.; Ludemann, F.; Botella, M.A.; Valpuesta, V.; Schwab, W. The strawberry fruit Fra a allergen functions in flavonoid biosynthesis. *Molecular Plant*, 2010, *3*, 113-124.

In: Berries: Properties, Consumption and Nutrition
Editor: Carlo Tuberoso
ISBN 978-1-61470-257-3

Chapter X

Problems and Methods to Improve the Market-Life of Berry Fruit

***Giovanna Giacalone*[*] *and Valentina Chiabrando*[‡]**
Dipartimento di Colture Arboree – Università di Torino,
Grugliasco (TO), Italy

Abstract

Berry fruit is highly perishable and it should be marketed soon after picking. When modern storage techniques are applied, fruit harvested in a particular season can be consumed some weeks later, decay is prevented and quality is ensured. In order to maximize storage life, fruit must have a high initial quality. The main factors, that limit the postharvest life of blueberries are excessive softening, water loss which results in fruit shrivelling, and the incidence of postharvest diseases (mainly caused by *Botrytis cinerea* and *Colletotrichum gloeosporioides*). Temperature management is the most critical postharvest factor, and for this reason, after harvesting, blueberries must be rapidly cooled and kept at temperatures close to 0°C for a maximum postharvest life. Cold storage, controlled atmosphere, modified atmosphere packaging, ozonation and innovative atmospheres have been used to extend the marketing season, reduce losses and increase profitability. However, the benefits of most of these treatments have been limited and often inconsistent. According to our experimental results, controlled atmosphere storage can maintain the quality and extend the storage life of blueberries. When added to refrigeration at close to 0°C, the controlled atmosphere maintained fruit firmness, the total soluble solids content and titratable acidity. Storage in plastic films reduced weight loss and slowed down the deterioration of the visual quality. In particular, berries packaged in micro-perforated (1mm ∅) and non-perforated films maintained their high quality attributes (high TSS content and titratble acidity)

[*] Dipartimento di Colture Arboree – Università di Torino, Via L. da Vinci 44, 10095 Grugliasco (TO), Italy, E-mail: giovanna.giacalone@unito.it.
[‡] Dipartimento di Colture Arboree – Università di Torino, Via L. da Vinci 44, 10095 Grugliasco (TO), Italy, E-mail: valentina.chiabrando@unito.it.

throughout the cold storage period. Non-perforated films maintained also berry crispness and a good intensity of flavour. Moreover, this treatment was the only one that reduced pathogen-induced decay during cold storage. The air treatment with ozone during the storage period was effective in reducing fungal decay, but little or no quality advantages were noted with the use of ozone on fruit firmness, soluble solids content or acidity.

Introduction

The postharvest storage of fruit crops is interesting because the metabolism continues, although the fruit is detached from the plant. The goal of postharvest storage technology is to manipulate the metabolism of fruit and vegetables during storage, in order to maximize quality and extend the market life.

Berries are fruit that must be harvested ready for consumption in order to achieve the maximum quality, in relation to flavour, colour, firmness and also the nutraceutical properties. As a consequence, berries are quite perishable and vulnerable to physiological deterioration. Fruit must be of high initial quality to maximize the storage life, and many factors are involved in fruit quality (cultivar, cultural practices, growing environment and harvest practices) [1].

The main characteristics related to the quality of ripe berry fruit are texture, flavour and colour.

Fruit firmness is an important component of the final quality of small fruit. Fruit softening is the result of over-ripening during postharvest conservation, which is shown by an increase in the cellular wall thickness between firm and ripe fruit; textural changes in fruit are thought to be, at least in part, a consequence of changes in the composition and architecture of the cell wall [2] and the result is a rapid decay and deterioration throughout the distribution process [3,4,5].

However, texture is not easy to define, in particular in small fruit like blueberries, because there is no common standardized method. This mechanical property affects not only the oral perception of the texture, and hence its eating quality, but also postharvest properties. Firmness depends on the microstructure of the fruit, and berry firmness may decrease, increase or remain unchanged during storage. This variation may be attributed to cultivar differences and/or their interaction with postharvest storage conditions. Moreover, berries are very susceptible to water loss, which results in a loss in gloss, fruit shrivelling and often an increase in firmness. The maximum permissible amount of water that can be lost (weight loss) from raspberries, blueberries and blackberries before they become unmarketable is 6% [6].

Changes in flavour and texture during berry storage can have a profound effect on consumer acceptability and can also influence the future fruit consumption.

For these reasons, techniques that manipulate the external environment are in use to improve the storability of berry fruit, these involve slowing the respiratory metabolism and other metabolic reactions, associated with quality retention [7].

In general, the storage life of fruit varies inversely with the rate of respiration. This is because respiration supplies the compounds that determine the rate of metabolic processes, which are directly related to quality parameters (firmness, sugar content, aroma, flavour). Commodities and cultivars with higher rates of respiration tend to have shorter storage-life than those with low rates of respiration [8]. Berry fruit has a high respiration rate and, as a consequence, a high deterioration rate. Cold storage, controlled atmosphere, modified atmosphere packaging, ozonation and innovative atmospheres have been used to extend the marketing season, reduce losses and increase profitability [9,10]. Storage temperature is the most important factor that can affect postharvest life. After the harvest, berry fruit must be cooled and kept close to 0°C for a maximum market life. However, each berry fruit has an optimum storage temperature, because of their different sensitivity to chilling injury. The removal of ethylene from the storage air may also reduce disease development in all berries. Moreover, the postharvest shelf-life of soft fruit is further shortened by infection with grey mould *Botrytis cinerea* [11]. Minimizing such deteriorative losses is of primary importance.

Recently, the packaging of highly perishable fruits in polymeric films with specific gas permeabilities, in combination with low temperature storage, has gained importance [12,13] because of the benefits of film packaging (maintenance of high relative humidity, reduction in water loss, improved sanitation due to a reduction in contamination of the product). The negative effect is an increased potential for water condensation within the package.

Another technique used to reduce the decay of fresh fruit and sanitize the produce is ozonation, but the results have been variable [14,15].

1. Cold Storage

Temperature management is the most effective tool to extend the postharvest life of berries. Low temperatures slow the metabolism and have a particular effect on the respiratory metabolism. Respiration is based on the reserves that are accumulated in the fruit during the growing season and respiration therefore reduces the eating quality (Table 1).

Table 1. Quality characteristics of raspberries at harvest and during storage (3 days) [16]

Raspberries	Harvest		Cold storage 3 days 1°C		Room storage 3 day 20°C	
	T.S.S. °*Brix*	Titratable acidity *meq/L*	T.S.S. °*Brix*	Titratable acidity *meq/L*	T.S.S. °Brix	Titratable acidity *meq/L*
Fairview	10.5	265	8.8	220	7.1	190
Skeena*	8.7	315	8.4	311	8.4	288
Gradina	9.6	216	8.2	237	6.5	194
Glen Prosen*	10.4	336	10.4	176	10.4	154
Meeker	9.9	272	9.5	240	8.1	215

* stored for 2 days..

Each 10°C decrease in temperature will reduce respiratory activity by a factor of 2 to 4 (Table 2) [17] with an evident benefit on the quality. Another problem is water loss. Fruit losses water when it is on the tree, but once harvested this water cannot be replaced by the tree and a weight loss therefore occurs. Low temperatures, in association with high relative humidity, reduce the water loss rate because of the reduction in the vapour pressure difference between the fruit and the surrounding air.

Table 2. Respiration Production rates (modified from [18])

Temperature	*mL CO_2/kg·hr*			
°C	blackberry	blueberry	cranberry	raspberry
0	11	3	2	12
10	31	9	4	49
20	78	34	9	100

An additional effect of cold storage is its influence on the rate of the growth and spread of pathogens: the lower the temperature, the slower the metabolism. Certain fungi that cause severe losses do not grow at low temperature [19]. Berry fruit is a rich source of phenolic compounds. The most important group of phenolics in berry fruit is flavonoids. The high antioxidant activities in berry fruit are generally attributed to phenolic compounds, such as anthocyanins. Phytonutrient levels usually decline when fruit starts to spoil and tissues begin to break down. Therefore, any postharvest treatment that is beneficial in maintaining the quality of fresh produce can also help maintain the antioxidant and nutritional values. Storage temperature, in addition to light and oxygen exposure, is one of the key factors that influence the stability of phenolic antioxidants in fruit during postharvest storage. Higher antioxidant capacity values have, in most cases, been maintained in fruit stored at 4 °C, instead of 25 °C. Therefore, keeping fruit under refrigerated storage seems to be the recommended choice [20]. Most berry crops, including blackberries, blueberries, and raspberries, are chilling tolerant and can be stored at -0.5 to 0°C, or slightly above their freezing points, to maintain their quality. Instead, cranberries are known to be chilling sensitive and can develop low-temperature breakdown after prolonged exposure to chilling temperatures [21].

Rapid cooling is essential in small fruit to maintain quality. Cooling fruit immediately after harvesting reduces water losses and the respiration heat. Berry fruit must be marketed quickly, with particular attention to maintaining cold chain during marketing.

Table 3. Optimum storage times and temperatures (modified from [18]).

Berry	temperature	time
blackberry	0±0.5°C	2-5 days
blueberry	0±0.5°C	1-2 weeks
cranberry	3±1°C	2-4 months
raspberry	0±0.5°C	2-5 days

2. Modified Atmosphere Packaging

Soft fruit, such as strawberries, raspberries, and blueberries, have a short postharvest shelf-life, which is exacerbated by infection with grey mould, *Botrytis cinerea* [11]. There is a fundamental need to minimize such deterioration losses at both the retail and home levels. Modified atmosphere packaging (MAP) has been shown to delay compositional changes associated with colour, firmness, flavour and nutritional quality, and reduce the water loss of fruit [22]. When packaged, berries continue to respire the trapped air until the CO_2 concentration rapidly approaches the critical 10-15% level necessary to inhibit *Botrytis* growth.

Recently, the packaging of highly perishable fruit in polymeric films with specific gas permeabilities, in combination with low temperature storage, has gained importance [13]. [24] defined modified atmosphere packaging (MAP) as "the initial alteration of the gaseous environment in the immediate vicinity of the product that permits the packaged product interactions to naturally vary their immediate gaseous environment".

The benefits of film packaging include the maintenance of high relative humidity and a reduction in water loss; improved sanitation due to a reduction in contamination of the product during handling; facilitation of brand identification and the provision of relevant information to the consumer. Instead, the negative effects include slowing down the cooling of the packaged products and an increased potential for water condensation within the package. Ideally, films should protect the fruit from mechanical damage, excessive drying and contamination. Packages should also provide safe stacking, efficient palletization, and easy storage in the warehouse or home, and assist in the display and sale of the fruit [25].

Only top quality fruit should be packed, since the fruit-to-package cost ratio is important in deciding the profit. One of the initial physiological effects of a modified atmosphere on the fruit metabolism is a decrease in respiratory intensity during the storage period, which involves a decrease in substrate consumption, CO_2 production, O_2 consumption and heat release.

MAP includes vacuum packaging, controlled atmosphere packaging and passive modified atmosphere packaging (Table 4) [23]. A modified atmosphere can be created inside a package either passively, through product respiration, or actively by replacing the atmosphere in the package with a desired gas mixture (the approach generally involves gas mixes confined to 5-15% CO_2, 2-5% O_2, with N_2 as the remainder). In the first method, as the fruit respires, the O_2 level decreases and the CO_2 level increases during storage [12].

Table 4. Different terminologies used in Modified Atmosphere Packaging techniques (modified from [23])

Terminologies	
Modified Atmosphere Packaging (MAP)	Replacement of air with a single gas or a mixture of gases. No further control over the initial composition
Controlled Atmosphere Packaging (CAP)	Proportion and type of gas mixture is controlled over the whole period of storage
Equilibrium Modified Atmosphere packaging (EMA)	Pack is flushed with gas or sealed without modification. The permeability of packaging and respiration of the product results in an equilibrium modified atmosphere
Vacuum Packaging (VP)	Product sealed in low gas permeability pack after part evacuation of pack results in changes in atmosphere during storage due to the altered metabolism of the product and microbial flora and gas permeation

In both cases, the package permeability must be compatible with the fruit respiration rate, and maintain an appropriate atmosphere for better conservation. High CO_2 and/or low O_2 levels in the micro-atmosphere around the commodities may extend shelf-life [26, 27], reduce fruit decay, delay senescence and delay softening [28]. However, excessively high levels of CO_2 and/or very low levels of O_2 can induce a transition from aerobic to anaerobic respiration, together with ethanol production, and a significant decline in the sensory quality and the development of off flavours.

Many types of plastic films are available for packaging, but relatively few have been used to wrap fresh fruit such us blueberries. Low-density polyethylene, polyvinyl chloride, and polypropylene are the main films that are used to package fruit and vegetables [13,22]. The selection of the proper MAP film with the appropriate water vapour, film permeability and gas transmission rates is essential for an optimum storage life. In general, a reduction in packaging film permeability is accompanied by an increase in the acceptability of the corresponding fruit [11]. The best quality of highbush blueberries, during long-term storage in different packaging materials, has been obtained in polyamide/polyethylene laminates [29].

Four commercially available films were evaluated for MAP in [30]: two micro-perforated films (0.3 mm and 1 mm in diameter), a non-perforated and a macro-perforated film (6 mm in diameter) during a highbush blueberry (cv Lateblue) postharvest storage period (4°C for 15 days). The benefits of small packages (consumer packs) were evaluated through chemical (total soluble solids content, titratable acidity and pH), visual (colour intensity, surface shine, firmness, intensity of odour, and overall appearance) and sensory (crispness, sweet taste, acidic taste, total flavour, and overall appreciation) evaluations. The results showed that the different packaging films significantly affected the chemical characteristics of the fruit during the postharvest storage period (Table 5).

Table 5 showed that the blueberries demonstrated the highest quality when packed in micro-perforated film (higher soluble solids content and titratable acidity). The berries stored in non-perforated film also gave better results than the control ones, and were significantly better than those in the macro-perforated film. The different packaging films also had a significant effect on the pH values: the blueberries packaged in macro-perforated film had the highest pH values (Table 5).

Moreover, the berries packaged with micro-perforated films 1 and 2 and the non-perforated film effectively controlled the loss in quality during shelf-life and had a higher colour intensity than the other samples. The non-perforated film also maintained berry crispness and a good intensity of flavour.

Table 5. Quality characteristics of blueberries stored under modified atmosphere packaging for 15 days [30]

Film type	*T.S.S. (° Brix)*	*Titratable acidity (meq/L)*	*pH*
Microperforated (0.3mm ∅) film	10.53 b	49.43 bc	3.44 b
Microperforated (1mm ∅) film	11.7 a	147.89 a	3.01 d
Non-perforated film	11.47 a	59.58 b	3.32 c
Macroperforated (6mm ∅) film	10.13 b	38.89 c	3.54 a
Control	11.16 b	60.25 b	3.39 bc

Means separated by Tukey's test. Means in columns with different letters are significantly different at p ≤ 0.05.

Table 6. Weight loss of blueberries stored under modified atmosphere packaging for 15 days

Film type	*1° day*	*2° days*	*3° days*	*4° days*	*5° days*	*6° days*	*7° days*	*8° days*	*9° days*	*10° days*	*11° days*	*12° days*	*13° days*	*14° days*
Microperforated (0.3mm ∅) film	0.03 n.s.	0.06 b	0.14 b	0.17 c	0.25 c	0.25 c	0.25 c	0.29 c	0.29 c	0.30 c	0.33 c	0.42 c	0.42 c	0.44 c
Microperforated (1mm ∅) film	0.45	0.80 ab	1.09 a	1.378 b	1.85 b	2.09 b	2.18	2.28 b	2.39 b	2.49 b	2.57 b	2.77 b	2.89 b	2.98 b
Non-perforated film	0.00	0.01 b	0.04 b	0.07 d	0.08 d	0.10 d	0.10 d	0.10 d	0.10 d	0.10 d	0.10 d	0.13 d	0.13 d	0.13 d
Macroperforated (6mm ∅) film	0.37	0.63 ab	0.88 b	1.13 b	1.53 b	1.74 b	1.88 b	1.99 b	2.11 b	2.23 b	2.31 b	2.55 b	2.63 b	2.76 b
Control	0.78	1.41 a	1.85 a	2.47 a	3.55 a	4.14 a	4.52 a	4.77 a	5.05 a	5.43 a	5.78 a	6.38 a	6.69 a	6.9 7 a

Means separated by Tukey's test. Means in columns with different letters are significantly different at p ≤ 0.05.

All the package films effectively reduced the loss in weight compared to the unwrapped control (Table 6). The control berries showed the highest loss in weight (7%) during the same storage period (15 days), due to transpiration and respiration. The macro-perforated film exhibited a higher fruit weight loss (3%) than the micro-perforated films and the non-perforated film 3 packaging systems. This loss became more evident and significant as storage continued.

Overall, the film packaging also reduced the incidence of *Botrytis cinerea* infection, compared to the control berries. Packaging the berries in microperforated and macro-perforated films reduced the total amount of fungal incidence to only 7.37% (film 1), 2.96% (film 2), and 19.4% (film 4), respectively, compared with 20.3% for the unwrapped control sample. Instead, the *Botrytis cinerea* infection was not observed in the case of the non-perforated film, which could be attributable to the presence of high CO_2 and low O_2. No major differences were observed between the effectiveness of the various micro-perforated and macro-perforated films that were used, but there was a significant difference in effectiveness for the non-perforated one.

In conclusion, the present study has demonstrated that if non-perforated and micro-perforated packaging films are used for blueberry packaging, it is possible to retain both the sensory and visual quality and also to reduce the development of post-harvest diseases.

3. Ozonation

Ozone, the tri-atomic form of oxygen, is a strong antimicrobial agent and may be an alternative antifungal agent in the storage of fruit. Ozone is a potent disinfecting agent, and the combination of cold storage and this gas may create new opportunities for the blueberry industry and in postharvest handling. Ozonation is a technology that can be used to reduce the decay of fresh fruit and vegetables and sanitize the produce [14]. Investigations into the effect of ozone on reducing decay have found that ozone can be used as an alternative postharvest fungicide, in addition to cold storage, to reduce the decay of blueberry fruit [31]. In lowbush blueberry, [32] found significant microbial reductions in all the samples treated with 1 ppm of ozone compared to the control berries. [33] concluded that ozone increases the storage life of rabbiteye blueberries and reduces weight loss and fruit decay.

In our study [34], we evaluated the evolution of berry (cv Bluecrop, Coville and Brigitta) quality, firmness and decay during a postharvest storage period (4 weeks). Two different storage conditions were compared: Traditional Storage (Normal Atmosphere, 3°C and 85% R.H) as a control and Innovative Storage (Normal Atmosphere, air enriched with ozone). The ozonation was created using AgroCare™, an environmental ozone generator. In order to evaluate the effect of the ozone treatments, the firmness of blueberry fruit was also determined, using a penetrometer test, which was performed in a Texture Analyzer TaxT2i® (Stable Micro System, UK).

The results have shown that ozone is an efficient inhibitor of postharvest modifications. The statistical testing of the data confirmed the significant difference between storage methods. In particular for Bluecrop (Figure 1); the berries stored for four weeks with a concentration of ozone in the atmosphere were not as sweet as the other samples. Moreover, the berries stored in ozone were less acid and were less firm than the samples stored in the Normal Atmosphere (3°C and 85% R.H) (Figure 1).

The atmospheric composition had no detectable effect on the total soluble solids content in Coville: there were no statistical differences ($p \leq 0.05$) between fruit stored in a normal atmosphere and that stored in the innovative way. As far as titratable acidity is concerned, the values for the innovative storage condition were higher (130.58 meq/L) than those found in the control (87.73 meq/L) at the end of the storage period. Moreover, the ozone treatment showed a significant effect on berry firmness: berries stored for four weeks in the atmosphere with ozone were firmer than the samples stored in a Normal Atmosphere (Table 6). No significant differences were found in cv Brigitta between the treatments, for any of the evaluated quality factors. Like Coville, Brigitta showed a high degree of firmness in the samples stored in the innovative conditions (Table 6).

As far as the effect of ozone storage on berry weight loss is concerned, the results showed that the different storage conditions did not differ significantly for each cultivar or for each picking date. The weight loss was not affected by the ozone air treatment.

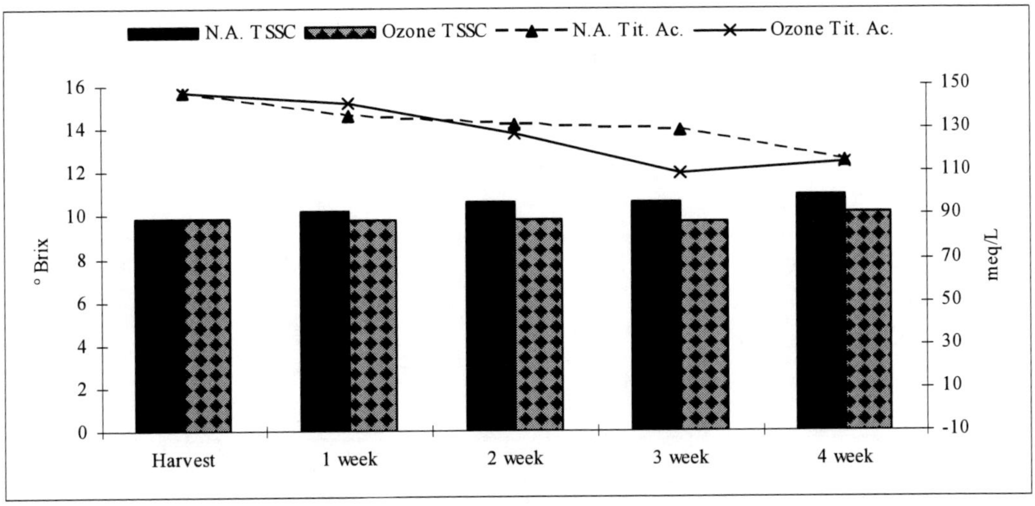

Figure 1. Total Soluble Solids content and titratable acidity during the postharvest storage period. Cv Bluecrop.

Table 6. Berry firmness (N) under two different storage conditions. Bluecrop, Coville and Brigitta cultivars

		BLUECROP		COVILLE		BRIGITTA	
		Normal Atmosphere	Ozone	Normal Atmosphere	Ozone	Normal Atmosphere	Ozone
Postharvest weeks	Harvest	1.48	1.48	1.54	1.54	1.53	1.53
	1 week	1.41	1.34	1.69	1.34	1.67	1.62
	2 week	1.32	1.30	1.67	1.95	1.63	1.69
	3 week	1.23	1.31	1.61	1.74	1.67	1.79
	4 week	1.24	1.17	1.67	1.83	1.55	1.60

Moreover, in order to evaluate the effect of ozone on controlling decay, the % of berries with *Botrytis cinerea* infection was calculated. *Botrytis cinerea* decay in the control was only apparent after 2 weeks of storage in Bluecrop and after 4 weeks of storage in Coville (Table 7). The results showed that ozone was effective at inhibiting the proliferation of Botrytis *cinerea*, and reducing the incidence of decay. For example, in Bluecrop, the incidence of *Botrytis cinerea* was lower after 28 storage days at 4 °C on blueberries exposed to 0.3 ppm ozone than on fruit exposed to ambient air.

Table 7. Incidence of *Botrytis cinerea* (% on weight) under two different storage conditions

		BLUECROP		COVILLE	
		Normal Atmosphere	Ozone	Normal Atmosphere	Ozone
	Harvest	0	0	0	0
	1 week	0	0	0	0
Postharvest weeks	2 week	2.33	0	0	0
	3 week	3.74	0	0	0
	4 week	7.48	1.50	6.21	0

4. Controlled Atmosphere

Controlled atmosphere storage (C.A.) is widely used to extend the storage and shelf-life of many kinds of fruit. In general, the reduction in the partial pressure of O_2 and the increase in that of CO_2 reduce the respiratory metabolism rate and minimize the changes in the physical and chemical attributes. Moreover, an elevated range of CO_2 is effective in suppressing many fungal decay organisms [4] and low O_2 has little impact on the growth of fungi [35].

Rabbiteye, highbush, and lowbush blueberries benefit from 10 to 15% CO_2 + 1 to 10% O_2 when kept at 5 °C or below [36,37,38]. Firmness and titratable acidity are maintained and decay decreases, with a shelf-life of up to 6 weeks. [39] found that the weight loss of the blueberry cultivar 'Duke' was minimized by a high rate of CO_2 in association with a low temperature (0-1°C). Berries stored at 6-12 kPa CO_2 maintained their firmness at acceptable values. They recommend storing highbush blueberries under high CO_2 levels of up to 12 kPa without O_2 reduction for a longer storage period of up to six weeks. Higher CO_2 levels of more than 12 kPa cannot be recommended, due to the negative impact on flavour, firmness, and acidity content. In our experience [40] the use of a C.A. (1 °C 3% O_2, 11% CO_2, for 60 days) lengthened the postharvest life of berries, which maintained their firmness, total soluble solids and titratable acidity content.

A 7 day storage of different red raspberry cultivars in controlled atmospheres (10% O_2+15% CO_2, 10% O_2+31% CO_2) suppressed rotting significantly [42] and kept the berry colour more attractive compared to storage in normal atmospheres. The total soluble solids were unchanged after storage, and the titratable acids decreased in all the analysed cultivars. The L-ascorbic acid levels were unchanged or slightly increased after a one-week storage period [42].

Raspberries benefit from 10 to 20% CO_2 + 5 to 10% O_2 [43]. C.A. storage slows respiration, ethylene production, softening, colour changes, and the growth of moulds. Levels of CO_2 > 20% can cause discoloration, softening, and off-flavor of raspberries [44]. Research indicates [45, 46] that red currant and gooseberry respond very well to C.A., whereas black currant only benefit slightly. The storage duration of red currant can be extended from 8 to 14 weeks, depending on the cultivar, using 1 °C, 18 to 20% CO_2 + 2% O_2. The storage duration of gooseberry can be extended from 6 to 8 weeks, using 1 °C, 10 to 15% CO_2 + 1.5% O_2. Increasing the CO_2 to 20% reduces the incidence of storage rot [45, 46] and lowering the O_2 reduces the respiration rate [47]. Compared to red currant and gooseberry, black currant does not respond as well to low O_2 and its storage can only be extended to 3 weeks, using 0 to 2 °C and 15 to 20% CO_2 [21].

Table 8. Quality parameters at the harvest and after C.A. (1 °C, 3% O_2, 11% CO_2) storage of Bluecrop, Coville and Lateblue cultivars [41]

		Bluecrop	Coville	Lateblue
T.S.S. (°Brix)	harvest	10.3	13.7	11.9
	60 days	9.4	12.7	9.4
Titrat. acidity (meq/L)	harvest	141	121	171
	60 days	145.5	173	248
pH	harvest	2.57	2.79	2.53
	60 days	2.54	2.68	2.55

5. 1-mcp Treatment

1-methylcyclopropene is an inhibitor of ethylene receptors that can affect ripening and senescence processes in fruit, vegetables and ornamental products [48,49]. 1-mcp is classified as a plant growth regulator and it induces beneficial effects, such as a delay in the physico-chemical changes related to the ripening process, as well as a reduction in decay and softening in many fruit and vegetables such as apples, kiwifruit, peaches, nectarines, plums and pears [50, 51, 52, 53]. Ethylene has little effect on the postharvest ripening of blueberries, [54] found little or no effect on blueberry quality when the fruit were treated with 1-mcp.

In order to evaluate 1-mcp effectiveness on blueberry fruit, we determined the change in fruit firmness, weight loss, soluble solids concentration and titratable acidity, as well as antioxidant activities, total phenolic and anthocyanin content, during long term storage in air and controlled atmosphere conditions [55]. The possibility of 1-mcp inhibiting the development of *Botrytis cinerea* during the postharvest storage period was also tested. After harvesting, blueberry fruit (cv Lateblue) was exposed to 1-mcp (0.3 and 0.6 $\mu l\ L^{-1}$). After the treatment, samples were stored in air at 0°C for 35 days and in a Controlled Atmosphere (3 kPa O_2 + 11 kPa CO_2) for 60 days.

Table 9. Effect of 1-mcp treatments on weight loss, total soluble solids content (TSS) and titratable acidity

	treatment	storage times (days at 0°C) 0	7	14	21	28	35
TSS (°Brix)	control	12.37 a	10.63 b	11.27 a	11.63 a	10.77 a	10.97 a
	1-mcp 0.3 μl L^{-1}	12.37 a	11.97 a	10.9 a	11.53 a	10.2 a	9.6 b
	1-mcp 0.6 μl L^{-1}	12.37 a	11 ab	10.6 a	10.47 b	10.9 a	9.97 ab
Titratable acidity (meq/L)	control	87.27 a	107.92 a	91.27 a	111.06 b	99.96 a	117.49 a
	1-mcp 0.3 μl L^{-1}	87.27 a	82 b	119.65 a	129.4 a	103.25 a	130.08 a
	1-mcp 0.6 μl L^{-1}	87.27 a	100.93 ab	111.77 a	115.6 b	98.63 a	126.08 a
Weigth loss (%)	control		2.05 a	2.83 a	3.12 a	3.78 a	4.4 a
	1-mcp 0.3 μl L^{-1}		1.87 ab	2.64 a	3.04 ab	3.62 b	4.22 a
	1-mcp 0.6 μl L^{-1}		1.72 b	2.41a	2.94 b	3.58 b	4.29 a

Means separated by Tukey's test. Means in columns with different letters are significantly different at $p \leq 0.05$.

The results have shown that blueberries treated with 1-mcp have a reduced weight loss during storage and a lower soluble solids content compared to untreated fruit (**Table 9**). A delay in the increase in the soluble solids content has been reported for pears [52] and plums [56] while the soluble solids content in apricots and plums was unaffected by 1-mcp treatments [57].

Titratable acidity increased during storage to a similar extent in all the treatments, but little or no significant effect of 1-mcp was observed on this parameter. Changes in berry weight (up to 4%) which occurred during the postharvest period may have influenced the titratable acidity values; it is possible that a portion of the increase in this variable during storage was due to water loss. These differences in effectiveness of 1-mcp on the quality parameters may be due to the different behaviour of the fruit, maturity stage or other experimental conditions, as suggested by [58]. Fruit firmness increased during storage and this increase was delayed by the application of 1-mcp, over the first few weeks of storage and was then quite stable until the end of the storage period (Figure 2).

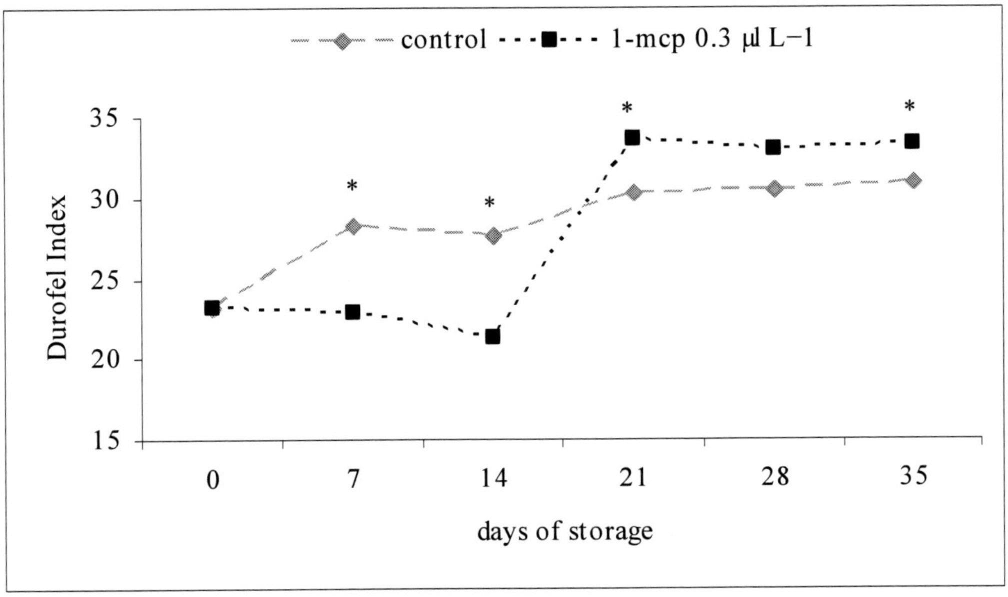

Means separated by Tukey's test. * = significantly different at $p \leq 0.05$.

Figure 2. Blueberry firmness stored under the normal atmosphere.

The antioxidant activity was relatively stable during air and C.A. storage and the effects of 1-mcp on the individual phytochemical groups were similar: no significant effect of 1-mcp treatment was observed on the anthocyanin content or on the total phenolic content.

The postharvest shelf life of blueberries is also limited by fungal decay. In the study by [55], the infection rate caused by *Botrytis cinerea* was very high and the 1-mcp treatments only reduced decay incidence in the first three weeks of storage. The presence of pathogens was expressed as a percentage of decayed fruit and is show in Table 10. Moreover, the incidence of *Botrytis cinerea* in fruit treated with 0.3 and 0.6 μl L^{-1} 1-mcp increased considerably with the storage time.

In conclusion, 1-mcp treatments have shown to partially control weight loss and decay development without any undesirable changes in the quality attributes, total sugars or acids after short and medium term cold storage, but these results are too inconsistent to recommend the use of 1-mcp in commercial applications.

Table 10. Incidence of *Botrytis cinerea* (%) during the storage period in the normal atmosphere (RA)

		storage times (days at 0°C)				
	treatment	7	14	21	28	35
incidence (%) of *Botrytis cinerea*	control	3.12	27.72	5.04	16.84	40.72
	1-mcp 0.3 μl L^{-1}	2.68	14.88	4.8	31.12	50.24
	1-mcp 0.6 μl L^{-1}	4.64	10.6	7.8	23.56	34.8

Conclusion

Cold storage, in association with high humidity, has a positive effect on berry fruit quality and extends postharvest life. Among the various types of berry fruit, highbush blueberry can be considered important because of the increase in consumers' demand and there is therefore a considerable need to maintain the quality and extend shelf-life. Blueberry can be stored for long periods, which vary according to the variety. Normal atmosphere storage (-0.5 to 1 °C; 85-90% RU) helps maintain acceptable quality levels for two to five weeks (depending on the cultivar).

C.A. can extend storage to over six weeks without any loss of fruit quality, but the extension of berry life is sometimes not the main effect and C.A. storage results in a better quality of the fruit. The use of modified atmosphere packaging is effective in retaining both the sensory and the sensorial quality and in reducing the development of post-harvest diseases, thanks to the use of non-perforated and micro-perforated packaging films. Moreover, storage in plastic films reduces weight loss and slows down visual quality deterioration.

Ozone treatments seem to be effective at inhibiting the proliferation of *Botrytis cinerea*, and reducing the incidence of decay, but few results have been found concerning the preservation of blueberry quality and the extension of postharvest life. 1-mcp treatments have shown to partially control weight loss and decay development, and no undesirable changes have been observed in quality attributes, total sugars or acids after short and medium term cold storage. However, these results are too inconsistent to recommend the use of 1-mcp for commercial application.

References

[1] Forney, C.F. Postharvest issues in blueberry and cranberry and methods to improve market-life. *Acta Horticulturae, ISHS*, 2008, *810*, 785-798.

[2] Brummell, D.A.; Harpster, M.H. Cell wall metabolism in fruit softening and quality and its manipulation in transgenic plants. *Plant Molecular Biology*, 2001, *47*, 311-339.

[3] Ballinger, W.E.; Kushman, L.J. Relationship of stage ripeness to composition and keeping quality of high bush blueberries. *Journal of the American Society for Horticoltural Science*, 1970, *95*, 239-242.

[4] Ceponis, M.J.; Cappellini, R.A. Reducing decay in fresh blueberries with controlled atmospheres. *HortScience*, 1985, *20*, 228-229.

[5] Sanford, K.; Lidster, P.D.; McRae, K.B.; Jackson, E.D.; Lawrence, R.A.; Stark, R.; Prange, R.K. Lowbush blueberry quality changes in response to mechanical damage and storage temperature. *Journal of the American Society for Horticoltural Science,* 1991, *116*, 47-51.

[6] DeEll, J. Postharvest handling and storage of berries. *Orchard Network Newsletter*, March 2005.

[7] Kalt, W.; Forney, C.F.; Martin, A.; Prior, R.L. Antioxidant capacity, vitamin C, phenolics, and anthocyanins after fresh storage of small fruits. *Journal of the Agricultural and Food Chemistry*, 1999, *47*, 4638–4644.

[8] Saltveit, M.E. Respiratory Metabolism. In: Gross, K.C.; Wang, C.Y. and M.E. Saltveit (eds.). *The Commercial Storage of Fruits, Vegetables, and Florist and Nursery Stocks*. Agriculture Handbook 66. U.S. Dept. of Agr., Agricultural Research Service, Washington, DC, 2004.

[9] Machado, N.P.; Franchini, E.R.; Ristow, N.C.; Coutinho, E.F; Cantillano, F.R.F.; Malgarim, M.B. Conservação pos-colheita de mirtilos "Florida", "Woodart" e "Bluegem" em atmosfera com oxigênio ionizado. *II Simposio Nacional do Morango e I Incontro de Pequenas Frutas e Frutas Nativas do Mercosul, Pelotas*. 2004.

[10] NeSmith, D.S.; Nunez-Barrios, A.; Prussia, S.; Aggarwal, D. Postharvest berry quality of six rabbie blueberry cultivars in response to temperature. *Journal of the American Pomological Society*, 2005, *59*, 13-17.

[11] Stewart, D.; Oparka, J.; Johnstone, C.; Iannetta, P.P.M.; Davies, H.V. Effect of modified atmosphere packaging (MAP) on soft fruit quality. Scottish Crop Research Institute, Annual report 1999, 119–124; http://www.scri.ac.uk/scri/file/ fullannualreports/ annual_report_1999.pdf.

[12] Day, B.P.F. Modified atmosphere packaging and active atmosphere packaging of fruit and vegetables. Proceedings of the International Symposium on Minimal Processing of Food, 14-15 April 1994, Majvik Kirkkonommi, Finland.

[13] Kader, A.A.; Watkins, C.B. Modified atmosphere packaging-toward 2000 and beyond. *HortTechnology*, 2000, *10*, 483-486.

[14] Forney, C.F.; Fan, L.; Hildebrand, P.M.; Song, J. Do negative air ions reduce decay of fresh fruits and vegetables? *Acta Horticulturae, ISHS*, 2001, *553*, 551-553.

[15] Palou, L.; Smilanick, J.L.; Crisosto, C.H.; Mansour, M. Effect of gaseosus ozone exposure on the development of green and blue moulds on cold stored citrus fruit. *Plant Disease*, 2001, *85*, 632-638.

[16] [Peano, C.; Baudino, M.; Bullano, F. Caratteri qualitativi di cinque cultivar di lampone rosso (*Rubus idaeus L.*) in prove di conservazione. *II Giornate Scientifiche*, 1994, 441-442.

[17] Thompson J.F.; Mitchell, F.G.; Kasmire R.F. Cooling horticultural commodities. In: Kader A.A. *Postharvest Technology of horticultural crops*. University of California Agriculture and Natural Resource publication 3311, 2002, 537.

[18] Mitcham, E.J.; Crisosto, C.H. Kader, A.A. Bushberry: blackberry, blueberry, cranberry, raspberry. Recommendations for Maintaining Postharvest Quality. *Postharvest Technology Research Information Center*, 2009.

[19] Lurie, S. *Temperature management*. Ed. Knee M. Fruit quality and its biological basis. Fruit technology and quality handbook from C.H.I.P.S. 2001.

[20] Piljac-Žegarac, J.; Šamec, D. Antioxidant stability of small fruits in postharvest storage at room and refrigerator temperatures. *Food Research International*, 2011, *44*, 345-350.

[21] Prange, R.K. Cranberry. In: Gross, K.C.; Wang, C.Y. and Saltveit M.E. (eds.). *The Commercial Storage of Fruits, Vegetables, and Florist and Nursery Stocks.* Agriculture

Handbook 66. U.S. Dept. of Agr., Agricultural Research Service, Washington, DC, 2004.

[22] Kader, A.A. Biochemical and physiological basis for effects of controlled and modified atmosphere on fruits and vegetables. *Food Technology*, 1986, *40*, 99-104.

[23] Philips, C.A. Review: Modified atmosphere packaging and its effects on the microbiological quality and safety of produce. *International Jounal of Science and Technology,* 1996, *31*, 463-479.

[24] Prince, T.A. Modified atmospheres packaging of horticultural commodities. *In controlled/Modified/Atmospheres/Vacuum Packaging Foods*, Brody, A.L. (Ed) Food Nutrition Press, Inc. Trumbull, C.T, 1989.

[25] Spayd, S.E.; Morris, J.R.; Ballinger, W.E.; Himelrick, D.G. Maturity standards, harvesting, and postharvest handling. In: Small Fruit Crop Management (G. J. Galletta and D. Himelrick, Eds.) Prentice Hall, Englewood Cliffs, N. J. pp. 28-50, 1990.

[26] Meir, S; Naiman, D; Akerman, M; Hyman, JY; Zauberman, G; Fuchs, Y. Prolonged storage of ''Hass'' avocado fruit using modified atmosphere packaging. *Postharvest Biology and Technology*, 1997, *12*, 51-60.

[27] Ding, C.K.; Chachin, K.; Ueda, Y.; Imahori, Y.; Wang, C.Y. Modified atmosphere packaging maintains postharvest quality of loquat fruit. *Postharvest Biology and Techonology*, 2002, *24*, 341-348.

[28] Kupferman, E.; Sanderson, P. Temperature management and modified atmosphere packing to preserve sweet cherry quality. *Tree Fruit Research and Extension Center*, 2001, http://postharvest.tfrec.wsu.edu/EMK2001B.pdf.

[29] Rosenfeld, H.J.; Haffner, K.; Sundell, A. Packaging trials with highbush blueberries (*Vaccinium corymbosum* L.). Postharvest treatment of fruit and vegetables - current status and future prospects. *Proceedings of the Sixth International Symposium of the European Concerted Action Program COST 94*, Oosterbeek, The Netherlands, 1998, 111-117.

[30] Chiabrando, V.; Giacalone, G. Studies on Shelf Life of ''Lateblue'' Highbush Blueberries. *Food Science and Technology International*, 2008, *14*, 199-205.

[31] Song, Y.; Fan, L.; Forney, C.F.; Jordan, M.A.; Hildebrand, P.D.; Kalt, W.; Ryan, D.A.J. Effect of Ozone treatment and controlled atmosphere storage on quality and phytochemicals in highbush blueberries. *Acta Horticolturae*, ISHS, 2003, 600, 417-423.

[32] Crowe, K.M.; Bushway, R.J.; Bushway, A.A. Evaluation of ozone as a single and synergistic oxidant for improvement of chemical and microbial safety of lowbush blueberries (*Vaccinium angustifolium*). *IOA Conference and Exhibition Valencia, Spain*, 2007, 1-11.

[33] Kim, T.J.; Silva, J.L.; Tokitkla, A.; Matta, F.B. Modified atmosphere storage influences quality parameters and shelf life of 'Tifblue' blueberries. *Journal of the Mississippi Academy of Sciences*, 2010, *55*, 143-148.

[34] Chiabrando, V.; Peano, C.; Beccaro, G.; Rolle, L.; Bounous, G. Postharvest quality of highbush blueberry (*Vaccinium corymbosum* L.) cultivars in relation to storage methods. *Acta Horticolturae,* ISHS, 2006, 715, 545-551.

[35] Brown, W. On the germination and growth of fungi at various temperatures, and in various concentrations of oxygen and carbon dioxide. *Annals of Botany*, 1922, *36*, 257-283

[36] Perkins-Veazie, P. *Raspberry*. Gross, K.C.; Wang, C.Y. and Saltveit M.E. (eds.). The Commercial Storage of Fruits, Vegetables, and Florist and Nursery Stocks. Agriculture Handbook 66. U.S. Dept. of Agr., Agricultural Research Service, Washington, DC, 2004.

[37] Smittle, D.A.; Miller, W.R. Rabbiteye blueberry storage life and fruit quality in controlled atmospheres and air storage. *Jounal of the American Society for Horticoltural Science*, 1998, *113*, 723-728.

[38] Prange, R.K.; Asiedu, S.K.; DeEll, J.R.; Westgarth, A.R. Quality of Fundy and Blomidon lowbush blueberries: Effects of storage atmosphere, duration and fungal inoculation. *International Journal of Plant Science*, 1995, *75*, 479-483.

[39] Harb, J.Y.; Streif, J. Controlled atmosphere storage of highbush blueberries cv 'Duke'. *European Journal of Horticultural Science*, 2004, *69*, 66-72.

[40] Chiabrando, V.; Giacalone, G.; Peano, C. Evoluzione delle caratteristiche qualitative dei frutti di mirtillo gigante americano in funzione delle modalità di conservazione. *Italus Hortus*, 2006, *13*, 114-117.

[41] Chiabrando, V. Comportamento strutturale e qualitative di diverse cultivar di mirtillo gigante Americano (*Vaccinium corymbosum* L.) in relazione alle modalità di conservazione. PhD thesis. 2006. Università di Torino.

[42] Haffner, K.; Rosenfeld, H.J.; Skrede G.; Wang, L. Quality of red raspberry Rubus idaeus L. cultivars after storage in controlled and normal atmospheres. *Postharvest Biology and Technology*, 2002, 24, 279-289.

[43] Perkins-Veazie, P. *Blueberry*. Gross, K.C.; Wang, C.Y., and Saltveit M.E. (eds.). The Commercial Storage of Fruits, Vegetables, and Florist and Nursery Stocks. Agriculture Handbook 66. U.S. Dept. of Agr., Agricultural Research Service, Washington, DC, 2004.

[44] Agar, I.T.; Streif, J. Effect of high CO_2 and controlled atmosphere (CA) storage on the fruit quality of raspberry. *Gartenbauwissenschaft*, 1996, *61*, 261-267.

[45] Batzer, U.; Helm, H.U. Lagerung von Beerenobst (Storage of small fruits). *Erwerbsobstbau*, 1999, *41*, 51-55.

[46] Thompson, A.K. *Controlled atmosphere storage of fruits and vegetables*. CAB Intl., Wallingford, UK, 1998.

[47] Robinson, J.E.; Browne, K.M.; Burton, W.G. Storage characteristics of some vegetables and soft fruits. *Annals of Applied Biology*, 1975, *81*, 339-408.

[48] Sisler, E.C.; Serek, M. Inhibitors of ethylene responses in plants at the receptor level: Recent developments. *Plant Physiology,* 1997, *100*, 577-582.

[49] Watkins, C.B.; Miller, W.B. 1-methylcyclopropene (1-MCP) based technologies for storage and shelf-life extension. *Acta Horticulturae*, 2005, *687*, 201-208.

[50] Boquete, E.J.; Trinchero, G.D.; Fraschina, A.A.; Vilella, F.; Sozzi, G.O. Ripening of 'Hayward' kiwifruit treated with 1-methylcyclopropene after cold storage. *Postharvest Biology and Technology*, 2004, *32*, 57-65.

[51] Liguori, G.; Weksler, A.; Zutahi, Y.; Lurie, S.; Kosto, I. Effect of 1-methylcyclopropene on ripening of melting flesh peaches and nectarines. *Postharvest Biology and Technology*, 2004, *31*, 263-268.

[52] Trinchero, G.D.; Sozzi, G.O.; Covatta, F.; Fraschina, A.A. Inhibition of ethylene action by 1-methylcyclopropene extends postharvest life of "Bartlett" pears. *Postharvest Biology and Technology*, 2004, *32*, 193-204.

[53] DeEll, J.R.; Murr, D.P.; Ehsani-Moghaddm B. Quality changes of "shiro" yellow plums in response to tretment with 1- methylcyclopropene. *Jounal of Food Quality*, 2008, *31*, 514–525.

[54] DeLong, J.M.; Prange, R.K.; Bishop, C; Harrison, P.A. The influence of 1-mcp on shelf-life quality of highbush blueberry. *HortScience*, 2003, *28*, 417-418.

[55] Chiabrando, V.; Giacalone, G. Shelf-life extension of highbush blueberry using 1-methylcyclopropene stored under air and controlled atmosphere. *Food Chemistry*, 2011, *126*, 1812-1816.

[56] Valero, D.; Martinez-Romero, D.; Valverde, J.M.; Guillen, F.; Castillo, S.; Serrano, M. Could the 1-MCP treatment effectiveness in plum be affected by packaging? *Postharvest Biology and Technology*, 2004, *34*, 295–303.

[57] Dong, L.; Lurie, S.; Zhou, H. Effect of 1-methylcyclopropene on ripening of 'Canino' apricots and 'Royal Zee' plums. *Postharvest Biology and Technology*, 2002, *24*, 135-145.

[58] Blankenship, S.M.; Dole, J.M. 1-Methylcyclopropene: a review. *Postharvest Biology and Technology*, 2003, *28*, 1-25.

In: Berries: Properties, Consumption and Nutrition
Editor: Carlo Tuberoso
ISBN 978-1-61470-257-3

Chapter XI

Berry Marketing: Overview of the Current Trends, Challenges and Future Opportunities to Connect Fresh Berry Producers and Consumers

Robert Verloop*

Naturipe Farms LLC, Estero Florida, USA

Abstract

The strength of today's global fresh "berry" industry can be attributed to a combination of factors. New production techniques, improved varieties (that taste great) and the growing scientific evidence of the health and nutritional benefits all contribute to build consumer appetite for berries.

Public and private health sector programs have developed consumer education campaigns stressing the importance of fruits and vegetables in our diet. This increased awareness of the "benefits of berries" along with higher quality, better tasting individual berry types has propelled berries to become the leading produce category in US retail supermarkets.

Berry growers and their sales and marketing teams cannot, however, take for granted this favorite fruit status. Consumer eating habits are fragile and ever shifting. Producers and their trading partners - retailers and restaurant operators, must never fall into the trap that there will always be high consumer demad for fresh berries. They must constantly explore how to be efficient and effective marketers, allowing for reasonable profits for those in the supply chain. All the while, the goal is to consistently satisfy the consumer's taste buds and ensure future purchasing.

This is not a passive exercise, engaged producers and marketers must find ways to build value (real and perceived), generate sales velocity (aligned with production and

* E-mail: rverloop@naturipefarms.com - Executive Vice President of Marketing Naturipe Farms LLC.

inventories) and perhaps most importantly, ensure viability (through sustainable farming and business practices).

1. Defining the Fresh Berry Marketplace

Over the last few years the fresh berry category, consisting primarily of strawberries, blueberries, blackberries, raspberries and assorted minor berry types, has become the leading fruit group at retail supermarkets. The strength of the fresh berry category in the USA is evident by comparing the dollar sales in the following retail sales data chart (Fresh Look Marketing / SymphonyIRI Group) [1]. The berries category accounts for 17.6% of total fruit dollar sales (Figure 1) and they saw a +4.6% increase (Table 1).

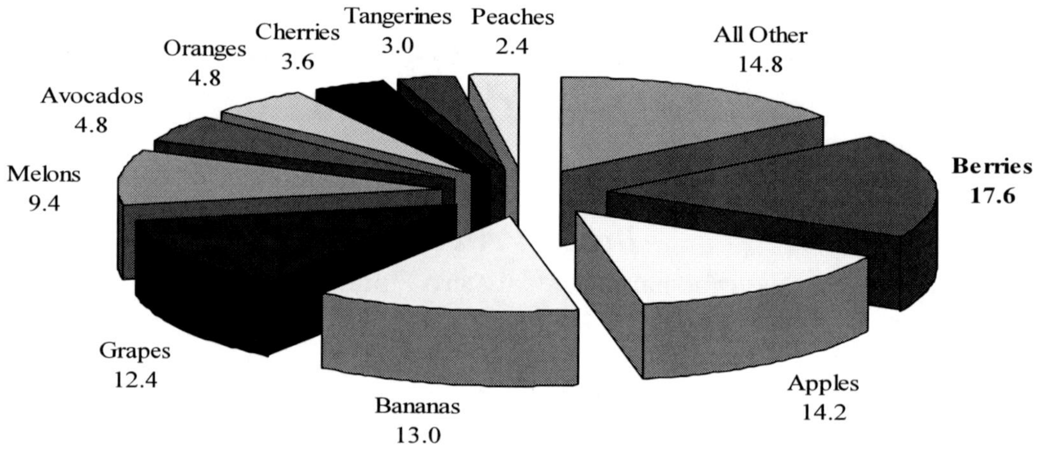

Figure 1. Total US fruit (% of dollar sales).

Table 1. Top 10 fruit categories (dollars) and change (%) in 52 weeks ending 1/2/11

Dollars	Current 52wks ($)	Change %
Berries	3,274,562,012	4.6
Apples	2,651,463,886	4.0
Bananas	2,423,972,538	-3.3
Grapes	2,303,759,231	-1.2
Melons	1,758,804,355	5.9
Avocados	890,213,197	9.1
Oranges	889,507,471	5.3
Cherries	668,288,250	1.1
Tangerines	558,228,537	29.5
Peaches	442,617,834	-2.7
Total Fruit	*18,630,097,785*	*3.5*

Source: Fresh Look Marketing [1].

Growers, sales and marketing teams and retailers can use industry category data to assess broad consumer trends. However in a large geographically diverse country such as the USA, there are many regional, demographic and psychographic consumer segments, as such the data must be used with caution.

Changes in the key performance indicators can be the result of other factors not related to the consumption demand, rather they can be the result of variables such as; size of the crop, the mix within a category and the supply dynamics of competing categories at retail. For example, poor weather in the growing regions will impact the amount of fruit available for sale and how a retailer promotes the category. The result may be a reduction in sales, but should not be interpreted as drop in consumer consumption habits.

Stakeholders in the berry marketplace agree that the category continues to be strong and will continue to expand. We will examine some of the dynamics that have propelled this expansion and why the berry future continues to be bright.

2. Learning from the Berry Category Leader

Strawberries continue to be the dominate berry in the USA (representing nearly 10% of the entire fruit category). Consumer appreciation for the three other major varieties continues to grow as evident in Figure 2 which depicts the current berry mix at retail.

Strawberry growers would point to improvements in production methods, expanded growing regions, new varieties, improved packaging and a balance between retail and foodservice (restaurant) sales. They have been long united to support industry wide efforts to conduct consumer marketing campaigns and raise awareness of the health properties, great taste and versatility of their products. They did not wait nor assume consumers would come to like their products; they proactively marketed the benefits of strawberries and engaged the trade to make strawberries a vocal point at retail displays and on restaurant menus.

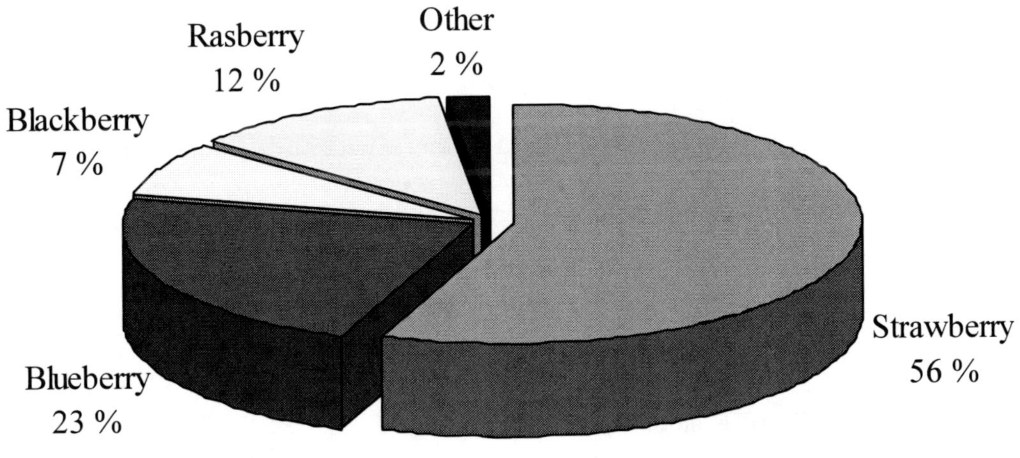

Figure 2. Berries breakdown (%) by variety.

3. Psychology of the Marketplace

When growers focus on the consumer experience (consistent, reliable, good taste, premium quality) they can influence the mindset of shoppers to be pre-disposed to have fresh berries on the shopping list. When consumers have positive eating experiences they are more likely to repurchased berries, sooner. Conversely, it is commonly accepted that when a consumer has a bad experience they will stay away from the category for 6-8 weeks, thinking that it's a "seasonal" thing.

What separates berries from many other produce categories is the positive media buzz that has been generated over the last 20 years about the nutritional and health benefits. Today's consumer is keenly aware that berries are healthy, taste good and are available all year long keeping berries top of mind. This did not happen by accident, trade associations such as the California Strawberry Commission [2] and the US Highbush Blueberry Council (USHBC) [3] have long invested in sound scientific nutrition research to highlight the benefits of eating berries. While not a "magic bullet" berries have steadily gained the respect and the support of the health and nutrition industry (Figure 3). These endorsements set a positive "psychology in the marketplace" and puts berries on the top of the shopping list.

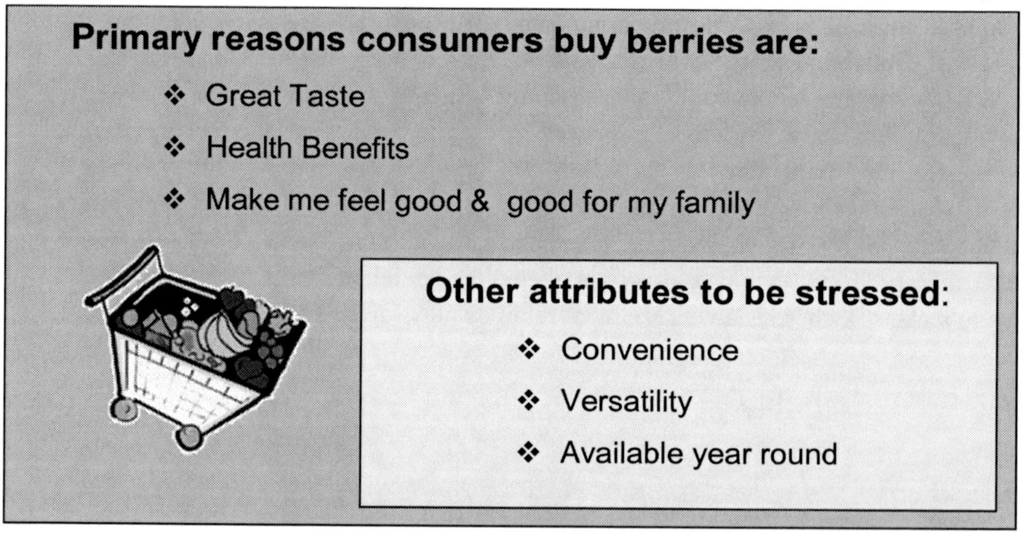

Figure 3. Main reasons for the buying of berries.

4. Marketing to the Senses

Consumers make the majority of food buying decisions based on taste and eating experience (Figure 4). The adjoining graphic from the USHBC study shows that taste (implied unique, flavor and texture) is still a primary trigger to purchase intent. Yet marketers need to understand the balance between functional benefits and emotional benefits and determine the right communication and marketing strategies to reach consumers. While we cannot ignore media stories about "Locally Grown", "Sustainability", "Air miles", "Carbon

Footprint" – the majority of purchase decision are influenced by satisfying the consumers senses – fresh, taste, appearance, texture, smell and enjoyment. In order to obtain long term viability, marketers must stay abreast of how these factors influence buying habits and the perception of real and perceived "value" to the consumer.

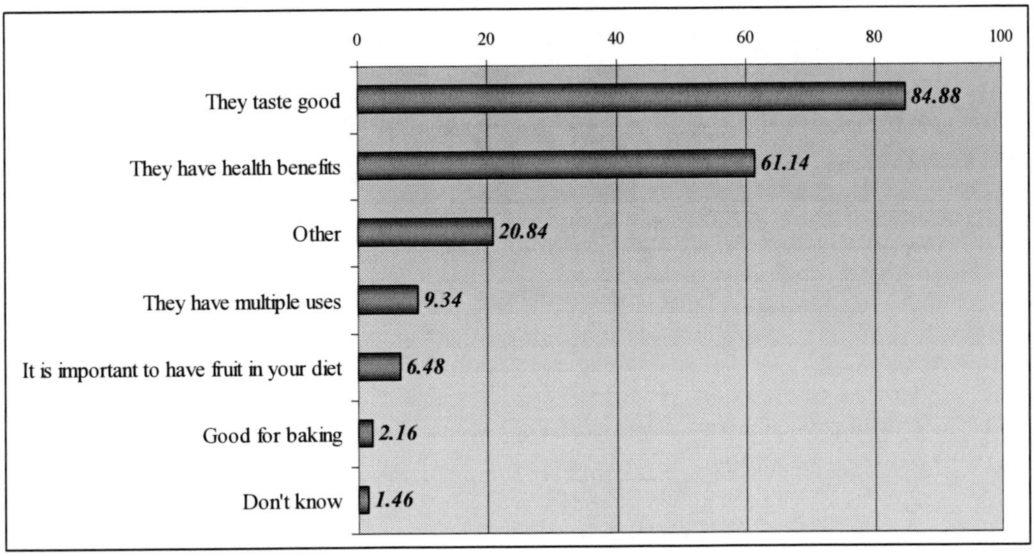

Figure 4. Principal purchase decisions (%) by consumers (modified from [3]).

5. The "4p's" of Marketing Fresh Produce: Product, Pricing, Promotions and Place

To sustain future growth for the fresh berry industry, stakeholders constantly make improvements in production techniques, packaging, product forms and supply chain management practices (Figure 5).

Progressive retailers and foodservice operators are focused on making the supply chain as smooth and efficient as possible. Having quality fresh berries is "table stakes" as are other basics such as proper food safety management practices and product traceability.

The focus on product innovation is at the core of the success of the global berry marketplace. For example: new packaging allowed consumers to receive farm stand quality berries on a year around basis. Protecting the integrity of the berries has allowed plant breeders to develop varieties that focus on taste enjoyment (and sufficient production per acre) versus the past practices that were perceived to be more concerned about the "ship-ability" of the berry.

Growers have also started to think differently about what they produce on their farms. An example is unfolding in today's global blueberry industry. Relatively unknown forty years ago as a fresh item, blueberries were consumed primarily as an ingredient in juice, jam, jelly, dried or another "further processed" items. The common varieties at the time were conducive for processing.

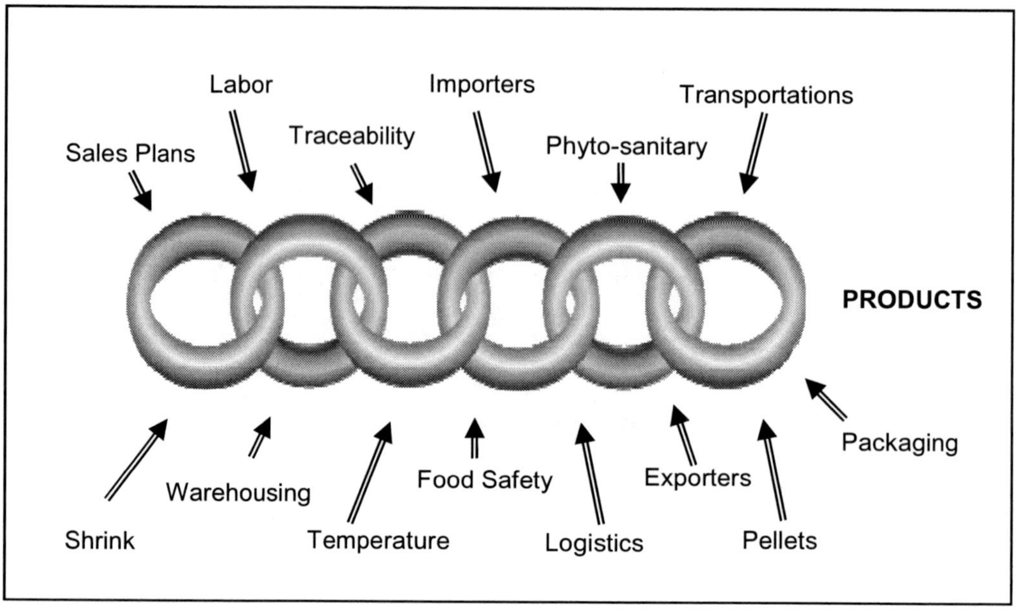

Figure 5. The produce supply chain.

It was not until the last twenty years that consumers started to seek out more fresh produce items, demanding (and paying a premium for higher quality fresh blueberries. Growers and plant breeders responded by developing new varieties that taste better, less variable and larger consistent berries. While some berry varieties are the result of plant breeding programs at public universities, larger innovative growers have funded private programs to develop their own proprietary varieties. This is where the marketers can have a significant impact - helping to understand consumer preferences, identify the triggers and barriers to purchase and to assit in removing the obstacles to increased consumption. Successful new varieties must consistently taste great and be available on a year 'round basis in order to appea to children, adults and restaurant chefs.

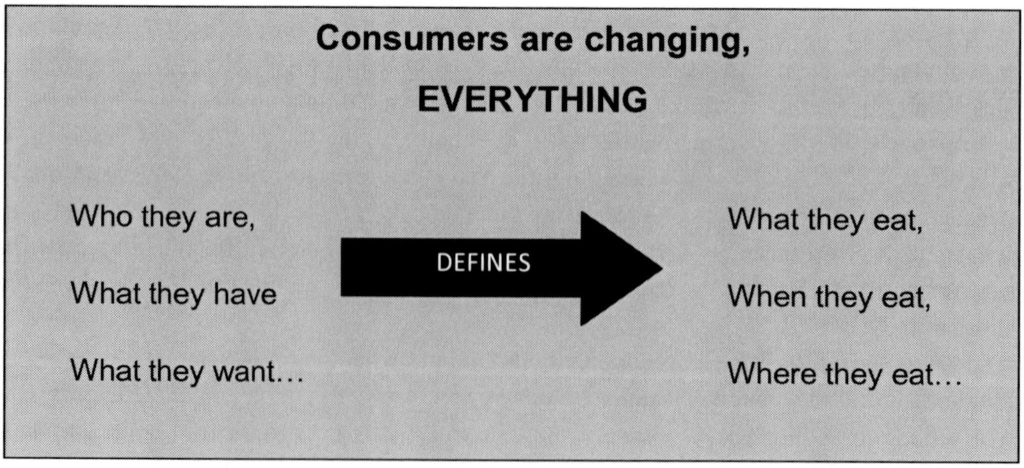

Figure 6. The most significant challenge in managing the growth of the berry category.

The graphic from strategic consulting firm The Hale Group [4] reported in Figure 6, simply communicates the most significant challenge growers, marketers, retailers and restaurant operators. Nothing is constant when it comes to consumer marketing. Pricing and promotion strategies are developed in collaboration between trading. Marketers are asked to provide more category development support and assist retailers to understand how they perform relative to others in the marketplace.

Producers are constantly challenged to anticipate trends and recommend how fresh berries can be positioned to be attractive to a broad base of consumers. It is imperative that producers understand the consumer trends so that their berries are readily available when the consumers are most likely to purchase or consume them. With all the challenges that come with distributing a fresh berry, there are also many benefits. Most importantly, fresh berries, when properly handled and delivered, remain a consumer favorite and meet the needs and demands of the ever changing consumer.

Successful consumer marketing, instore merchandising and sales promotions, will attract consumer to the berry display and create an appealing reason to purchase berries on a frequent basis. A common list of Best Practices follows:

Berry Merchandising "Best Practices"

- Position the berry display towards the front of the produce department under refrigeration.
- Carry all varieties at all times, organic in special or adjacent section.
- Use color breaks to attract attention and stimulate impulse sales.
- Utilize secondary displays located at the front of department or lobby during promotional and key seasonal periods to trigger un-planned purchases.
- Incorporate co-marketing products and tie-ins adjacent to the main and secondary displays (rule is twice as many berries as tie-ins).
- Clear and attractive signage for each item on the display will help consumer find the berries and influence inpulse purchasing. Utilize recipes for usage ideas and to show the verstility of berry (good for all day parts).
- Merchandise category in front of department on weekends even when not on promotion.
- As seasonal volume increases increase the display size of the larger packs to drive volume sales.

Progressive growers will develop new channels of distribution to match projected increases in production, especially in blueberries, blackberries and raspberries. Understanding where the consumers are spending their food dollars can provide insight as to the places where growth may come from in the future. The following graphics provide insight into the size of the retail and foodservice channels (Figure 7) and how they differ in the selling and marketing approaches (Figure 8). Branded produce companies are increasingly moving from the traditional commodity sales approach, to embrace programs selling in both of these channels. This expanded view of the foodservice marketplace requires a fresh new approach from packaging to product specifications to mastering the culinary and menu development process (something that escapes the majority of produce marketers and sellers).

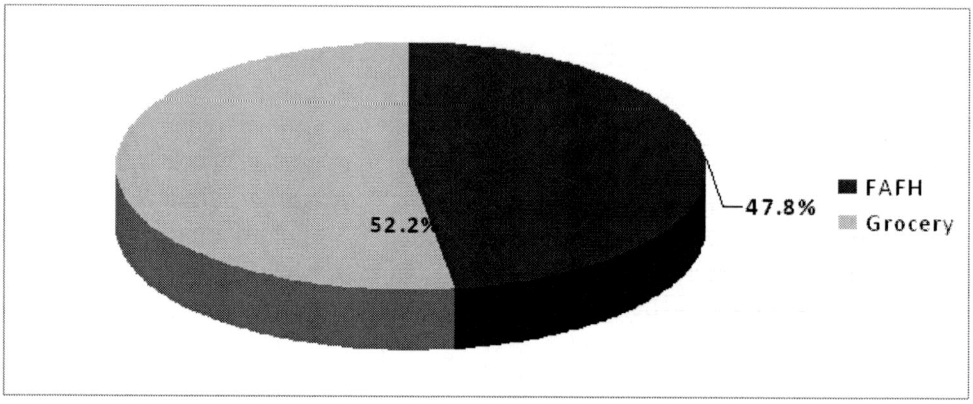

Figure 7. Share of consumer food 2009. FAFH: Foods that are consumed Away From Home (Data: Culinary Sales Support. Inc. (CSSI) Inc, January 2010, [5]).

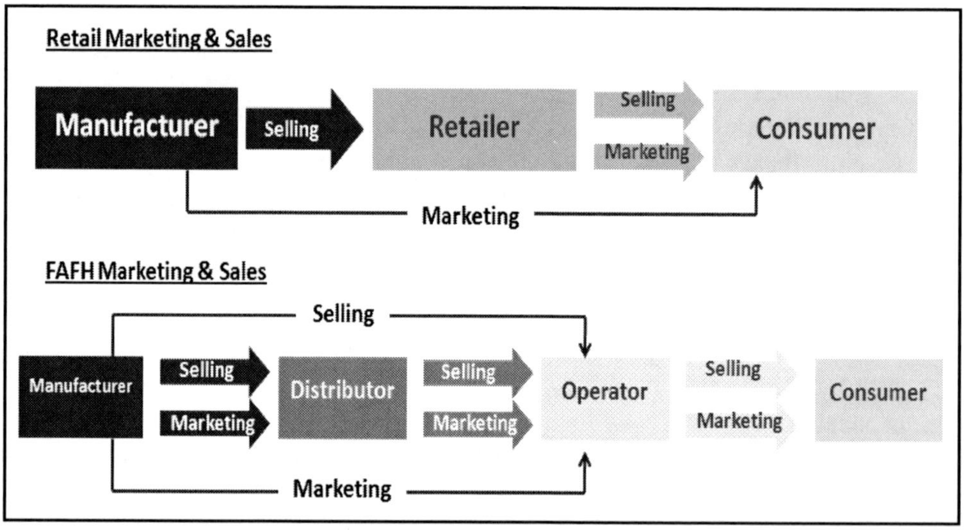

Figure 8. (Culinary Sales Support. Inc. (CSSI) Inc, January 2010, [5]).

6. Innovations

Beyond health and taste, consumers are seeking convenience and consistent quality and above all products must be safe. New technologies such as the following example address opportunities to improve consumer affinity and loyalty with berry products. As example, in the fall of 2010, Naturipe Farms [6] announced the development of Berry Quick Fresh Blueberries Snacks, using new processing technologies and USDA & FDA approved biodegradable products that do not harm the berries nor the environment.

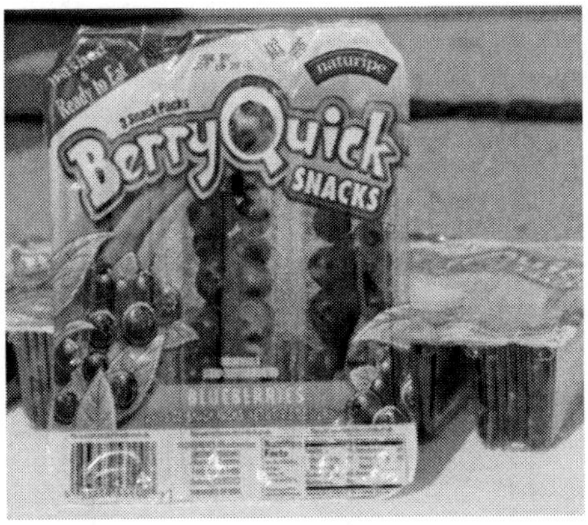

FEATURES	BENEFITS
Unique to foodservice	Brings multiple new opportunities for menu innovation
Long shelf-life	Freshest taste; minimized waste for maximum profit
Pre-washed	Alleviates food safety concerns
Ready-to-eat	Saves on labor; pour and serve, or open and eat
Multiple uses	Versatile as a filling, topping, side or snack
Numerous packaging options	Convenient to store, handle and eat
Healthiest fruit	Multiple health benefits not found in other fruits
Highest quality blueberries	No bruising or punctures; fresh taste
Flavorful	Tartness and/or sweetness spices up any menu
Great appearance	Vibrant color adds excitement to any application
Traceable	Ensures quick response should questions arise
Distribution	Currently USA. Future expansion in South America, Asia & EU

This triple inspected and triple-washed proprietary process gently cleanses the blueberries leaving them free of residues and allergens and does not require treatment with wax or preservatives. The patented single serve packaging maintains the taste, vitality and vigor of each berry which results in a practical shelf life of 3 weeks or more when properly refrigerated. The convenient packaging is ideal for consumers as single serve, washed, ready to eat blueberries. They can also be used by chefs and restaurant operators as pre-portioned packs which improve back of the house operational efficiencies and allow the development of new blueberry menu applications.

Conclusions

Consumer demand for healthy, superior tasting fresh berries will continue to drive growers to improve all aspect from field to fork. The advent of new varieties, new packaging and promotional vehicles sets up a bright future for this category. With new production acreage coming into full maturity over the next five years there is a growing need to expand channels of distribution, increase consumer demand and purchase frequency and product innovation. The fresh berry category will continue to be a leader of the retail produce departments and the opportunities for new growth in the foodservice channel offer many exciting new ways to reach consumers.

References

[1] Fresh Look Marketing (FLM) - *http://www.freshlookmarketing.com/*
[2] California Strawberry Commission - *http://www.calstrawberry.com/*
[3] US Highbush Blueberry Council (USHBC) - *http://www.blueberry.org/ushbc.htm*
[4] The Hale Group - *http://www.halegroup.com/phpwcms/*
[5] Culinary Sales Suport. Inc. – contact: *liz.diakonow@culisales.com*
[6] Naturipe Farms - *http://www.naturipefarms.com/*

Index

A

B

C

D

E

F

G

H

I

J

K

L

M

N

O

P

Q

R

S

V

W

Y